BEHAVIORAL NEUROLOGY

100 MAXIMS

Volume 1 in the Series
100 Maxims in Neurology
Series Editor
Roger J Porter MD

BEHAVIORAL NEUROLOGY
100 MAXIMS

Orrin Devinsky

Chief, Department of Neurology, Hospital for
Joint Diseases, New York University School of
Medicine, New York.

Edward Arnold
A division of Hodder & Stoughton

LONDON   MELBOURNE   AUCKLAND

For my wife and best friend, Deborah

© 1992 Orrin Devinsky

First published in Great Britain 1992

British Library Cataloguing in Publication Data

Devinsky, Orrin
 Behavioural Neurology: 100 Maxims. – (100
 Maxims in Neurology Series)
 I. Title II. Series
 616.8

ISBN 0 340 53619 5

Whilst the advice and information in this book is believed to be
true and accurate at the date of going to press, neither the author
nor the publisher can accept any legal responsibility or liability
for any errors or omissions that may be made. In particular (but
without limiting the generality of the preceding disclaimer) every
effort has been made to check drug dosages; however, it is still
possible that errors have been missed. Furthermore, dosage
schedules are constantly being revised and new side effects
recognised. For these reasons the reader is strongly urged to
consult the drug companies' printed instructions before
administering any of the drugs recommended in this book.

Typeset in Linotron Palatino by
Rowland Phototypesetting Ltd,
Bury St Edmunds, Suffolk
Printed in Great Britain for Edward Arnold, a division of Hodder
and Stoughton Limited, Mill Road, Dunton Green, Sevenoaks,
Kent TN13 2YA by St Edmundsbury Press Ltd, Bury St Edmunds,
Suffolk and bound by Hartnolls Ltd, Bodmin, Cornwall.

Foreword to the 100 Maxims in Neurology series

This first volume of the *100 Maxims* series is the culmination of five years of planning and perseverance. Such labour has proved necessary to create a unique series of books in neurology.

The origin of the series lies in the early 1980s, when I began thinking about how a firm grasp of the fundamentals of diagnosis and treatment of epilepsy could benefit a physician confronted by this difficult disorder. In 1984, thanks to the generosity of Lord Walton of Detchant, my own book, *Epilepsy: 100 Elementary Principles* was included in his prestigious series *Major Problems in Neurology*. The second edition (WB Saunders) was published in 1989.

The real challenge, however, was to create an entire series on the notion that physicians like – in so far as is possible – to have concrete rules to guide their diagnosis and therapy. Even the best doctors, those with great knowledge and sensitive insight, lean on their experience of what has proven to be correct and what has not. Thus was born the *100 Maxims in Neurology* series. The neurological disorders that we have chosen for this series lend themselves to 100 guiding principles for diagnosis and treatment. Discipline on the part of the authors has been necessary in order to reach, but not to exceed, this number. The books are intended to be monographs, although a few will combine the expertise of as many as three authors. Each book will be well referenced to make certain that the opinions expressed can be fortified by further reading.

The concept of '100 Maxims' is a specific service to the reader; each author is forced to say unequivocally what is important (and, by exclusion, what is less important). The ideal list of maxims comes from the author's own experience, as well as from recognition of those errors of diagnosis and treatment made most frequently. The format requires that the author be committed to a specific plan of action. Even though the text generally 'qualifies' the maxim, each maxim stands on its own as a declarative statement. Most textbooks are much less concrete in their recommendations regarding diagnosis and therapy. In summary, *100 Maxims* obliterates the curious dichotomy of the professor who is highly specific in verbal recommendations to students but enormously cautious in book chapters on the same subject!

I am grateful to many, but most especially to my wife, Candace, who has continuously supported my efforts, and to the editorial staff of Edward Arnold Publishers, without whose encouragement and perseverance this series could not have been created.

Roger J Porter
1991

Foreword to Behavioral Neurology: 100 Maxims

The *100 Maxims in Neurology* series begins with a book which addresses one of the most difficult areas in neurology – the interface of the mind and the brain. *Behavioral Neurology: 100 Maxims* by Orrin Devinsky MD is the fruit of an astounding effort by a single author; I am delighted that his book is the first volume in our series.

The book is logically constructed, beginning with the elementary mental status assessment. Dr Devinsky moves immediately to demystify the jargon so prevalent in discussions of behavioral neurology, clarifying everything from subcortical lesions to multimodal association cortex. 'Localize the lesion,' admonishes the author, as he makes the signs of behavioral investigation nearly as precise as clonus at the ankle. Localization of the lesion then becomes the driving force of the book. Erudition on confusional states is followed by similar elucidation on amnesia. The aphasia discussion is especially complete, and will be of use to all of us who occasionally struggle with aphasia and such related concepts as alexia, agraphia and apraxia. Dr Devinsky moves from the visual system to the right hemisphere to the individual lobes. Specific neurological problems – stroke, trauma, epilepsy, movement and sleep disorders – lead to the last chapters on iatrogenesis and psychiatric diseases.

Dr Devinsky has fully accomplished the goal of elucidating, in a straightforward manner, the most difficult and imprecise of neurological subjects. True to the *100 Maxims* series, he has set forth, for the practicing physician, the 100 most important rules of diagnosis and therapy. For those rules which are occasionally broken, and most are, the insightful qualifications and explanations of the text combine clarity with easy reading. Dr Devinsky has made behavioral neurology more approachable for us all. I will refer frequently to his text for advise and counsel.

Roger J Porter
1991

Acknowledgments

Norman Geschwind kindled my interest in behavioral neurology during medical school. This book reflects his spirit and enthusiasm.

Roger Porter's encouragement and counsel allowed me to start and complete this project.

Lou Caplan and Marty Samuels have read through most of these pages in draft. Their generous criticisms and suggestions were extremely helpful. Other colleagues who have offered valuable assistance in specific areas include David Bear, Frank Benson, Robert Cancro, Enrico Fazzini, Ed Feldmann, Jordan Grafman, Bob Green, Bonnie Levin, and Ken Perrine.

Frances Taylor, BJ Hessie, and Lawrence Davis provided editorial assistance. Nicholas Dunton, Diane Leadbetter-Conway and the staff at Edward Arnold have been a pleasure to work with.

Preface

The study and teaching of behavioral neurology remain in their infancy. Although Hippocrates recognized the brain as the seat of behavior in the 5th century BC, the exploration of brain–behaviour relationships did not begin in earnest until more than 2000 years later, with the pioneering explorations of such founders as Charcot, Broca, Hughlings Jackson, Korsakov, Babinski, Liepman, Papez and Wernicke.

The neurology of behavior has since emerged as an important discipline. As the arena for studying how the brain subserves cognition, emotion and consciousness, behavioral neurology straddles the boundaries of numerous, more established disciplines – extending from the most fundamental explorations of molecular biology to the broadest questions of philosophy. Certainly, it has shared in the dramatic advances of recent decades – a period of revolution for the basic and clinical neurosciences.

Yet our knowledge is still remarkably limited. We test what we have tests for, focus on those behaviors we have some knowledge of, and ignore those deficits we have not been taught to recognize. Some of the most critical behavioral problems that accompany stroke and dementia – personality change, irritability, loss of will power, impulsiveness – remain poorly defined, their therapy ignored. Even the simple act of looking into another person's eyes – a behavior that is indeed altered by brain disorders – has received little attention, despite being one of the most eloquent and expressive events in human communication.

This book has modest goals. It is intended to be a concise introduction to behavioral neurology, focusing on the essential elements of diagnosis and therapy. Behavioral neurology – the effort to understand the relationship between the brain and behavior – is inherently fascinating. I have tried to create a balance between the vivid prose that can best portray normal and abnormal behavioral patterns and the format of *Maxims*, aiming most of all for a succinct and focused description. My more ambitious hope, however, is to stimulate at least one person to explore further the neurology of behavior, especially those regions that remain uncharted.

Orrin Devinsky
1991

Contents

Chapter 1 Mental status assessment and localization of behavioral functions

Chapter 2 Delirium (confusional state) and dementia

Chapter 3 Aphasia

Chapter 4 Amnesia

Chapter 5 Alexia, agraphia and apraxia

response to commands and results from
disconnection or destruction of dominant
hemisphere association areas

Chapter 6 Disorders of visual processing

Chapter 7 Right hemisphere disorders

Chapter 8 Frontal lobe disorders

common with large midline or bilateral dorsofrontal
lesions

Chapter 13 Epilepsy

Chapter 14 Movement disorders

Chapter 15 Sleep disorders

Chapter 16 Iatrogenic mental disorders and systemic illnesses

Chapter 17 Psychiatric disorders

1

Mental Status Assessment and Localization of Behavioral Functions

1. The mental status examination has an undeservedly bad reputation and should never be omitted from the neurological examination

It is as inappropriate to omit the mental status examination as it is to ignore muscle strength or reflexes. Indeed, mental status evaluation is the first component of the neurological examination and it can be critical to the correct interpretation of other findings. For example, a patient with delirium and brisk doll's eyes is likely to have hepatic encephalopathy; recent onset of short-term memory impairment accompanied by olfactory hallucinations and fever suggests herpes simplex encephalitis. Furthermore, to label aphasia as dementia because language was not systematically tested is as grave an error as mislabelling upper motor neuron facial weakness as 'Bell's palsy' because upper extremity drift and reflex asymmetries were not sought. The following case illustrates how this can occur.

> A 70-year-old multimillionairess was admitted to an inpatient neurology service with the diagnosis of dementia. She had been well until 18 months earlier when the New York city police discovered her wandering the streets in the middle of the night; she appeared to be 'psychotic'. She was admitted to a nearby hospital and treated with chlorpromazine. Later, discharged without medication, she remained 'confused and bizarre'. She was followed for 18 months by an attending neurologist and was again admitted to the hospital, this time to exclude possible intentional poisoning by a relative for financial gain. Her speech was pressured, fluent and well-articulated, but was peppered with neologisms and paraphasias and made no sense. When asked, 'Where are you?', She replied 'Where are, where are . . . yes, well of course I was . . .'. 'Is it true that helicopters in South America eat their young?', she was asked. 'Those children . . . always eating', she replied. The question, 'Do two pounds of flour weigh more than one?' brought her response, 'Flour, I love flowers'.

This woman had Wernicke's aphasia, not dementia. A screen of language function with testing of comprehension would have made the correct diagnosis possible 18 months earlier (Maxim 34).

In addition, recent advances in our understanding of brain–behavior relationships and the recognition that neurobehavioral disorders are frequent and treatable also mandate that the physician no longer avoid the mental status examination.

However, many physicians – even neurologists – mistakenly regard the mental status examination as difficult, ambiguous, time-consuming, better left in the hands of a psychiatrist or psychologist and, worst of all, irrelevant. It is, or should be, none of the above.

One needs only to read a detailed neuropsychological evaluation or watch a lengthy obsessive language examination to conclude that the resident or practicing neurologist has no time to be fussing over higher functions. A mental status screen, however, can be performed in only three minutes. The essentials of diagnosis and classification are straightforward and can be mastered with practice.

The components of the mental status examination are separable and can be individually tested and correlated with the anatomical location. However, the pieces must be viewed in the context of the whole. Behavior patterns cannot be neatly dissected into discrete units; the fundamental diagnostic process is a systematic and synthetic evaluation of signs and symptoms rather than pattern recognition. The differential diagnosis is then refined further by searching for the presence or absence of specific corroborative features.

Findings from the mental status examination must be synthesized with each other and with findings from neurological and general medical examinations. For example, an anxious, diaphoretic patient with tachycardia, brisk reflexes, tremor, exophthalmos and thyromegaly is easily diagnosed as hyperthyroid, when one synthesizes the diverse mental, neurological and medical symptoms.

As the patient states the chief complaint, the examiner runs through a mental checklist (Maxim 3; Table 3.1): appearance (neat or disheveled), affect (labile, depressed), level of consciousness (alert, lethargic) and ability to speak clearly and present an orderly, coherent history. By the time the medical history ends, the examiner may need only to supplement the observations with a few tests. In addition, a good bedside assessment of mental status can be completed in 15 to 20 minutes with experience (Strub and Black, 1985).

Finally, there are cases in which a more thorough mental status examination must be performed. This is often the case in patients with known or suspected brain lesions and acute psychiatric disorders erupting from a normal behavioral baseline.

References

Strub RL, Black FW. *The Mental Status Examination in Neurology*. Philadelphia: FA Davis Company, 1985.

2.   *The neurologist's law – 'localize the lesion' – also applies to mental function*

In behavioral neurology, the area of neural dysfunction as well as the pathogenesis must be determined. Localization is an integrative process that systematically explores anatomical sites in which a lesion may cause specific behavioral change and synthesizes findings from the medical history and neurological examination with functional neuroanatomy to identify the pathological focus or foci.

Because identifying a disorder's pathogenesis requires separate, but overlapping, data and analysis, it is natural to want to integrate information on etiology and localization to help fill in the missing pieces. However, it is better to separate these diagnostic entities, so that an error in one area will not lead to an error in the other.

The approach to localization of complex behavior, such as language, is similar to that of other neurological disorders. In evaluating arm weakness, for example, the neurologist systematically begins by exploring the most peripheral (i.e. muscle) and ends by testing the most central portions (i.e. primary and association motor cortex) of the motor system. *Incorrect localization often results from placing the lesion too centrally* and failing to consider more peripheral (e.g. neuromuscular junction) or intermediate (e.g. plexus, spinal cord) sites. Similarly, in evaluating behavioral changes it is wise to begin more peripherally before moving to the cortex or subcortex. Speech problems may be caused not only by left perisylvian lesions, but by drugs, metabolic disorders, vocal cord lesions or recurrent laryngeal nerve palsies. Likewise, impaired visual recognition may result not only from a lesion of the visual association cortex, but also from eye and optic nerve injuries.

Signs and symptoms must be considered in the context of the associated deficits. For example, dysarthria accompanied by diplopia and facial numbness suggests a brainstem lesion, but dysarthria accompanied by non-fluent speech with phonemic (literal) paraphasias (spoken syllabic substitution errors such as 'slat' instead of 'slack' or 'boot' instead of 'book'; Maxim 30) and right-sided weakness of the face and arm indicates a lesion in the left frontal lobe.

Computed tomography and magnetic resonance imaging of the brain have permitted almost immediate correlation of clinical and anatomical data, allowing both the clinician and researcher the opportunity to refine the localization process. However, overly precise localization of cognitive functions is a common pitfall.

The limitations of the localization process constitute one of the most durable controversies in behavioral neurology. On the one hand, the extreme view conceptualizing an equipotential cerebral cortex is ludicrous (Lashley, 1929). At the same time, however, complex behaviors are more difficult to quantify and localize accurately than elementary neurological functions (e.g. motor control of the left thumb) and one cannot map personality to a small cube of frontal or temporal lobe.

Neuroimaging studies have seduced us into another pitfall of the localization process – assuming that when a function is disrupted, the area in which the lesion is found subserves that function. As Hughlings Jackson admonished us, lesions and deficits – not functions – can be localized on the cerebral map (Jackson, 1878). Our understanding of human cognition and emotion comes largely from pathologic studies, not normal physiology. The intellectual leap between lesion and function site is not trivial. Behavioral disorders after focal lesions result, in part, from preserved areas of brain (Maxims 9 and 10).

A useful theoretical aid to achieving the happy medium between too precise localization and overgeneralization is the network approach of directed attention. Put forth by Mesulam (1981, 1990), it serves as an important model for such cognitive processes as language, memory and visuospatial function. The network theory postulates that complex behaviors are not subserved by isolated centers but by sets of distributed regions that form integrated functional systems. These functional systems, in turn, are determined by neural interconnections (Mesulam, 1985). Mesulam summarized the network approach's general principles:

> 1. Complex functions are represented within distributed interconnected sites that collectively constitute an integrated network for each function.
> 2. Individual cerebral areas each contain the neural substrate for several sets of behaviors and may, therefore, belong to several partially overlapping networks.
> 3. Lesions confined to a single region are likely to result in multiple deficits.
> 4. Different aspects of the same complex function may be impaired as a consequence of damage to one of several cortical areas or their interconnections.

This network approach is helpful in understanding such neurobehavioral disorders as subcortical aphasia (Maxims 11 and 34), particularly when one seeks to define the nature of deficits or predict the extent of recovery. Although language functions are located primarily in the left hemisphere of most people (Maxim 24), subcortical areas are interconnected with language areas and are important for activation and coordination of cortical functions. Thus, subcortical lesions can disrupt language functions. However, since other subcortical and cortical areas frequently 'replace' the work done by the damaged subcortical areas, many cases of subcortical aphasia are transient.

Finally, when determining how precisely to localize a function, one should also note that the degree to which specific behaviors and behavioral deficits can be localized depends on many factors, including age, handedness, the time course and nature of the pathological process, and previous brain insults. For example, a slow-growing, massive right frontotemporal glioma in a young woman may present over months with only subtle personality changes or headaches, while a small Wernicke's area infarct in an elderly woman can devastate language comprehension in moments.

References

Jackson H. On affections of speech from disease of the brain. *Brain* 1878; **1**: 304–30.

Lashley KS. *Brain Mechanisms and Intelligence*. Chicago: University of Chicago Press, 1929.

Mesulam M-M. A cortical network for directed attention and unilateral neglect. *Ann Neurol* 1981; **10**: 309–25.

Mesulam M-M. *Principles of Behavioral Neurology*. Philadelphia: FA Davis Company, 1985, p. 57.

Mesulam M-M. Large-scale neurocognitive networks and distributed processing for attention, language, and memory. *Ann Neurol* 1990; **28**: 597–613.

3.   *The observation and history of the patient's behavior are the most important aspects of mental evaluation*

Diagnoses and therapeutic opportunities are often missed because important clues are never observed or sought. An adolescent with labile emotions and paranoia whose upper lip is drawn tightly over the teeth and whose mouth is open with a fixed smile should be evaluated for Wilson's disease, as well as primary psychiatric disease. A patient whose dinner plate is clean on the right side but barely touched on the left side may have a right parietal lesion and left-sided neglect. Similarly, lack of motor and verbal spontaneity suggests depression or frontal lobe disorders.

Observation begins when you first meet the patient. How does he greet you (eye contact, speech)? Is he distracted by novel stimuli? Is his mood appropriate for the situation? The physician should quickly run through a series of behavioral observations (Table 3.1).

There are several reasons why behavioral problems are easily overlooked:

- Most people tend to minimize problems, especially behavioral ones.
- Some patients are not fully aware of their problem.
- The duration of patient contact for most physicians is limited.
- Behavioral problems are often intermittent or situation-dependent.

Vital behavioral information can often be gained through interviews with family or friends, who have the advantage of more extensive and diverse

Table 3.1 Behavioral observation.

General appearance
Degree of illness, distress or pain
State of consciousness
Age – does appearance match chronology?
Body habitus – obese, anorexic, wasting
Facial expression
Hygiene – skin, hair, teeth, feet, ? unilateral neglect
Dress – cleanliness, ? unilateral neglect

Interpersonal relation
Eye contact
Emotional contact – engaged and interested, withdrawn
Anxiety/anger/suspiciousness
Appropriateness of behavior

Activity
Spontaneity (motor/verbal) and delay in initiation
Level of motor activity – hyper versus hypo
Restlessness/akathisia
Asymmetry of movement – facial expression, extremities
Abnormal movements
    Dystonic posture
    Tics
    Tremors
    Facial grimaces/dyskinesias

Affect*
Normal
Labile with prominent fluctuations
Apathetic and unconcerned
Inappropriate (e.g. patient talks about sad subject and appears elated)

Mood†
Normal – includes mild sadness and happiness
Dysphoric – depression, anxiety, irritability
Euphoric – implies pathologic elation, as in mania
Labile – relates to congruence between situation and expressed emotion
    (e.g. patient talks of father's death while smiling)

Language
Spontaneous speech – fluency, prosody and articulation
Paraphasias, neologisms
Repetition
Perseverations (pathological repetitions), palilalia

Thought and ideation
Loose associations; ability to maintain a coherent stream of thought
Paranoid ideation (suspiciousness)
Illusions (misperceptions of stimuli)
Hallucinations
Delusions (false beliefs)

---

* Affect refers to the behavioral pattern that expresses emotion (subjectively
experienced feeling state).
† Mood is a pervasive and sustained emotion.

contact with the patient. In addition, nursing and ancillary medical personel (e.g. physical therapist) may have important insights.

An alert patient who provides a clear and organized account of the present illness usually does not have a major neurobehavioral disorder. However, there are important exceptions to this rule, and this is where physicians most often err. In fact, the patient who seems normal on first appearance may suffer from serious cognitive or emotional disorders. Even standard intelligence quotient testing may fail to uncover major cognitive lacunes. The famous patient, HM, had bilateral temporal lobectomies and was left with a severe, permanent loss of short-term memory, but his

Table 3.2 Behavioral history.

Chief complaint (include age, sex, handedness, duration)

Present illness
Premorbid baseline
Onset of behavioral change – precipitating factors
Progression/recurrence
Interventions (e.g. medication)
Current level of behavioral disability
Associated behavioral symptoms
    Cognitive (e.g. memory, language)
    Affective (e.g. depression, mania)
    Alteration of consciousness
    Hallucinations/illusions
    Anxiety/phobias
    Paranoia/delusions
    Changes in social functions
Associated neurological symptoms
Pending litigation

Past history
Prior central nervous system insult or disease
Prior psychiatric disorder/hospitalization
Prior medical/surgical disorder
Alcohol or illicit drug use
Sexual orientation/HIV status

Prescribed medications

Social history
Educational background (highest grade or year of schooling completed
    and academic success)
Vocational background (layoffs, changes)
Marital/relationship status

Family history
Neurologic/psychiatric/medical disorders
? Adopted/consanguineous
If patient is left-handed or ambidextrous - ? family history

postoperative IQ was 13 points higher than before surgery! (Milner, 1966).

The patient with memory loss may confabulate, filling in memory gaps with the best or most plausible answer. One should corroborate details if memory impairment is suspected. Patients with psychiatric impairment may be aware of their problems but attempt to hide them (e.g. delusions, paranoia, depression, obsessions and compulsions). The decision to survey specific symptoms in these patients must be based on behavioral observations and the history obtained from the patient and others. However, in asking about sensitive issues, such as suspiciousness, one must phrase the questions in a non-judgmental way.

The behavioral history is summarized in Table 3.2.

References

Milner B. Amnesia following operation on the temporal lobes. In: *Amnesia* (Whitty CWM and Zangwill OL, eds). Oxford: Butterworths, 1966, pp. 109–33.

4.   *Mental status examination is systematic and hierarchical*

Unlike the physical and neurological examinations, in which test sequences may vary with personal preference, mental status evaluation must proceed within a hierarchical framework. This is because the assessment of certain functions is critically dependent upon the integrity of other functions. One cannot assess praxis after comprehension, because normal comprehension is required for praxis. One cannot test memory before attention, because patients must be attentive for meaningful memory assessment.

The mental status examination should test, in the following order: (1) level of consciousness; (2) attention (Maxims 6, 50 and 62); (3) orientation to person, place and time; (4) language (Chapter 3); and (5) memory (Chapter 4). The components of mental status examination are summarized in Table 4.1.

Consciousness may be divided into two elementary components: arousal, the degree of alertness or wakefulness; and content, the sum of cognitive and affective processes (Plum and Posner, 1980). Mental status testing begins with arousal because the entire content of consciousness is critically dependent upon it. Arousal state is stratified into six levels: (1) hyperalertness, (2) alertness, (3) somnolence, (4) obtundation, (5) stupor and (6) coma.

Hyperalertness may be seen in mania, acute psychosis, agitation and anxiety. The arousal level is excessive; there may be motor hyperactivity, frequent scanning eye movements, distractability with sharply focused attention for brief periods, and increased sympathetic activity.

Table 4.1   Mental status examination.

Level of consciousness
Attention
Orientation
Person/place/time
Language
   Spontaneous speech
   Comprehension
   Confrontation naming
   Repetition
   Reading
   Writing
Memory
   Immediate
   Short term (verbal, visual)
   Long term
Fund of information
Constructional skills
Calculations
Right–left orientation
Geographic orientation
Finger gnosis
Praxis
Similarities/proverbs
Frontal sequential tasks (alternating sequences)

Alertness is the normal state of wakefulness when behavioral function is optimal.

Somnolence refers to a lethargic, drowsy or sleepy state in which a person will be lulled into sleep if not stimulated. Recognizing somnolence is important; it may foreshadow progressive decline of consciousness. For example, somnolence may be the initial behavioral change in treatable, but potentially lethal, disorders, such as subdural hematoma. Because somnolence is accompanied by decreased attention and cognitive function, the assessment of higher cognitive functions, such as memory and arithmetic skills, in such patients is unreliable.

Obtundation is a transitional state between lethargy and stupor. The obtunded patient has mental blunting that cannot be fully overcome with stimulation and is lethargic and confused. It is often more helpful to decide if a patient is somnolent or stuporous, because obtundation is a relatively vague description.

Stupor is a state of depressed consciousness in which the unresponsive, sleeping patient can be aroused only with constant, vigorous stimulation. The patient never rises above a lethargic or obtunded condition. The content of consciousness cannot be accurately assessed in stupor.

Coma is a state in which neither spontaneous nor evoked arousal occurs.

Table 4.2   Glasgow Coma Scale.

Parameter	Response	Score
Eyes		
Open	Spontaneously	4
	To verbal command	3
	To pain	2
No response		1
Best motor response		
To verbal command	Obeys	6
To painful stimulus	Localizes pain	5
	Flexion (withdrawal)	4
	Flexion – abnormal (decorticate)	3
	Extension (decerebrate)	2
	No response	1
Best verbal response	Oriented, converses	5
	Disoriented, converses	4
	Inappropriate words	3
	Incomprehensible sounds	2
	No response	1
Total		3–15

Eyes remain closed and noxious stimuli provoke no verbal response, only primitive withdrawal movements at best. Acute coma often evolves into a vegetative state, a subacute or chronic condition characterized by sleep–wake cycles and spontaneous eye opening without cognitive or affective functions (Levy *et al.* 1978). Whether the vegetative state is classified as a chronic coma or a non-comatose condition of arousal without awareness is a matter of semantics.

The Glasgow Coma Scale is a system for classifying comatose patients and is based on three categories of responses: eye opening, motor and verbal (Table 4.2) (Jennett and Teasdale, 1981). This coma scale correlates closely with outcome: the lower the total score, the worse the long-term prognosis for functional recovery (Jennet and Teasdale, 1981). In coma, it is also extremely important to assess the pupillary responses, ocular movements and respiration (Plum and Posner, 1980).

Coma must be distinguished from akinetic mutism, the locked-in syndrome and catatonia. In *akinetic mutism* (Maxim 27), the patient appears awake and his eyes may follow the examiner, but he lacks spontaneous motor and verbal responses (Cairns *et al.*, 1941). There is bowel and bladder incontinence, and response to noxious stimuli is incomplete (Devinsky *et al.*, 1987). Akinetic mutism has been reported following bilateral damage to the frontal lobes, including the cingulate and orbital gyri and the septal area, and small lesions of the paramedian reticular formation in the diencephalon and midbrain (Nielsen and Jacobs, 1951; Barris and Schuman, 1953; Cravioto et al., 1960; Kemper and Romanul, 1967; Skultety, 1968; Freemon, 1971).

The *locked-in state* (Maxim 27) is characterized by tetraplegia and mutism with preserved cognition due to de-efferentation of lower cranial nerve, truncal and appendicular muscles caused by lesions (most often infarction) in the ventral pons or midbrain. Patients can usually communicate by blinking or moving their eyes volitionally (Plum and Posner, 1980).

Catatonia is characterized by a dramatic decrease in spontaneous movements and activity and reactivity to the environment. Catatonia is often accompanied by resistance to movement and cataleptic rigidity – in which limbs may be placed in a position that will be maintained (American Psychiatric Association, 1987). Catatonia can result from both organic and psychiatric causes.

Merely classifying arousal according to the above six grades does not fully describe the behavioral diversity seen in practice and more complete information is often required to identify changes in patient condition. If the level of consciousness is not normal (alert), provide additional descriptive information and define the maximal level of behavioral responsiveness and the intensity of stimulation required for arousal. For example, 'The patient is stuporous; he responds to moderate sternal rubbing with eye opening and grunting, and with more vigorous stimulation he pulls away the examiner's hand. Within 30 seconds after cessation of stimulation he is unresponsive to voice'. Also, when evaluating the level of consciousness and other mental functions, record the patient's responses ('drowsy, does not know the date') instead of recording negative statements ('patient is not alert').

References

American Psychiatric Association. *Diagnostic and Statistical Manual of Psychiatry* (3rd edition, revised). Washington, DC: American Psychiatric Association Press, 1987, p. 196.

Barris RW, Schuman HR. Bilateral anterior cingulate gyrus lesions. *Neurology* 1953; **3**: 44–52.

Cairns H, Oldfield RC, Pennybacker JB et al. Akinetic mutism with an epidermoid cyst of the third ventricle. *Brain* 1941; **64**: 273–90.

Cravioto H, Silberman J, Feigin I. A clinical and pathologic study of akinetic mutism. *Neurology* 1960; **10**: 10–21.

Devinsky O, Lemann W, Evans AC, Moeller JR, Rottenberg DA. Akinetic mutism in a bone marrow transplant recipient following total body irradiation and amphotericin B chemoprophylaxis. A positron emission tomographic and neuropathologic study. *Arch Neurol* 1987; **44**: 414–17.

Freemon FR. Akinetic mutism and bilateral anterior cerebral artery occlusion. *J Neurol Neurosurg Psychiat* 1971; **34**: 693–8.

Jennett B, Teasdale G. Management of head injuries. Philadelphia: FA Davis Company, 1981, pp. 77–84.

Kemper TL, Romanul FCA. State resembling akinetic mutism in basilar artery occlusion. *Neurology* 1967; **17**: 74–80.

Levy DE, Knill-Jonmes RP, Plum F. The vegetative state and its prognosis following nontraumatic coma. *Ann NY Acad Sci* 1978; **315**: 293–306.

Neilson JM, Jacobs LL. Bilateral lesions of the anterior cingulate gyri. *Bull Los Angeles Neurol Soc* 1951; **16**: 231–4.

Plum F, Posner JB. The diagnosis of stupor and coma. Philadelphia: FA Davis Company, 1980, p. 3.

Skultety FM. Clinical and experimental aspects of akinetic mutism. *Arch Neurol* 1968; **19**: 1–14.

5. *Neuropsychological testing is an elaboration of the mental status examination*

Bedside mental status testing is limited by time, environment (often noisy), qualitative analysis and materials. Neuropsychological evaluation permits a more complete and quantitative assessment of cognitive functions. However, neuropsychological testing *does not replace* bedside screening of mental status.

Before obtaining a neuropsychological consultation, formulate the questions that should be addressed. The neuropsychological examination is not an amorphous, global procedure that yields a composite picture of brain function. The preceding bedside mental status testing should have included a broad survey of mental functions and, together with the behavioral history, will identify impaired areas needing further elaboration on formal testing.

There is no practical battery of neuropsychological tests that will suit the needs of all patients. Although most neuropsychologists have a standard screening battery of baseline tests, supplemental testing is often required to characterize a deficit fully. For example, if the patient's chief complaint is impaired memory for recent events, the examination can focus on the various stages in the memory process as well as other disorders that may secondarily impair memory (e.g. attention deficits) or be confused with amnestic disorders (e.g. depression). Also, some disorders such as abulia and sleepiness produce global mental dysfunction.

Neuropsychological testing employs a series of tests and provides an analysis of brain function that must be integrated with the clinical history. Areas in which neuropsychological testing is helpful are summarized in Table 5.1. The principal indications for obtaining neuropsychological testing are (1) localizing areas of cerebral and cognitive dysfunction, and (2) quantification of cognitive strengths and weaknesses. As with any 'quantitative–subjective' test (and most tests are when you include the interpretation), one must be cautious when applying the results. The same raw scores may give rise to quite different interpretations depending on the training and bias of the psychologist and the setting or reason for referral (e.g. litigation). Furthermore, since the interpretation reflects a synthesis of the test scores and clinical history, erroneous clinical information (e.g. from the patient or family) or misleading laboratory studies (e.g. overinterpreted EEG) can be perpetuated and magnified.

Comprehensive neuropsychological batteries include the Halstead–Reitan and Luria–Nebraska (Halstead, 1947; Reitan, 1955; Russell *et al.* 1970; Swiercinsky, 1978; Adams, 1980; Golden, 1981; Stambrook, 1983). The Halstead–Reitan battery was developed to identify patients with brain damage with a psychometric approach, but it is excessively long, includes many global tasks and inadequately covers language and memory. Supplemented with linguistic and memory tests, the Halstead–Reitan battery is useful but even more lengthy. The Luria–Nebraska battery is a standardized format of Luria's clinical neurology approach using Christensen's tests (Christensen, 1979) with normative data. Although it has good breadth, it lacks depth in specific areas. Its reliability and specificity for identifying patients with brain damage and cognitive dysfunction remain controversial (Spiers, 1981).

Many neuropsychologists now use a composite of discrete tests. The Wechsler Adult Intelligence Scale-Revised (WAIS-R) is the standard test for intellectual function for patients between 16 and 75 years of age (Wechsler, 1981). The Full Scale intelligence quotient (IQ) reflects global functions and is calculated from the Verbal and Performance (non-verbal) scale scores. Verbal subtests include Information, Digit Span, Vocabulary,

Table 5.1 Indications for neuropsychological testing.

Indication	Comment
Organic versus functional disorder	Identifies areas of cerebral involvement often not observed on routine testing; inconsistent patterns suggest a psychogenic disorder
Post-stroke, head trauma, cranial neurosurgery	Determines extent and degree of cognitive deficit, identifies areas of preserved function for rehabilitation
Prior to brain tumor or AVM resection	Determines localization of cognitive functions and predicts deficit, which often extends beyond the lesion site. Intracarotid sodium amytal (ISA) test for side of language dominance and memory function. Can predict cognitive areas at risk in surgery
Dementia	Presence and severity
Epilepsy surgery	Ideally, lateralization and localization of cognitive deficits should be the same as the seizure focus. ISA test (see above)
Litigation	Determines the extent of cognitive impairment

Table 5.2   Neuropsychological and behavioral tests.

Intellectual/executive/frontal lobe tests

Wechsler scales (WAIS-R, WISC-R)
Multiple aspects of intellectual functioning
Verbal scale
  Information, Digit Span, Vocabulary, Arithmetic, Comprehension,
  Similarities
Performance scale
  Picture Completion, Picture Arrangement, Block Design, Object
  Assembly, Digit Symbol

Wisconsin card sorting test
Assesses cognitive flexibility, maintenance of set, and concept formation in
  a problem-solving task. Sensitive to frontal lobe dysfunction

Stroop test
Assesses cognitive flexibility, inhibition of competing response sets,
  cognitive speed. Patient reads a list of words, a list of colors and a list of
  color words printed in discordant ink

Trail making test
Part of Halstead–Reitan battery. Assesses psychomotor speed, cognitive
  flexibility. Part A: connect randomly dispersed numbers. Part B:
  alternately connect randomly dispersed numbers and letters

Wide range achievement test-revised
Academic achievement test: reading, arithmetic, spelling

Memory

Wechsler memory scale-revised
Five indexes scored from various subtests: General Memory, Attention,
  Verbal Memory, Non-verbal Memory, Delayed Recall. Subtests include
  general information/orientation, three mental control tasks, recognition
  memory for geometric figures, immediate and delayed drawing of
  geometric designs, immediate and delayed recall of two paragraphs, and
  verbal and non-verbal paired associate learning tasks

Rey complex figure test
Copy and immediate and delayed recall of a complex geometric figure

Buschke selective reminding test
Verbal learning task of 12 words over 12 trials. Scores separate storage from
  retrieval

Rey auditory verbal learning test
Verbal learning task of 15 words repeated over five trials. A distractor
  (separate) list is read after the initial five trials, followed by free recall and
  delayed recall and recognition of words from the original list. It assesses
  learning and interference effects

Supraspan tests
Learning of long digit spans and visual spans (greater than the patient's
    usual span) over repeated trials. Sensitive to hippocampal functions,
    possibly with lateralizing significance (verbal versus non-verbal)

Language

Boston naming test
Visual confrontation naming of 60 line drawings

Word fluency
Generation of words beginning with 'F', 'A' and 'S' in one minute. Sensitive
    to left hemisphere impairment, especially frontal

Token test
Assesses comprehension of propositional language by response to
    commands (e.g. 'Put the white circle on top of the blue square')

Boston diagnostic aphasia examination
Battery of numerous language tasks. Normed on aphasic populations.
    Includes tests of nearly all areas of language functioning

Non-verbal, spatial

Hooper visual organization test
Assesses non-constructional visual perception and synthesis. Patient
    identifies line drawings which have been cut up and rearranged

Judgment of line orientation test
Measure of spatial relations. Patient matches target line at a certain angle
    to a sunburst array of other lines

Rey complex figure test
Copy a complex figure. Sensitive to neglect and constructional disorders

Facial recognition test
Matching heavily shadowed faces. Assesses passive (i.e.
    non-constructional) perceptual integration

Sensation/perception
  Perceptual and sensory examination
  From Halstead–Reitan battery. Visual fields; extinction to double
      simultaneous stimulation in visual, auditory and tactile modalities; finger
      agnosia; graphesthesia; right/left orientation; and stereognosis

Motor
  Grooved pegboard
  Test of motor dexterity involving rapid placement of grooved pegs into
      holes on a board
  Dynomometer
  From Halstead–Reitan test. Quantification of grip strength.
  Finger oscillation (tapping) test
  From Halstead–Reitan battery. A test of fine motor dexterity.
      Multiple trials of 10 second periods of rapidly pressing telegraph-type key

Praxis
Tasks of limb-kinetic, ideomotor, ideational and buccofacial praxis.

Personality

MMPI:–2
Three validity scales, 10 clinical scales, usually interpreted by profile
    patterns rather than individual scale elevations

MCMI-II (Millon)
Similar to MMPI (T–F questions) but shorter. Oriented more to DSM-IIIR
    personality disorders

Rorschach
'Ink blot test.' Some score it formally with deviations from normative
    populations and concordance with clinical groups; others form dynamic
    interpretations from content and sequence of responses. Especially
    sensitive to psychotic or borderline disorders

Bear-Fedio inventory (temporal lobe questionnaire)
Test of traits assessing dimensions of the 'temporal lobe epilepsy interictal
    personality syndrome' Specificity of this inventory is controversial.

Arithmetic, Comprehension and Similiarites. Performance subtests include
Picture Completion, Picture Arrangement, Block Design, Object Assembly
and Digit Symbol. The Wechsler Intelligence Scale for Children-Revised
(WISC-R) is used for patients aged 6 to 15 years and the Wechsler Preschool
and Primary Scale for Intelligence-Revised (WPPSI-R) is used for children
under the age of 6 years. Neither the WAIS-R nor WISC-R tests memory
functions.

The Wechsler Memory Scale (WMS; Wechsler, 1973) is the most widely
used test for evaluation of memory and provides a statistically age-adjusted
memory quotient (MQ) (Wechsler, 1973). There are several features concerning the WMS that should be noted: (1) inclusion of non-memory tests
(i.e. orientation and attention) into the MQ, which can produce an over-
estimation of memory ability; (2) an emphasis on verbal memory; (3) a lack
of delayed recall (failure to assess retention); and (4) inadequate separation
of verbal from non-verbal memory in the MQ. Many neuropsychologists
add a 30 minute delayed recall paradigm following recall of two stories
(verbal) and visual designs (non-verbal) to test retention (Russell, 1975). A
revision of the WMS has been released (Wechsler, 1987) which rectifies
some of these problems, including separate indices for attention, visual
and verbal memory, and delayed recall, as well as general memory.

A review of all major neuropsychological tests is beyond the scope of
this book. Table 5.2 summarizes some of the commonly used tests. The
interested reader is referred to the other books and articles that provide a
more extensive review of this subject (Benton *et al.*, 1983; Kimura and
McGlone, 1983; Weintraub and Mesulam, 1985; Lezak, 1988).

References

Adams KM. In search of Luria's battery: A false start. *J Consult Clin Psychol* 1980; **48**: 511–16.

Benton AL *et al*. *Contributions to Neuropsychological Assessment: A Clinical Manual*. Oxford, New York: Oxford University Press, 1983.

Christensen AL. *Luria's Neuropsychological Investigation* (2nd edition). Copenhagen: Munksgaard; Los Angeles: Western Psychological Services, 1979.

Golden CJ. A standardized version of Luria's neuropsychological tests. In: *Handbook of Clinical Neuropsychology* (Filskov SB, Boll TJ, eds). New York: Wiley-Interscience, 1981, pp. 608–42.

Halstead W. *Brain and Intelligence: A Qualitative Study of the Frontal Lobes*. Chicago: University of Chicago Press, 1947.

Kimura D, McGlone J. *Neuropsychology Test Procedures*. London: DK Consultants, 1983.

Lezak MD. *Neuropsychological Assessment*. Oxford, New York: Oxford University Press, 1988.

Reitan R. Investigation of the validity of Halstead's measures of biological intelligence. *Arch Neurol Psychiat* 1955; **48**: 475.

Russell EW. A multiple scoring method for the assessment of complex memory functions. *J Clin Psychol* 1975; **43**: 800–9.

Russell EW, Neuringer C, Goldstein G. *Assessment of Brain Damage: A Neuropsychological Key Approach*. New York: John Wiley, 1970.

Spiers PA. Have they come to praise Luria or bury him? The Luria–Nebraska Battery controversy. *J Consul Clin Psychol* 1981; **49**: 331

Stambrook M. The Luria-Nebraska Neuropsychological Battery: A promise that may be partly fulfilled. *J Clin Neuropsychol* 1983; **5**: 247–69.

Swiercinsky D. *Manual for the Adult Neuropsychological Evaluation*. Springfield, IL: Charles C Thomas, 1978.

Wechsler DA. *Wechsler Memory Scale*. New York: The Psychological Corporation, 1973.

Wechsler DA. *Wechsler Adult Intelligence Scale-Revised (WAIS-R)*. New York: The Psychological Corporation, 1981.

Wechsler DA. *Wechsler Memory Scale-Revised*. New York: The Psychological Corporation, 1987.

Weintraub S, Mesulam M-M. Mental status assessment of young and elderly adults in behavioral neurology. In: *Principles of Behavioral Neurology* (Mesulam M-M, ed.). Philadelphia: FA Davis Company, 1985, pp. 71–123.

6.   *Attention, the ability to maintain a coherent stream of thought, is a prerequisite for higher cognitive functions*

William James (1890) wrote 'Everyone knows what attention is. It is the taking possession by the mind, in clear and vivid form, of one out of what seem several simultaneous possible subjects or trains of thought. Focalization, concentration, of consciousness are its essence. It implies withdrawal from some things in order to deal effectively with others . . . .'.

The level of consciousness must be determined before attention is assessed. The lethargic, obtunded or stuporous patient cannot be attentive. However, a patient may be alert but inattentive. The vegetative state, for example, is characterized by an alert appearance without attentive or cognitive powers.

Attention is the foundation for higher cognitive functions. The ability to sustain attention, or vigilance, is necessary for complex behaviors, such as understanding and remembering a story. Therefore, *attention must be tested before other cognitive functions*. Failure of an inattentive patient to perform serial seven subtractions from 100 sheds no light on arithmetic skills.

Specific testing of attention is usually not necessary in a patient who is not distractible and who can provide a detailed, clear and thoughtful account of his problem. However, the patient who is distractible, gets lost in his train of thought, answers questions with nods and yes/no responses, or complains of difficulty with concentration, memory or other cognitive functions deserves formal tests of attention. Further, if mental status deficits are identified, inattention should be considered as a possible contributing factor.

Diminished attention is the hallmark of delirium. Although the delirious patient may be hyperalert, somnolent or obtunded, he is also distractible and inattentive. Any novel stimulus, for example, a beeper, person passing in the hall or outside construction noise, will distract the inattentive subject and cause the patient's center of focus to shift as if he is watching a ping-pong match.

Attentional mechanisms may be directed diffusely or unilaterally:

Diffuse attentional deficits

The diffusely distributed attentional system surveys the internal and external environments for important novel or changing stimuli. Anatomically, this system includes the ascending reticular activating system (ARAS), thalamus, limbic system and neocortex. The ARAS and thalamic relays are essential for arousal. Limbic, primary and association sensory areas, and higher order (multimodal, heteromodal) association areas all contribute to the attentional network, particularly the parietal and frontal lobes, which are especially important in selective attention (Roland, 1982; Posner *et al.*, 1984; Mesulam, 1985).

The diffusely distributed functions can be tested using digit repetition and number-tapping. Digit repetition measures attention to a verbal stimulus and the ability to maintain attention during repetition of the number sequence. In this test, the patient is asked to repeat a series of random digits, beginning with three digits and then progressively adding a digit until he makes an error, or correctly repeats seven digits. It is important to avoid presenting the digits in a logical sequence (e.g. 3–2–1 or 1–3–5–7) or grouped, as in a telephone number (e.g. 753–1249). The examiner should slowly state the numbers with a consistent pause of approximately one second between them and without inflection or breaks. The normal adult can repeat six or seven digits forward; repeating three or four digits backwards is a more difficult task that requires more cognitive processing (Spitz, 1972). A sample sequence of digit repetition is:

    3 – 8 – 2
    5 – 2 – 9 – 4
    2 – 6 – 1 – 8 – 3
    7 – 4 – 9 – 5 – 2 – 8
    4 – 9 – 1 – 3 – 5 – 2 – 7

The number-tapping test assesses vigilance by asking the patient to tap his index finger each time he hears a target number. Numbers are presented at the uniform rate of approximately one per second. Inattentive subjects will often commit omission errors, tapping correctly for the first one or two target numbers, but failing to tap with subsequent target stimuli. Perseveration errors, in which the patient continues to tap with subsequent non-target numbers, are characteristic of patients with frontal lesions (Maxim 54). A sample sequence of numbers (target number equals 4) is:

    1 – 11 – 14 – 3 – 4 – 6 – 2 – 17 – 11 – 4 – 4 – 12 –
    19 – 3 – 15 – 5 – 1 – 8 – 15 – 14 – 7 – 4 – 10 – 7

Significant language comprehension deficits may render digit repetition and the number-tapping test invalid as measures of attention and vigilance.

Unilateral attentional deficits.

The unilaterally directed attentional system is subserved by the contralateral hemisphere. Unilateral neglect is most common after right parietal injury and is characterized, in these cases, by failure to attend to left-sided stimuli or by extinction of the left-sided stimulus with bilateral stimulation (Maxims 62 and 63) (Critchley, 1953; Denny-Brown and Chambers, 1958). However, neglect also occurs with left parietal or non-parietal (frontal, cingulate or subcortical) lesions (Heilman et al., 1983). Unilateral neglect (inattention or extinction) can be tested with double simultaneous stimulation in visual, tactile, or less often, auditory modalities. However, it may be difficult to differentiate homonymous hemianopsia from unilateral neglect. In these cases, it is best to test the visual fields in a very dark room, using a small penlight. Patients with visual neglect see the penlight in the blind hemifield, and those with hemianopsia do not.

References

Critchley M. *The Parietal Lobes*. Sevenoaks: Edward Arnold, 1953.
Denny-Brown D, Chambers RA. The parietal lobe and behavior. *Assoc Res Nerv Ment Dis* 1958; **36**: 35–117.
Heilman KM, Watson RT, Valenstein E, Damasio AR. Localization of lesions in

neglect. In: *Localization in Neuropsychology* (Kertesz A, ed.). Orlando, FL: Academic Press, 1983, pp. 455–70.

James W. *The Principles of Psychology*. New York: H Holt and Company, 1890, pp. 403–4.

Mesulam MM. Patterns in behavioral neuroanatomy: Association areas, the limbic system, and hemispheric specialization. In: *Principles of Behavioral Neurology* (Mesulam MM, ed.). Philadelphia: FA Davis Company, 1985.

Posner MI, Walker JA, Friedrich FJ, Rafal RD. Effects of parietal injury on covert orienting of attention. *J Neurosci* 1984; **4**: 1863–74.

Roland PE. Cortical regulation of selective attention in man. A regional cerebral blood flow study. *J Neurophysiol* 1982; **48**: 1059–78.

Spitz HH. Note on immediate memory for digits: Invariance over the years. *Psychol Bull* 1972; **78**: 183.

7.   The cerebral hemispheres are anatomically and functionally divided into four lobes

Brodmann's (1910) schema, which remains most popular today, identified 47 cytoarchitecturally distinct areas of the human cerebral cortex (Fig. 7.1), while von Economo (1929) distinguished 109 areas and Vogt and Vogt (1919) recognized more than 200. We now recognize that a true functional and anatomical map of the cortex must consider not only the types of cells and fibers, but also the receptors, neurotransmitters, neuropeptides and connections.

Even the division of cerebrum into motor and sensory areas is an oversimplification since these, too, are interconnected. Activity in a sensory area can modify function in a motor area. For example, a painful stimulus applied proximal to an area involved by focal motor seizures can occasionally prevent further seizure spread. On the other hand, electrical stimulation of sensory areas may cause movement, as when stimulation of occipital visual areas triggers contralateral conjugate eye movements.

Although precise anatomical and functional subdivisions of the brain remain elusive, the gross separation of four cerebral lobes has been a universal starting point. The two obvious landmarks on the lateral cerebral surface are the central sulcus and the Sylvian fissure. Figures 7.2–7.4 show the four cerebral lobes from the lateral, medial and inferior views and their subdivisions.

The *frontal lobe* lies anterior to the central sulcus and includes the primary motor cortex (BA 4); the premotor or secondary motor area (BA 6, 8), the supplementary motor area (medial portion of BA 6); frontal eye fields (BA 8); Broca's area (BA 44, 45), and the prefrontal cortex (BA 9, 10, 11 and 12). The extensive prefrontal cortex includes the majority of the superior, middle and inferior frontal gyri of the dorsolateral cortex, as well as the orbital (BA 11, 12) and medial frontal (BA 32) and anterior cingulate (BA 24) gyri. Disorders associated with frontal lobe lesions are summarized in Table 7.1.

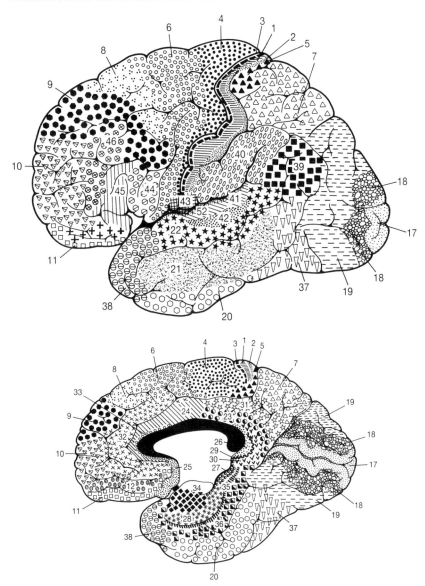

Fig. 7.1   Brodmann's cytoarchitectural map of the human brain. After Brodal.

The *parietal lobe* lies behind the central sulcus. The primary somesthetic cortex (BA 1, 2 and 3) is situated on the posterior bank of this sulcus, with the somesthetic association cortex (BA 5) lying immediately behind the primary cortex. The secondary somesthetic cortex (BA 43) is a small area located inferior to the primary sensorimotor cortex. The posterior parietal lobe is divided into superior (BA 7) and inferior (BA 39 and 40) lobules. The inferior parietal lobule is divided into the supramarginal and angular gyri. Disorders associated with parietal lobe lesions are summarized in Table 7.2.

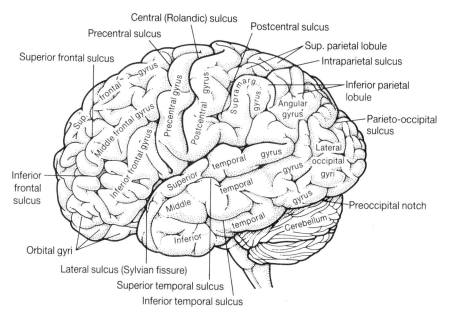

Fig. 7.2 Lateral surface of the brain showing the four cerebral lobes.

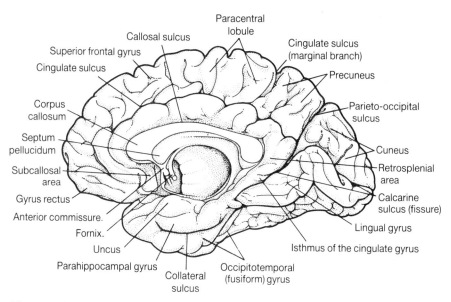

Fig. 7.3 Medial surface of the brain showing the four cerebral lobes.

Table 7.1 Disorders associated with frontal lobe lesions.

Primary motor cortex
Weakness (maximal in distal muscles, fine movements)
Increased tone (spasticity) – mild

Motor association cortex
Weakness (maximal in proximal muscles)
Increased tone (spasticity)
Buccofacial apraxia (left side)
Sympathetic (callosal) apraxia (left side)
Grasp reflex

Supplementary motor area
Grasp reflex
Impaired rapid alternating movements
Transient transcortical motor aphasia (left side)
Transient impairment of motor initiation

Broca's area (left hemisphere)
Broca's aphasia
Dysprosody (also occurs with right-sided lesions)

Prefrontal area

Left
Inability to plan and execute multistepped processes
Transcortical motor aphasia
Depression

Right
Left-sided extinction and neglect
Blunted or labile affect
Impersistence
Reduplication
Disinhibition
Confabulation
Depression
Alien hand sign

Bilateral
Abulia
Inability to plan and execute multistepped processes
Dysprosody
Blunted and labile affect
Depression
Disinhibition and loss of social graces
Incontinence
Catatonia
Perseveration
Confabulation

The *temporal lobe* lies inferior to the Sylvian fissure and its posterior and superior aspects are continuous with the parietal and occipital lobes. The lateral temporal lobe is divided into superior, middle and inferior gyri (BA 20, 21, 22, 37, 38, 41 and 42). The primary auditory cortex or Heschl's gyrus (BA 41) and auditory association cortex (BA 42 and 22), which includes Wernicke's area, both lie in the posterosuperior aspect. The remainder of the lateral temporal lobe is association cortex, much of which has connections with the limbic and visual system. The medial temporal lobe is part of the limbic system and includes the amygdala, hippocampus, and para-hippocampal and fusiform (occipitotemporal) gyri. Limbic areas are concerned with emotion and memory (Maxims 58 and 61). Disorders associated with temporal lobe disorders are summarized in Table 7.3.

The *occipital lobe* lies posterior to the temporal and parietal lobes and consists mainly of visual cortex: primary visual or striate cortex (BA 17)

Table 7.2   Disorders associated with parietal lobe lesions.

Primary somatosensory cortex
Impairment of cutaneous and proprioceptive (joint position) sensation
Impairment in ability accurately to localize pain and temperature
    sensations

Secondary somatosensory cortex
Impairment in fine sensory discrimination (changes in weight, texture,
    temperature, separation of two points)

Parietal association cortex

Left (1–4 = Gertsmann's syndrome; 1–9 = angular gyrus syndrome)
1.   Agraphia
2.   Acalculia
3.   Finger agnosia
4.   Right/left disorientation
5.   Alexia
6.   Conduction aphasia
7.   Anomic aphasia
8.   Constructional apraxia
9.   Impaired proverb and similarities–differences interpretation
10.   Apraxia (ideomotor)
11.   Extinction and neglect of right-sided stimuli (uncommon)

Right
Extinction and neglect of left-sided stimuli
Visuospatial disorders
Geographic disorientation
Constructional apraxia
Dressing apraxia
Impersistence

and visual association cortex (BA 18 and 19). Disorders associated with occipital lobe lesions are summarized in Table 7.4.

The *insula* (Figure 8.1) is the cortical area lying deep within the Sylvian fissure and covered by inferolateral frontoparietal and superolateral temporal cortex. Its functions remain poorly understood, although electrical stimulation of the insula produces visceral sensory and motor phenomena, including nausea, vomiting, changes in blood pressure and heart rate (Penfield and Jasper, 1954; Penfield, 1958). Lesions in the area of the left insula may cause conduction aphasia, but this deficit probably results in injury to subjacent fibers interconnecting auditory association and Broca's areas or to adjacent temporoparietal language cortex or subcortical fibers (Damasio and Damasio, 1983).

Cerebral white matter contains myelinated axons. There are three principal fiber groups: (1) association fibers that interconnect cortical areas within the same hemisphere (Fig. 7.5); (2) commissural fibers that connect corresponding areas of the two hemispheres (Maxim 52; Fig. 52.1); and (3)

Table 7.3   Disorders associated with temporal lobe lesions.

Primary auditory cortex (Heschl's gyrus)
Unilateral lesions cause no hearing impairment
Bilateral lesions cause cortical deafness (rare)

Auditory association cortex/Wernicke's area

Left
Wernicke's aphasia
Conduction aphasia

Right
Impaired music perception
Sensory dysprosodia

Bilateral – unilateral disorders and auditory agnosia

Lateral temporal non-auditory cortex
Agitated delirium (right)
Synesthesia
Impairment of associating auditory and visual stimuli with emotional
    valence

Medial (limbic) cortex
Short-term memory (verbal greater on left, visuospatial on right)
Decreased or increased aggression
Emotional disorders
Depression
Mania (usually right-sided lesions)
Hallucinations/illusions
Kluver–Bucy syndrome (bilateral anterior lesions)

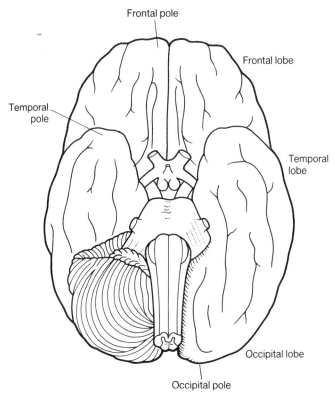

Fig. 7.4   Inferior surface (base) of the brain showing three cerebral lobes.

Table 7.4   Disorders associated with occipital lobe lesions

Primary visual (striate) cortex
Contralateral homonymous hemianopsia – unilateral lesions
Cortical blindness – bilateral lesions

Visual association cortices

Left
Alexia
Color anomia
Right hemiachromatopsia*

Right
Palinopsia
Left hemiachromatopsia*

Bilateral
Visual agnosia
Prosopagnosia (inferomesial)
Balint's syndrome† (oculomotor apraxia, simultanagnosia, optic ataxia)

---

*Lesions are inferior and usually extend to the temporal lobe.
†Lesions are usually superior and often extend to the parietal lobes.

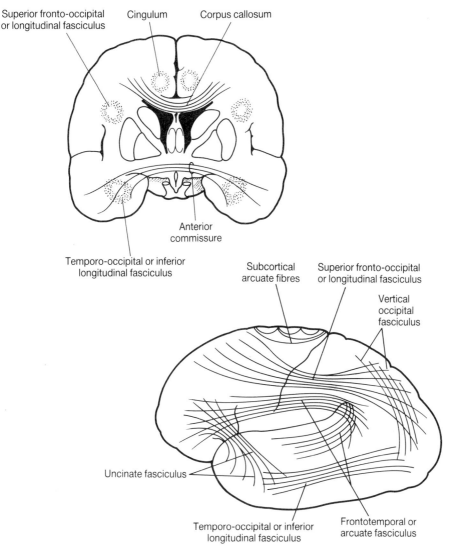

Fig. 7.5 The important association and commissural fiber bundles.

projection fibers that connect the cerebral cortex with the brainstem and spinal cord; these fibers pass in the corone radieta and internal capsule. Other white matter fiber collections include the arcuate fibers, which connect adjacent gyri of nonassociation cortex, and the geniculocalcarine tract.

References

Brodmann K. Feinere anatomie des grosshirns. In: *Lewandowsky's Handbuch der Neurologic* (volume 5). Leipzig: JA Barth, 1910, pp. 206–307.
Damasio H, Damasio AR. The localization of lesions in conduction aphasia. In:

Localization in Neuropsychology. New York: Academic Press, Inc., 1983, pp. 231–43.

Penfield W. Functional localization in temporal and deep Sylvian areas. *Res Publ Assoc Nerv Ment Dis* 1956; **36**: 210–26.

Penfield W, Jasper H. *Epilepsy and the Functional Anatomy of the Human Brain.* Boston: Little, Brown, and Company, 1954, pp. 424–37.

Vogt C, Vogt O. Allgemeine ergebnisse unserer hirnforschung. *J Psychol Neurol* 1919; **25**: 279–461.

von Economo C. *The Cytoarchitectonics of the Human Cerebral Cortex.* Oxford: Oxford University Press, 1929.

8.   *Multimodal (heteromodal) association cortex is the brain substrate for cognitive functions*

The human cerebral cortex can be divided into four functional types: (1) *limbic–paralimbic areas*; (2) *primary sensory or motor areas*, called idiotypic cortex; (3) *specific association areas*, both unimodal or motor, and (4) *multimodal association areas* (Fig. 8.1).

Limbic and paralimbic areas are critical for emotion, motivation, instinct, visceral processes, sexual and social relations, attention and memory. Limbic areas, which are connected with hypothalamic and paralimbic areas, include the amygdala, hippocampus, septum and cingulate gyrus. Paralimbic areas, which are connected with limbic and heteromodal association areas, include the temporal pole, parahippocampal gyrus, anterior insula and caudal orbitofrontal gyrus. The limbic lobe or *le grand lobe limbique*, as coined by Broca in 1878, refers to a ring of gray matter on the medial aspects of the hemisphere. The anatomical justification for denoting the limbic lobe and functional justification for the limbic system has been questioned (Brodal, 1981). However, these terms are embedded in our clinical and scientific framework, and they are useful, despite their limitations.

Primary sensory areas are the first cortical areas to receive modality-specific (e.g., visual, auditory) input; they perform initial processing of such data. The sensory input is organized by criteria specific to its modality. For example, somatosensory input is organized by body part, visual input by

Fig. 8.1 Distribution of functional zones in relation to Brodmann's map of the human brain. The boundaries are not intended to be precise. AA, auditory association cortex. AG, angular gyrus. A1, primary auditory cortex. CG, cingulate cortex. INS, insula. IPL, inferior parietal lobe. IT, inferior temporal gyrus. MA, motor association cortex. MPO, medial parieto-occipital area. MT, middle temporal gyrus. M1, primary motor area. OF, orbitofrontal region. PC, prefrontal cortex. PH, parahippocampal region. PO, paraolfactory area. PS, peristriate cortex. RS, retrosplenial area. SA, somatosensory association cortex. SG, supramarginal gyrus. SPL, superior parietal lobule. ST, superior temporal gyrus. S1, primary somatosensory area. TP, temporopolar cortex. VA, visual association cortex. V1, primary visual cortex. Reproduced with permission from Mesulam and the publisher, F.A. Davis. xx

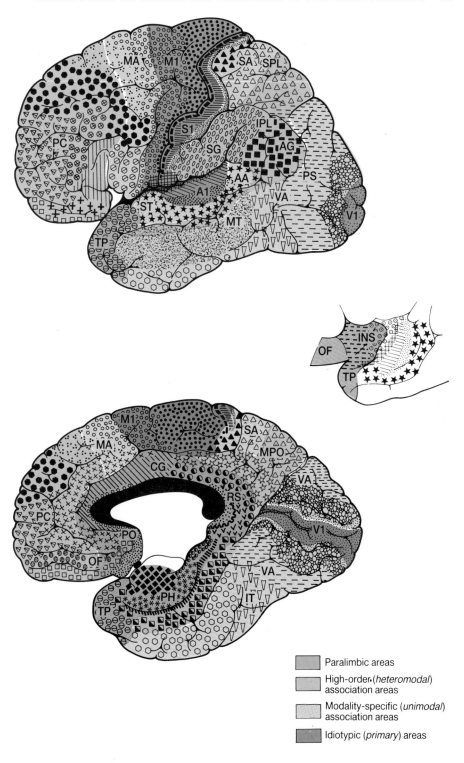

areas in the visual field, and auditory input by tone and spatial location. Secondary sensory areas lie adjacent to primary areas and are intermediate between primary and unimodal-specific sensory association areas in both cytoarchitecture and function.

Unimodal-specific sensory association areas perform additional analysis and processing of sensory information and communicate this higher order information to multimodal association cortex.

The primary motor area sends efferents in the corticospinal tract to control skeletal muscle activity. The supplementary motor area is analogous to secondary sensory areas and is important in the initiation of movement. The motor-specific association (premotor) area shares features of sensory unimodal association cortex, with connections to both primary motor cortex and multimodal cortex, and are important for sensorimotor integration and complex movements (Halsband and Freund, 1990). These functions include regulation of motor exploration; ocular scanning, a function located in the frontal eye fields (BA 8); motor programs for speech, located in Broca's area (BA 44, 45), and such complex hand movements as piano playing. In addition, motor-specific association areas are probably involved in initiation, learning, planning and inhibition of complex movements (Brinkman and Porter, 1983; Lüders *et al.*, 1983; Lesser *et al.*, 1984).

Multimodal association cortex areas are present in the frontal, parietal and temporal lobes (Fig. 8.1). These areas receive input from multiple sensory and motor association cortices and perform higher order analysis, integration and synthesis of sensorimotor data. Therefore, these areas of multimodal association cortex are cognitive, rather than sensorimotor, in nature (Mesulam, 1985). Furthermore, multimodal association cortex areas are not tied to one sensory modality or motor function and have important input and output to paralimbic and limbic areas. These connections from multimodal cortex to limbic areas help assess the emotional relevance of stimuli and complex situations, providing the pathway for conceptual ideas, e.g. 'Joe hit your father', to modify mood and affect. On the other hand, connections from limbic areas to multimodal association cortex areas enable emotions to modify cognitive processes. For example, feelings of fear or paranoia can trigger intent scanning of the visual field in search of threatening stimuli.

References

Brinkman C, Porter R. Supplementary motor area and premotor area of monkey cerebral cortex: Functional organization and activities of single neurons during performance of a learned movement. In: *Motor Control Mechanisms in Health and Disease* (Desmedt JE, ed.). New York: Raven Press, 1983.

Broca P. Anatomie comparée des circonvolutions cérébrales; le grand lobe limbique et la scissure limbique dans la serie des mammiferes. *Rev Anthropolol Series 2* 1878; 1: 384–498.

Brodal A. *Neurological Anatomy in Relation to Clinical Medicine.* Oxford, New York: Oxford University Press, 1981, pp. 689–90.

Halsband U, Freund HJ. Premotor cortex and conditional motor learning in man. *Brain* 1990; **113**: 207–22.

Lesser RP, Lüders H, Dinner DS, Hahn J, Cohen L. The location of speech and writing functions in the frontal language area: Results of extraoperative cortical stimulation. *Brain* 1984; **107**: 275–91.

Luders H, Lesser RP, Dinner DS, Morris HH, Hahn J. Inhibition of motor activity elicited by electrical stimulation of the human cortex. *Epilepsia* 1983; **24**: 519.

Mesulam M-M. Patterns in behavioral neuroanatomy: Association areas, the limbic system, and hemispheric specialization. In: *Principles of Behavioral Neurology* (Mesulam M-M, ed.). Philadelphia: FA Davis Company, 1985, pp. 1–70.

9. *Positive symptoms reflect activity of preserved, but often dysfunctional, nervous tissue*

Reynolds (1861) introduced the concept of positive and negative neurological symptoms as being the excess or negation of vital properties, respectively. Positive symptoms are abnormal, 'superimposed' behaviors that presumably reflect overactivity of neural function and include sensations, such as hallucinations; movements, as in clonic jerking or chorea; and thoughts, such as paranoid delusions. Negative symptoms are due to a reduction or loss of neurological function, for example, weakness, blindness, confusion or coma. Jackson (1875, 1881) postulated that negative symptoms result from dissolution of neural function while positive symptoms are caused by activity or hyperactivity of 'lower' centers that are normal, except 'figuratively speaking, for insubordination from loss of control'. Thus, under Jackson's theory, the lesion *per se* does not directly produce 'extravagant conduct', delusions or misidentification of a nurse as a wife. Consider, for example, a man with a left hemisphere lesion who makes semantic paraphasias. The inability to name a table correctly is a negative symptom. The incorrect choice, 'chair', represents a positive symptom. Jackson argued that the wrong utterance is produced by activity from only a fragment of the nervous arrangements for speech. He postulated that complex mental states are always the product of healthy nerve tissue, that is, positive phenomena.

Similarly, Kraeplin's (1919) early description of dementia praecox focused on loss of mental functions, or dementia, but both he and Bleuler (1950) recognized an extensive group of more acute, positive phenomena that included aggressive behavior, delusions, and hallucinations and illusions in all sensory modalities. These phenomena are most likely to occur early in the course of illness. Positive symptoms are also common in bipolar and anxiety disorders (Silberman *et al.*, 1985). In schizophrenia, negative symptoms include affective flattening, impoverished thought and speech, loss of motivation, inability to experience pleasure (anhedonia) and impaired attention. Based on these observations, Crow (1980) suggested that schizophrenia may represent two overlapping syndromes. Patients with the first syndrome have a more acute course characterized by prominent delusions and hallucinations, preserved intellect and a good response to neuroleptics. The etiology in these patients, Crow postulated, is dopaminergic hyperactivity. In contrast, patients with the second syndrome have a more chronic course with intellectual deterioration, diminished spontaneity and affect, and a poor response to neuroleptics. The presumed etiology in this latter group is neuronal loss.

While psychiatrists have thus adopted the concept of positive and negative symptoms, it has largely been abandoned by neurologists (Berrios, 1985). This is ironic, as the concept emerged from the study of behavior during and after seizures.

Part of this reticence may lay in the fact that, in neurologic disorders, the distinction between positive and negative symptoms is often blurred. However, employing this concept can yield insight into the functions of lesioned and preserved areas during neurobehavioral examination. The positive symptoms or hallucination and repetitive involuntary movements illustrate this benefit well.

Hallucinations may result from excitation or occur as release phenomena following lesions in any part of the sensory pathway. Electrical stimulation of the cerebral cortex, limbic and diencephalic areas can elicit simple and formed hallucinations and illusions; these events are typically paroxysmal and transient, and they have significant value in localizing lesions. On the other hand, release hallucinations are often more prolonged, less stereotyped and can often be modified by purposeful acts (e.g. changing the direction of gaze). Although they have less localizing value than excitatory hallucinations, they tend to appear in the portion of the sensory field with impaired sensation. Their postulated mechanism is a loss of normal inhibitory mechanisms that causes 'overactivity or release' of otherwise normal nervous tissue. Thus, these positive symptoms – release hallucinations – result from a loss of normal function. Causes of release hallucinations include sensory deprivation, which can cause hallucinations in all modalities (Bliss and Clark, 1962), and focal cerebral or peripheral sensory lesions, which may cause hallucinations in visual, auditory, tactile, vestibular or olfactory modalities (Hecaen and Ropert, 1959; Cogan, 1973; Cascino and Adams, 1986). In addition, the most likely mechanism of hallucinations in migraine and ischemia is release phenomenon.

Another positive symptom, repetitive involuntary movements, as in shaking, jerking or swinging of an extremity, may result from transient hemodynamic ischemic episodes (Yanagihara et al., 1985). These non-epileptic movements are associated with occlusion or high-grade stenosis of the contralateral carotid artery and the upright position.

Negative symptoms in neurology are functional losses resulting from destruction or physiologic inhibition of neuronal aggregates or white matter fibers. The symptoms can affect any sensory modality, strength, coordination or thought and affect. Hemiparesis resulting from a stroke in the contralateral primary motor cortex or internal capsule is a classic negative symptom. As one moves from primary motor and sensory modalities to intellect and emotion, subtleties emerge between positive and negative symptoms. For example, loss of mental flexibility and organizational skills after frontal lesions can be viewed as simply functional losses or negative symptoms. However, if perseverations (abnormal repetitions) are present, these positive symptoms can 'produce' negative symptoms such as an inability to shift sets.

The heuristic value of conceptualizing symptoms as positive or negative may be greatest for complex behaviors with brain disease. We neurologists tend to think that 'lesions cause symptoms' since persons without lesions do not have symptoms. Jackson correctly recognized that formulation as too simplistic. Neurobehavioral correlates of localized lesions tell us not only about the functions of involved areas, but also about the functions of preserved areas, including those with and without prominent connections to the lesional zone.

References

Berrios GE. Positive and negative symptoms and Jackson: A conceptual history. *Arch Gen Psychiat* 1985; **42**: 95–7.

Bleuler E. *Dementia Praecox or the Group of Schizophrenias*, (J Zinkin, transl.). New York: International University Press, 1950.

Bliss EL, Clark LD. Visual hallucinations. In: *Hallucinations* (West LJ, ed.). New York: Grune and Stratton, 1962.

Cascino GD, Adams RD. Brainstem auditory hallucinosis. *Neurology* 1986; **36**: 1042–7.

Cogan DG. Visual hallucinations as release phenomena. *Albrecht von Graefes Arch Klin Exp Ophthalmol* 1973; **188**: 139–50.

Crow TJ. Molecular pathology of schizophrenia: more than one disease process? *Br Med J* 1980; **280**: 1–9.

Hecaen H, Ropert R. Hallucinations auditives au cours du syndromes neurologiques. *Ann Med Psychol* 1959; **1**: 257–306.

Jackson JH. On temporary mental disorders after epileptic paroxysms. *West Riding Lunatic Asylum Med Rep* 1875; **5**: 105–29.

Jackson JH. Remarks on dissolution of the nervous system as exemplified by certain post-epileptic conditions. *Med Press Circ* 1881; **1**: 329–32.

Kraeplin E. Dementia praecox and paraphrenia (Barclay RM, Robertson GM, transl.). Edinburgh: Churchill Livingstone, 1919.

Reynolds JR. *Epilepsy: Its Symptoms, Treatment and Relation to Other Chronic Convulsive Diseases*. London: John Churchill, 1861, pp. 8–10.

Silberman EK, Post RM, Nurnberger J, Theodore W, Boulenger JP. Transient sensory, cognitive and affective phenomena in affective illness: A comparison with complex partial epilepsy. *Br J Psychiatr* 1985; **146**: 81–9.

Yanagihara T, Piepgras DG, Klass DW. Repetitive involuntary movement associated with episodic cerebral ischemia. *Ann Neurol* 1985; **18**: 244–50.

10.   *Diaschisis is dysfunction in cerebral areas remote from the destructive lesion*

Von Monakow (1914) introduced the term diaschisis to describe interruption of brain function in areas connected to a cerebral area that has been injured. Diaschisis, therefore, is secondary dysfunction in areas 'remote' from the circumscribed lesion. In general, dysfunction is maximal in areas that have the strongest interconnections with the lesion site. The concept of diaschisis remains controversial, however, largely due to confusion over its definition.

Diaschisis is derived from the Greek word meaning 'shocked throughout'. Von Monakow described four principal features of diaschisis:

1. The shock must be limited to a localized brain area.
2. Initial symptoms result from loss of excitatory input (not loss of active inhibition) among areas interconnected with the injured nervous structure.
3. The loss of function usually appears quite suddenly (e.g. following stroke), but may also occur in a gradually progressive form (e.g. in those with tumors), which Von Monakow termed 'slowly creeping diaschisis'.
4. Clinical deficits undergo gradual resolution in well-defined phases. However, as Von Monakow recognized, in some cases the shock's effects cannot be 'repaired' or 'compensated', and the diaschisis (dysfunction) is permanent.

Von Monakow described three main types of diaschisis, based on the anatomical pathways involved:

1. Diaschisis cortico-spinalis, or *spinal diaschisis*: impaired function of spinal cord motor cells following a motor cortex lesion which results in weakness.
2. Diaschisis associativa, or *intrahemispheric diaschisis*: impaired function of intact cortical areas resulting from injury to interconnected, ipsilateral cerebral areas.
3. Diaschisis commissuralis, or *interhemispheric diaschisis*: impaired function of intact cortical areas resulting from injury to interconnected, contralateral cerebral areas. For example, 'massive lesions of commissural fibers in the left hemisphere will interrupt dynamically the points of entry and exit of fibers in the cortex of the right hemisphere, which will impair a number of more complicated nervous processes [apraxia, aphasia, agnosia]' (Von Monakow, 1914).

The definition and principal anatomic subtypes of diaschisis put forth by Von Monakow have undergone some changes. Loss of inhibitory, as well as excitatory, input can produce dysfunction at remote sites. Also, brainstem, diencephalic and striatal lesions can impair function at remote sites; i.e. *subcortical diaschisis*.

The loss of reflexes that complicates acute spinal shock following spinal injury is a useful, albeit simplistic, model of cerebral diaschisis. In humans, a lesion that interrupts descending facilitory input causes transient loss of spinal reflexes (Barnes *et al.*, 1962). In monkeys, however, metabolic studies using ^{14}C-deoxyglucose have demonstrated intriguing changes in spinal cord glucose utilization above and below the level of the cord transection (Schwartzman et al., 1983). The observation of hypometabolic spinal areas adjacent to hypermetabolic regions, for example, suggests that functional changes remote from the lesion may result from loss of inhibitory as well as excitatory inputs. Unfortunately, use of measures that are less precise than those employed in such metabolic studies may yield a combination of hypo- and hypermetabolic zones, falsely suggesting 'no change'. Electrophysiological data, derived from electroencephalographic and evoked potential studies, also lack precise anatomical correlates. It is not suprising, therefore, that recent clinical and animal studies of diaschisis – examining metabolic and, less often, electrophysiological changes following stroke – provide conflicting and inconclusive data (Glassman and Malamut, 1976; Slater et al., 1977; Meyer et al., 1979; Feeney and Baron, 1986; Wise et al., 1986; Lagreze et al., 1987; Dobkin et al., 1989).

Subcortical injuries can disrupt function at remote sites. Interruption of fibers passing from the brainstem to the diencephalon and cerebral cortex can cause coma and depress cerebral blood flow and oxygen consumption (Lassen, 1959; Plum and Posner, 1980). Thalamic strokes cause a reduction of ipsilateral cerebral blood flow and metabolism (Pawlik et al., 1985; Baron et al., 1986; Pappata et al., 1990). Failure to activate specific cortical areas may explain certain linguistic and other cognitive deficits following thalamic lesions. Similar metabolic changes in the frontal cortex have been observed after striatal lesions (Laplane et al., 1989). These observations suggest that the mechanism by which subcortical lesions produce behavioral changes is, at least in part, reliant on secondary changes in cortical function (Maxim 11).

The metabolic effects of cortical lesions on ipsilateral cortical areas (i.e. intrahemispheric diaschisis) are usually subtle and may reflect other factors, including ischemia or independent 'remote' lesions, increased intracranial pressure, undercutting of the subcortical white matter, and diffusion of toxins from the necrotic area (Astrup et al., 1981; Baron, 1985; Feeney and Baron, 1986). Metabolic studies in animals suggest that, although ipsilateral cortical diaschisis occurs, it is not a critical factor in the pathogenesis of behavioral deficits (Deuel and Collins, 1984; Hosokawa et al., 1985). Although diaschisis may contribute to reduced blood flow and metabolism in adjacent and remote ipsilateral cortical areas, as well as to such clinical deficits as aphasia, the evidence to support such a role remains unconvincing (Soh et al., 1978; Gibbs et al., 1984; Samson et al., 1985).

Interhemispheric (transcallosal) diaschisis is supported by metabolic, electrophysiological and clinical studies (Kempinsky, 1958; Slater et al., 1977; Meyer et al., 1979; Pappius, 1981; Caselli, 1991). While cerebral blood flow is often depressed contralateral to a stroke, some studies have suggested that several factors other than diaschisis may contribute to this change (Feeney and Baron, 1986; Wise et al., 1986). However, more recent studies, using magnetic resonance imaging, measures of cerebral blood flow and positron emission tomography, suggest that diaschisis is an important factor in the pathogenesis of metabolic depression contralateral to cortical strokes (Lagreze *et al.*, 1987; Dobkin *et al.*, 1989). Sympathetic apraxia (Maxim 43) and impairment of somesthetically mediated object recognition after extensive right hemisphere infarction (Caselli, 1991) are clinical examples of interhemispheric diaschisis.

Among the cases in which diaschisis has been postulated to explain dysfunction, stroke is the most common mechanism of injury. However, slowly progressive lesions such as tumors may also cause diaschisis (Riese, 1958; Von Monakow, 1914).

Metabolic and clinical changes resulting from diaschisis involve loss of both excitatory and inhibitory cells and fibers. The wealth of interconnections between the lesional area and other cortical and subcortical areas may determine how easily the clinical, metabolic and electrophysiological correlates of diaschisis can be detected.

For Von Monakow, diaschisis was a refutation of the purist localization theories that were in vogue at the turn of the 20th century:

> The generally accepted theory according to which aphasia, agnosia, apraxis etc. are due to destruction of narrowly circumscribed appropriate praxia, gnosia and phasia centres, must be finally discarded on the basis of more recent clinical and anatomical studies. It is just in the case of these focal symptoms that the concept of complicated dynamic disorders in the whole cortex becomes indispensible.
>
> (Von Monakow, 1914)

However, localized cerebral functions and diaschisis are not mutually exclusive; they are both compatible with the concept of integrated functional networks (Maxim 2; Mesulam, 1990).

The importance of diaschisis lies beyond its capacity to explain behavioral deficits observed in clinical practice; diaschisis may provide insights into the process of functional recovery and therapy (Meyer *et al.*, 1980; Yamaguchi *et al.*, 1980). For example, future neurological therapy may focus on areas that are structurally intact but functionally impaired, and restorative neurology may seek to reverse the process of diaschisis.

References

Astrup J, Siesjo P, Symon L. Thresholds in cerebral ischemia. The ischemic penumbra. *Stroke* 1981; **12**: 723–5.

Barnes CD, Joynt RF, Shottelius BA. Motor neuron resting potentials in spinal shock. *Am J Physiol* 1962; **203**: 1113–16.

Baron JC. Positron tomography in cerebral ischemia: a review. *Neuroradiology* 1985; **27**: 509–16.

Baron JC, D'Antona R, Pantano P, Serdaru M, Samson Y, Bousser MG. Effects of thalamic stroke on energy metabolism of the cerebral cortex. *Brain* 1986; **109**: 1243–59.

Casselli RJ. Bilateral impairment of somesthetically mediated object recognition in humans. *Mayo Clin Proc* 1991; **66**: 357–64.

Dobkin JA, Levine RL, Lagreze HL, Dulli DA, Nickles RJ. Evidence for transhemispheric diaschisis in unilateral stroke. *Arch Neurol* 1989; **46**: 1333–6.

Deuel RK, Collins RC. The functional anatomy of frontal lobe neglect in the monkey: clinical and quantitative 2-deoxyglucose studies. *Ann Neurol* 1984; **15**: 521–9.

Feeney DM, Baron JC. Diaschisis. *Stroke* 1986; **17**: 817–29.

Gibbs JM, Wise RJ, Leenders KL, Jones T. Evaluation of cerebral perfusion reserve in patients with carotid artery occlusion. *Lancet* 1984; **i**: 311–14.

Glassman RB, Malamut DL. Recovery from electroencephalographic slowing and reduced evoked potentials after somatosensory cortical damage in cats. *Behav Biol* 1976; **17**: 333–54.

Hosokawa S, Kato M, Aiko Y, Shima F. Altered local cerebral glucose utilization by unilateral frontal cortical ablations in rats. *Brain Res* 1985; **343**: 8–15.

Kempinsky WH. Experimental study of distal effects of acute focal injury. *Arch Neurol Psychiat* 1958; **79**: 376–89.

Lagreze HL, Levine RL, Pedula KL, Nickles RJ, Sunderland JJ, Rowe BR. Contralateral flow reduction in unilateral stroke: evidence for transhemispheric diaschisis. *Stroke* 1987; **13**: 527–8.

Laplane D, Levasseur M, Pillon B, Dubois B, Baulac M, Mazoyer B, Dinh ST, Sette G, Danze F, Baron JC. Obsessive-compulsive and other behavioral changes with bilateral basal ganglia lesions. *Brain* 1989; **112**: 699–725.

Lassen NA. Cerebral blood flow and oxygen consumption in man. *Physiol Rev* 1959; **39**: 183–238.

Mesulam M-M. Large-scale neurocognitive networks and distributed processing for attention, language, and memory. *Ann Neurol* 1990; **28**: 597–613.

Meyer JS, Naritomi H, Sakai F, Ishihara N, Grant P. Regional cerebral blood flow, diaschisis, and steal after stroke. *Neurol Res* 1979; **1**: 101–19.

Meyer JS, Sakai F, Yamaguchi F, Yamamoto M, Shaw T. Regional changes in cerebral blood flow during standard behavioral activation in patients with disorders of speech and mentation compared to normal volunteers. *Brain Lang* 1980; **9**: 61–77.

Pappata S, Mazoyer B, Tran Dinh S, Cambon H, Levasseur M, Baron JC. Effects of capsular or thalamic stroke on metabolism in the cortex and cerebellum: a positron emission tomography study. *Stroke* 1990; **21**: 519–24.

Pappius HM. Local cerebral glucose utilization in thermally traumatized rat brain. *Ann Neurol* 1981; **12**: 157–62.

Pawlik G, Herholz K, Beil C, Wagner R, Wienhard K, Heiss WD. Remote effects of focal lesions on cerebral blood flow and metabolism. In: *Functional Mapping of the Brain in Vascular Disorders* (Heiss WD, ed.). Berlin: Springer-Verlag, 1985, pp. 59–83.

Plum F and Posner JB. *The Diagnosis of Stupor and Coma*. Philadelphia: FA Davis, 1980.

Riese W. The principle of diaschisis. *Internat Rev Med* 1958; **171**: 73–82.

Samson Y, Baron JC, Bousser MG, Rey A, Derlon JM, David P, Comoy J. Effects of extra-intracranial arterial bypass on cerebral blood flow and oxygen metabolism in humans. *Stroke* 1985; **16**: 606–16.

Schwartzman CD, Eidelberg E, Alexander GM, Yu J. Regional metabolic changes in the spinal cord related to spinal shock and later hyperreflexia in monkeys. *Ann Neurol* 1983; **14**: 33–7.

Slater R, Reivich M, Goldberg H, Banka R, Greenberg J. Diaschisis with cerebral infarction. *Stroke* 1977; **8**: 684–90.

Soh K, Larsen B, Skinhoj E, Lassen NA. Regional cerebral blood flow in aphasia. *Arch Neurol* 1978; **35**: 625–32.

Von Monakow C. *Diaschisis* (1914 article translated by Harris G). In: *Brain and*

Behavior I: Mood States and Mind (Pribam KH, ed.) Baltimore: Penguin, 1969, pp. 27–36.

Wise R, Gibbs J, Frackowiak R, Marshall J, Jones T. No evidence of transhemispheric diaschisis after human cerebral infarction. *Stroke* 1986; **17**: 853–61.

Yamaguchi F, Meyer S, Sakai F, Yamamoto M. Case reports of three dysphasic patients to illustrate rCBF responses during behavioral activation. *Brain Lang* 1980; **9**: 145–8.

11. *Subcortical lesions can produce 'cortical' deficits*

It is a common but incorrect assumption that all complex behavioral functions are subserved by cells and circuitry housed in the neocortex. This misconception rests on two false premises: (1) highly organized behavior that can be learned, modified and creatively adapted to a specific environmental situation is restricted to humans and perhaps the great apes, and (2) communications between the cortex and subcortex are essentially one-way: the cortex tells the lower centers what to do. Many animals with a relatively poorly developed neocortex (e.g. rat, fox, lion and poodle) demonstrate highly complex behaviors and have outsmarted humans on more than one occasion.

The neurobehavioral relationship between 'higher' and 'lower' centers is not a one-way street. The boy with a hypothalamic hamartoma who curses viciously at his mother and then pushes her down (Plum and Van Uitert, 1978; Berkovic *et al.*, 1988); the woman with a left mesial temporal metastasis from breast carcinoma who develops psychosis (Malamud, 1967); and the man with progressive supranuclear palsy who is intellectually slowed and no longer able to keep up with his job (Albert *et al.*, 1974) are all examples of how lesions 'below' the neocortex can profoundly disrupt complex behavior, despite a relatively intact neocortex. Furthermore, subcortical white matter is the communication system that cortical regions use to receive and send information to other cortical and subcortical areas. White matter lesions can therefore severely disrupt function in the neocortex, limbic cortex and subcortical nuclei.

The anatomy and physiology of the cortex and subcortex are intricately interwoven. Cortical and subcortical areas that are richly interconnected are associated with strikingly similar clinical findings when either one is destroyed. The following examples illustrate this neuroanatomic–behavioral relationship:

  1. Bilateral destruction of striatal areas that have reciprocal connections with prefrontal regions causes a 'frontal lobe syndrome' (Laplane *et al.*, 1989).

  2. Lesions in right thalamic and striatal areas that are connected with right parietal association cortex cause left-sided neglect (Damasio *et al.*, 1980; Watson *et al.*, 1981; Ferro *et al.*, 1987).

  3. Lesions of the bilateral hippocampus, mammillary bodies or dorsomedial

nuclei of the thalamus cause severe short-term memory loss (Squire, 1982). Interconnections between the hippocampus and mammillary bodies (i.e. fornix) and the mammillary bodies and anterior thalamic nuclei (i.e. mamillothalamic tract) form part of the Papez circuit (Maxims 36 and 61).

4. Akinetic mutism results from large bifrontal lesions that include cingulate gyri, as well as from subcortical lesions that disrupt the medial forebrain bundle, which carries ascending catecholaminergic fibers to the frontal lobes (Maxim 27) (Barris and Schuman, 1953; Ross and Stewart, 1981).

Table 11.1 summarizes the neurobehavioral findings that occur with subcortical or non-neocortical lesions.

Lesion localization is usually possible by analysis of associated signs and symptoms. Depressed level of consciousness may indicate a diffuse process with increased intracranial pressure or a diencephalic or brainstem lesion. Hemiparesis equally involving the face, arm and leg most likely indicates a capsular lesion. Loss of pain and temperature sensation to the same degree as loss of joint position sensation is most likely to be due to a subcortical or peripheral lesion rather than a cortical lesion. Thus, the

Table 11.1   Neurobehavioral disorders with non-neocortical lesions.

Speech and language
Mutism – cingulate, medial forebrain bundle, diencephalon
Dysarthria – pyramidal and extrapyramidal cortex or tracts, cerebellum,
   lower motor neuron
Aphasia – subcortical white matter, striatum, thalamic

Short-term memory
Hippocampus, fornix, basal forebrain (septum, hypothalamus),
   diencephalon (mammillary bodies, dorsomedial nucleus)

Dementia
Multiple subcortical white or gray matter lesions, thalamus,? basal ganglia

Frontal lobe syndrome (judgment/planning/social graces)
Bilateral striatal, brainstem nuclei that synthesize biogenic amines

Emotion
Limbic system, hypothalamus, thalamus, medial forebrain bundle,
   brainstem nuclei that synthesize biogenic amines

Depression
Left anterior subcortex, basal ganglia, substantia nigra/ventral tegmental
   area

Unilateral neglect
Subcortical white matter, basal ganglia, thalamus

Attention
Midline brainstem and diencephalon, hypothalamus, striatum

Delirium
Thalamus, multiple subcortical gray or white matter areas

---

neurobehavioral findings must be integrated with general medical and segmental neurological examinations.

References

Albert ML, Feldman RG, Willis AL. The sub-cortical dementia of progressive supranuclear palsy. *J Neurol Neurosurg Psychiat* 1974; **37**: 121–30.

Barris RW, Schuman HR. Bilateral anterior cingulate gyrus lesions: Syndrome of the anterior cingulate gyri. *Neurology* 1953; **3**: 44–52.

Berkovic SF, Andermann F, Melanson D, Ethier RE, Feindel W, Gloor P. Hypothalamic hamartomas and ictal laughter: evolution of a characteristic syndrome and diagnostic value of magnetic resonance imaging. *Ann Neurol* 1988; **23**: 429–39.

Damasio AR, Damasio H, Chui HC. Neglect following damage to frontal lobe or basal ganglia. *Neuropsychologia* 1980; **18**: 123–32.

Ferro JM, Kertesz A, Black SE. Subcortical neglect: Quantitation, anatomy, and recovery. *Neurology* 1987; **37**: 1487–92.

Laplane D, Levasseur M, Pillon B, Dubois B, Baulac M, Mazoyer B, Dinh ST, Sette G, Danze F, Baron JC. Obsessive-compulsive and other behavioral changes with bilateral basal ganglia lesions. *Brain* 1989; **112**: 699–725.

Malamud N. Psychiatric disorder with intracranial tumors of the limbic system. *Arch Neurol* 1967; **17**: 113–23.

Plum F, Van Uitert R. Nonendocrine diseases and disorders of the hypothalamus. In: *The Hypothalamus* (Reichlin S, Baldessarini RJ, Martin JB, eds). New York: Raven Press, 1978, pp. 415–73.

Ross ED, Stewart RM. Akinetic mutism from hypothalamic damage: Successful treatment with dopamine agonists. *Neurology* 1981; **31**: 1435–9.

Squire LR. The neuropsychology of human memory. *Ann Rev Neurosci* 1982; **5**: 241–73.

Watson RT, Valenstein E, Heilman KM. Thalamic neglect: possible role of the medial thalamus and nucleus reticularis in behavior. *Arch Neurol* 1981; **38**: 501–6.

2
Delirium (Confusional State) and Dementia

12. *Confusion and clouding of consciousness are the hallmarks of delirium*

Delirium is a transient mental disorder characterized by impairment of attention, increased autonomic (principally sympathetic) activity, global disturbance of cognitive function, disorientation and alterations of the sleep – wake cycle and psychomotor activity (Lipowski, 1980a,b). The onset of delirium may be acute or subacute; symptoms usually fluctuate, and periods of suprising lucidity may be present. The cause is most often diffuse derangement of cerebral function from systemic or intracranial insults, as described in Maxim 13.

Although no age group is exempt from delirium, it is most common in the elderly. Acute confusion may be a more common initial feature of physical illness in the old than fever, pain or tachycardia (Hodkinson, 1976). Between one-third and one-half of the hospitalized elderly are likely to be delirious at some point during admission (Lipowski, 1983). Patients who experience delirium are twice as likely to die within a month of hospitalization than non-delirious patients of the same age (Hodkinson, 1973).

DSM-III-R diagnostic criteria for delirium are presented in Table 12.1 (American Psychiatric Association, 1987). The most common and consistent feature of delirium is a disorder of attention characterized by distractibility and difficulty in focusing or sustaining attention. Alertness may be reduced or enhanced.

Delirious patients also often have a relatively global disturbance of cognitive function, which impairs perception, memory (most prominently recent memory), abstract thought and maintenance of an ordered sequence of directed behavior. The patient's speech may be incoherent and perseverative, circumlocutious and devoid of content. Language testing reveals marked dysgraphia, mild word-finding difficulties and verbal paraphasias (Geschwind and Chedru, 1972). Approximately half of delirious patients

Table 12.1 DSM-IIIR diagnostic criteria for delirium.

Reduced ability to maintain attention to external stimuli (e.g. questions must be repeated because attention wanders) and to shift attention appropriately to new external stimuli (e.g. perseverates answer to a previous question)

Disorganized thinking, as indicated by rambling, irrelevant, or incoherent speech

At least two of the following:

Reduced level of consciousness, e.g. difficulty keeping awake during examination

Perceptual disturbances: misinterpretations, illusions, hallucinations

Disturbance of sleep-wake cycle with insomnia or daytime sleepiness

Increased or decreased psychomotor activity

Disorientation with respect to time, place or person

Memory impairment, e.g. inability to learn new material, such as the names of several unrelated objects after five minutes or to remember past events

Clinical features develop over a short period of time (usually hours to days) and tend to fluctuate over the course of the day

Either 1 or 2:

1. Evidence from the history, physical examination or laboratory tests of a specific organic factor (or factors) judged to be etiologically related to the disturbance

2. In the absence of such evidence, an etiological organic factor can be presumed if the disturbance cannot be accounted for by any non-organic mental disturbance, e.g. manic episode accounting for agitation and sleep disturbance

---

American Psychiatric Association, 1987 (with permission)

experience hallucinations, which are most often visual or auditory (Lipowski, 1980b).

Disorders of the sleep–wake cycle and psychomotor activity are extremely common in delirium, frequently taking the form of daytime somnolence and nocturnal insomnia. Nightmares and vivid dreams during sleep, and dream-like mentation while awake can also occur. In addition, delirium often develops, and is usually worse, at night.

Dramatic variations in psychomotor activity are common in delirious patients. While some patients display motor hyperactivity with agitation, incessant movements, and increased autonomic activity, others are apathetic or catatonic, and others shift from hypo- to hyperkinesis. The most challenging diagnostic problem is the quiet confusional state. These patients are only recognized by mental status testing.

Finally, the affective state of the delirious patient ranges from neutral to the extremes of depression or, less often, euphoria. Fear and anger may occur, often in response to threatening hallucinations or persecutory delusions, triggering attempts to escape or fight that can endanger the patient and others.

References

American Psychiatric Association. *Diagnostic and Statistical Manual of Mental Disorders.* (3rd edition, revised). Washington, DC: American Psychiatric Association Press, 1987, p. 103.

Geschwind N, Chedru F. Disorders of higher cortical function in acute confusional states. *Cortex* 1972; **8**: 395–411.

Hodkinson HM. Mental impairment in the elderly. *J R Coll Physic* 1973; **7**: 305–17.

Hodkinson HM. *Common Symptoms of Disease in the Elderly.* Oxford: Blackwell Scientific Publication, 1976, p. 24.

Lipowski ZJ. Delirium updated. *Comprehen Psychiat* 1980a; **21**: 190–6.

Lipowski ZJ. *Delirium: Acute Brain Failure in Man.* Springfield, Ill: Charles C Thomas Publications, 1980b.

Lipowski ZJ. Transient cognitive disorders (delirium, acute confusional states) in the elderly. *Am J Psychiat* 1983; **140**: 1426–36.

13. *Delirium is often caused by a life-threatening, but treatable disorder*

Once the clinical syndrome of delirium is recognized, the cause must be identified. Acute or subacute mental changes usually result from underlying cerebral or systemic disorders. Table 13.1 details the organic causes of delirium (Morse and Litin, 1969; Hodkinson, 1973; Mesulam, 1976; Lipowski, 1983; American Psychiatric Association, 1987). A transient cognitive disorder should never be attributed to psychosocial stress alone (Lipowski, 1983).

The common causes of delirium include (1) prescription and non-prescription drugs, (2) cardiovascular and pulmonary disorders, (3) infections, (4) metabolic encephalopathies, and (5) focal and diffuse brain lesions. Most of these etiological agents require specific treatment.

Among the many drugs that can trigger delirium, anticholinergics, opioids, psychotropics, digitalis and cimetidine are common offenders. Alcohol intoxication, alcohol withdrawal and phencyclidine intoxication also frequently cause delirium.

Cardiopulmonary disorders can trigger a decrease in cerebral blood flow or oxygenation, producing transient cognitive disturbances. Cerebrovascular causes of delirium include transient ischemic attacks, stroke and chronic subdural hematomas.

Infections and metabolic encephalopathies are among the most treatable but potentially devastating causes of delirium.

Diffuse central nervous system insults, including trauma, such as in

Table 13.1   Organic causes of delirium.

Drug intoxication
Prescription: anticholinergic agents, sedative-hypnotics, digitalis
   preparations, cimetidine, opiates, lithium, antiepileptic drugs,
   salicylates, corticosteroids
Ethyl and methyl alcohol
Cocaine, phencyclidine
Abused inhalants: gasoline, glue, nitrous oxide

Poisons
Industrial toxins: carbon disulphide, organic solvents, methyl chloride and
   bromide, organophosphate insecticides, heavy metals, carbon monoxide
Plants and mushrooms

Drug withdrawal
Alcohol
Sedative-hypnotic drugs
Amphetamine, cocaine

Metabolic disorders
Hypoxia, severe anemia
Hypoglycemia
Hepatic, renal, pancreatic, pulmonary insufficiency
Disorders of fluid and electrolyte balance
   Dehydration, water intoxication
   Alkalosis, acidosis
   Hyper- and hyponatremia; hyper- and hypokalemia; hyper- and
      hypocalcemia; hyper- and hypomagnesemia
Porphyria
Carcinoid syndrome

Nutritional disorders
Avitaminosis: nicotinic acid, thiamine, B_{12}, folate
Hypervitaminosis: intoxication by A or D

Hormonal disorders
Hyperinsulinism
Hypo- and hyperthyroidism
Hypopituitarism
Hypo- and hypercortisolism
Hypo- and hyperparathyroidism

Infections
Systemic: pneumonia, bacteremia, septicemia, hepatitis, SBE etc.
CNS: meningitis, encephalitis, abscess, neurosyphilis, slow viruses

Head trauma

Epilepsy
Ictal and postictal states

Vascular disorders
Transient ischemic attack and stroke: thrombotic, embolic, vasculitic
Migraine
Cardiac: myocardial infarction, congestive heart failure, arrhythmias

Intracranial tumors
Primary CNS
Metastatic
Infectious: abscess, parasitic cyst
Subdural hematoma

CNS degenerative disorders
Alzheimer's disease
Metachromatic leukodystrophy
Parkinson's disease
Progressive supranuclear palsy
Multiple sclerosis

Physical agents
Heatstroke
Radiation
Electrical trauma

Autoimmune
Serum sickness
Food allergy

---

head injury or long bone fracture with fat embolism, radiation, electrical injury, postictal state and meningeal carcinomatosis, also cause confusional states.

Factors that may predispose to acute confusion or delirium include sleep and sensory deprivation, severe fatigue and stress, age over 60 years, pre-existing brain damage such as in dementia, and addiction to ethanol or other drugs.

In addition, delirium often develops in the surgical patient (Mesulam and Geschwind, 1976). Operative causes include anesthesia (e.g. nitrous oxide narcosis), hypotension, hypoxia and alterations in volume status. Postoperative causes include electrolyte and acid–base abnormalities, hypoglycemia, anemia, hypotension, hemorrhage, infection, medications, sleep and sensory deprivation, alcohol withdrawal and stroke. Physical examination, careful review of the anesthesiologist's operative record and postoperative medications, and blood gas and electrolyte measurements will almost always reveal the pathogenesis of delirium.

The differential diagnosis of delirium includes disorders associated with rapid changes in mentation, including stroke, depression, mania, psychosis and conversion disorder. Delirium can dominate the clinical presentation in focal strokes, obfuscate other, possibly slight, neurological deficits and lead to misdiagnosis of toxic or metabolic encephalopathy, postictal states, or psychiatric illness. Delirium has been reported as a prominent manifestation of strokes in the anterior (Amyes and Nielsen, 1955), middle (Mesulam *et al.*, 1976; Caplan *et al.*, 1986; Mori and Yamadori, 1987), and posterior (Horenstein *et al.*, 1967; Devinsky *et al.*, 1988) cerebral arteries.

These strokes are often misdiagnosed on presentation. Diagnostic errors are particularly common when hemiparesis or other obvious focal deficits do not accompany behavioral changes. The non-dominant middle cerebral artery is most often involved: delirium occurs in almost half of patients with this type of stroke (Mesulam *et al.*, 1976; Mori and Yamadori, 1987). Patients frequently display agitation and, in some patients, psychosis accompanied by suspiciousness, paranoid delusions and hallucinations occurs as a presenting (Price and Mesulam, 1985) or delayed (Levine and Finkelstein, 1982) manifestation. Strokes in the right middle cerebral artery can also cause hemianopsia, neglect, constructional apraxia and sensori-motor deficits.

Patients with infarcts of the posterior cerebral artery are more likely to develop delirium if the onset is acute and there is simultaneous involvement of both arteries (Symonds and MacKenzie, 1957). Unilateral infarcts are more likely to produce confusional states when they affect the dominant hemisphere (Devinsky *et al.*, 1988).

Traditionally, the principal manifestations of posterior cerebral artery infarction have been considered to be visual field loss and hemisensory deficit. When the dominant hemisphere is involved, patients may have alexia without agraphia and anomia most severe for colors (Adams and Victor, 1985). Less often, such infarcts result in hemiplegia, transcortical sensory aphasia, memory impairment, release hallucinations in the blind part of the visual fields, visual agnosia and third nerve palsy during the acute stage. Thalamic pain syndrome and such movement disorders as cerebellar ataxia, tremor and choreoathetosis can develop after weeks or months (Fisher, 1986; Mori and Yamadori, 1987; Devinsky *et al.*, 1988).

Infarcts of the anterior cerebral artery may also be associated with delirium, as well as sexually inappropriate behavior (Amyes and Nielsen, 1955). Thalamic strokes, also, can produce delirium, as well as personality changes and disorders of language and memory. Among these patients, delirium is most frequent in those with anteromedial thalamic lesions (Graff-Radford *et al.*, 1984; Santamaria *et al.*, 1984).

In summary, delirium may result from cortical or subcortical strokes and most commonly occurs when the right middle cerebral artery distribution is involved.

Fluent aphasia, which results from lesions in dominant posterior temporal or parietal lobes, may be mistaken for delirium, because it usually has a rapid onset and is not associated with focal symptoms, such as hemiparesis. In such cases, it helpful to note that paraphasias and neologisms are more common with fluent aphasias than with delirium, and prominent comprehension deficit is the hallmark of Wernicke's aphasia.

Dementia is easily confused with delirium. The most important clue to differential diagnosis is the temporal evolution of symptoms: in dementia, it is usually insidious, while it is usually rapid in delirium. In the elderly patient, however, things are not this simple. Indeed, delirium is often superimposed on dementia in the elderly. The insidious onset of cognitive decline may not be appreciated by family or friends, who may instead bring the patient to medical attention when infection or pulmonary disease gives rise to a sudden deterioration in mental status. While attention is always impaired in delirium, attention is preserved during the earliest stages of the most common dementing disorder, Alzheimer's disease (Maxim 17). Furthermore, a patient with known dementia may experience both delirium and depression. The differential diagnosis of delirium and dementia is summarized in Table 13.2.

A thorough medical history, physical and neurological examinations, and laboratory studies can identify the cause of delirium in about 90 percent of cases (Lipowski, 1983). Important tests include blood electrolytes, liver and renal function tests, white and red blood cell counts, urinalysis, blood cultures, blood gas measurement, electrocardiogram, chest X-ray, toxic substances screen, lumbar puncture, electroencephalography (EEG), and computed tomography or magnetic resonance imaging of the head. The EEG is a very sensitive indicator of diffuse cerebral function and typically shows a bilateral slowing of background activity that correlates with the degree of cognitive impairment in delirium (Engel and Romano, 1959).

After treating the underlying cause, provide symptomatic and supportive care. Good nutrition, fluid and electrolyte balance, and a non-threatening environment must be provided. Rooms should be well-lit and contain some familiar objects, as well as a clock and calendar for orienta-

Table 13.2 Differential diagnosis of delirium and dementia*.

Feature	Delirium	Dementia
Onset	Rapid, often at night	Insidious
Duration	Hours to weeks	Months to years
Course	Fluctuates over 24 hours; often worse at night	Relatively stable
Awareness	Impaired	Usually normal
Alertness	Fluctuates	Usually normal
Orientation	Impaired (especially for time)	Impaired or intact
Memory	Immediate and recent memory impairment; fair fund of knowledge	Recent memory impairment; variable loss of long term memory
Perception	Visual and auditory illusions common	Usually normal
Sleep–wake cycle	Impaired; often reversal of normal day–night cycle	Fragmented sleep
Electroencephalogram	Diffusely slow	Normal or diffusely slow

*Modified from Lipowski, 1973 (with permission).

tion. Medical and nursing staff should be supportive and help to reorient the patient. Use of hypnotics should be limited because they can exacerbate confusion. However, low doses of 25–50 mg diphenhydramine or of a short-acting benzodiazepine, such as 15–30 mg temazepam, may be used when needed. For significant agitation, haloperidol is an effective drug with minimal anticholinergic effects; usual doses range from 0.5 to 4.0 mg, given 2–3 times daily either orally or intramuscularly.

References

Adams RD, Victor M. *Principles of Neurology.* New York: McGraw-Hill International Book Company, 1985.

American Psychiatric Association. *Diagnostic and Statistical Manual of Mental Disorders* (3rd edition, revised). Washington, DC: American Psychiatric Association Press, 1987, p. 103.

Amyes EW, Nielsen JM. Clinicopathologic study of vascular lesions of the anterior cingulate region. *Bull LA Neurol Soc* 1955; **20**: 112–30.

Caplan LR, Kelly M, Kase CS, Hier DB *et al.* Infarcts in the inferior division of the right middle cerebral artery: Mirror image of Wernicke's aphasia. *Neurology* 1986; **36**: 1015–20.

Devinsky O, Bear D, Volpe BT. Confusional states following posterior cerebral artery infarction. *Arch Neurol* 1988; **45**: 160–3.

Engel GL, Romano J. Delirum, a syndrome of cerebral insufficiency. *J Chronic Dis* 1959; **9**: 260–77.

Fisher CM. Unusual vascular events in the territory of the posterior cerebral artery. *Can J Neurol Sci* 1986; **13**: 1–7.

Graff-Radford NR, Eslinger PJ, Damasio AR, Yamada T. Nonhemorrhagic infarction of the thalamus: Behavioral, anatomic, and physiologic correlates. *Neurology* 1984; **34**: 14–23.

Hodkinson HM. Mental impairment in the elderly. *J R Coll Physic* 1973; **7**: 305–17.

Horenstein S, Chamnberlain W, Conomy J. Infarctions of the fusiform and calcarine regions: Agitated delirium and hemianopia. *Trans Am Neurol Assoc* 1967; **92**: 85–9.

Levine DN, Finkelstein S. Delayed psychosis after right temporoparietal stroke or trauma: Relation to epilepsy. *Neurology* 1982; **32**: 267–73.

Lipowski ZJ. Transient cognitive disorders (delirium, acute confusional states) in the elderly. *Am J Psychiat* 1983; **140**: 1426–36.

Mesulam M-M, Geschwind N. Disordered mental states in the postoperative period. *Urol Clin N Am* 1976; **3**: 199–215.

Mesulam M-M, Waxman SG, Geschwind N, Sabin TD. Acute confusional states with right middle cerebral artery infarctions. *J Neurol Neurosurg Psychiat* 1976; **39**: 84–9.

Mori E, Yamadori A. Acute confusional state and acute agitated delirium: Occurrence after infarction in the right middle cerebral artery territory. *Arch Neurol* 1987; **44**: 1139–43.

Morse RM, Litin EM. Postoperative delirium: A study of etiologic factors. *Am J Psychiat* 1969; **126**: 388–95.

Price BH, Mesulam M. Psychiatric manifestations of right hemisphere infarctions. *J Nerv Ment Dis* 1985; **173**: 610–14.

Santamaria J, Blesa R, Tolosa ES. Confusional syndrome in thalamic stroke. *Neurology* 1984; **34**: 1618.

Symonds C, MacKenzie I. Bilateral loss of vision from cerebral infarction. *Brain* 1957; **80**: 415–55.

14. *Dementia is an acquired, persistent loss of cognitive and social functions*

The line between 'a touch of senility' and dementia is arbitrary and often reflects the degree of interference with relationships, social activities or work. The normal aging process is associated with some mild cognitive losses and slowing of mental functions. However, many persons 80 years of age and older are quite sharp mentally and function well in demanding occupations. Therefore, *significant loss of mental functions in the elderly should always be considered abnormal and investigated.*

Dementia is defined as global deterioration of cognitive and intellectual functions that is usually associated with personality changes and severe enough to impair personal or occupational performance. In order to diagnose dementia, the current *Diagnostic and Statistical Manual of Psychiatry* IIIR (American Psychiatric Association, 1987) requires evidence of short- and long-term memory loss and at least one of the following: (1) impaired abstract thinking, such as the inability to find similarities between related words or difficulty defining words or concepts; (2) impaired judgment and planning; (3) language, praxis, recognition or visuospatial disorder; or (4) personality change. Cummings and Benson (1986) offer different diagnostic criteria, requiring sustained loss or change of at least three of the following: (1) cognition, or ability to manipulate old information; (2) memory, or ability to learn new or retrieve old information; (3) visuospatial function, including constructional and topographic abilities; (4) language; and (5) alterations in personal behavior. However, in employing any diagnostic definition, the exact criteria fulfilled are not as important as *the presence of a global and sustained loss of mental functions that is disabling to the person.* Therefore, if a patient can compensate fully for mild memory loss and difficulty with calculations using a note pad and calculator, the patient is not demented.

In most cases of dementia, the loss of mental functions is progressive, occurring at a steady but gradual pace, as in Alzheimer's disease, or in discrete steps, as in multi-infarct dementia. However, non-progressive dementia can occur acutely or subacutely after insults such as in encephalitis, anoxia, head trauma or massive demyelination. During the early stages of progressive dementia, intellectual loss and behavioral change often have a patchy distribution. Symptoms are most often observed by family members, friends and coworkers, but may be reported by patients. In many cases, however, the patient is unaware of or vigorously denies any problem.

Memory loss is often the initial and most prominent disorder in dementia. On mental status testing, deficits are usually identified in several areas. These areas include attention, language (i.e. naming, comprehension of complex sentences and paragraphs), calculations, perception, praxis, dressing, ability to follow sequential three-step commands (e.g.

'Touch your left thumb to your right ear, close your eyes, stick out your tongue'), problem solving, judgment and abstract thinking. Behavioral changes are prominent and include irritability, agitation, fearfulness, social avoidance, and verbal and physical aggressiveness.

Cortical atrophy, as demonstrated computed tomography (CT) or magnetic resonance imaging (MRI) of the brain, is not dementia. As the brain ages, it simply shrinks. Indeed, spry and ingenious elderly minds may have prominent cortical atrophy, and moderately demented patients can have only slight atrophic changes. The intuitive notion that brain size correlates with intelligence has plagued man's conceptualization of intelligence. More is usually, but not always, better. Cro-Magnon skulls are larger than those of modern man (Gould, 1981). Although cortical atrophy is not synonymous with dementia, demented patients with Alzheimer's disease or multiple infarcts generally have increased cortical and subcortical atrophy when compared with age-matched controls (Soininen *et al.*, 1982). Furthermore, in those with Alzheimer's disease, brain atrophy and ventricular dilatation, as measured by quantitative CT, usually correlate with intellectual impairment (Creasey *et al.*, 1986).

Originally, dementia referred to progressive, irreversible decline in mental functions. However, dementia is now defined functionally and is known to accompany reversible and treatable disorders, as well as relentless degenerative diseases. In fact, treatable causes of dementia account for approximately 10 to 20 percent of all cases.

Dementia is graded into three levels of severity according to the patient's level of function (see DSM-IIIR; American Psychiatric Association, 1987).

Mildly demented patients are able to live independently with reasonable hygiene, nutrition and judgment despite significant impairment in cognitive, social or work activities. These patients often have psychiatric abnormalities, including changes in personality and affect and, less often, psychotic symptoms (Rubin and Kinscherf, 1989).

Moderately demented patients are not safe in a completely unsupervised setting. They are likely to ignore important aspects of hygiene, eat a very limited diet, drive unsafely and they often have difficulty with finances, which makes them vulnerable to aggressive sales people (Friedland *et al.*, 1988).

Severely demented patients function at an extremely low level, which makes activities of daily living, such as shopping, eating or bathing difficult or impossible. They require continuous supervision.

Dementia must be distinguished from focal cerebral disorders, such as aphasia and amnesia. Small, critically placed lesions in such regions as Wernicke's area can be devastating, leaving the patient with a language comprehension deficit that secondarily impairs a wide range of congitive functions. Such patients are not demented. Left-sided angular gyrus (inferior parietal lobe) lesions cause aphasia, alexia, agraphia, acalculia, right–left disorientation and constructional disturbances that may simulate dementia (Benson *et al.*, 1982). Similarly, bilateral or dominant hemisphere temporal lobe lesions may profoundly disrupt short-term memory to cause amnesia, but not dementia.

In contrast to delirium, which it superficially resembles, dementia is usually not associated with clouded sensorium and is not transient (Table 13.2). Attentional deficit is always present in delirium and often absent in early dementia. Acute onset, illusions, hallucinations and disruption of sleep–wake cycles are also much more commonly seen in delirium. Other psychiatric disorders that may be confused with dementia are discussed in Maxim 15.

In Western societies, dementia is approaching epidemic proportions (Plum, 1979). The prevalence of severe dementia increases from less than 1 percent between the ages of 65 and 70 years to over 15 percent after the age of 85 years (Terry and Katzman, 1983). Furthermore, in the USA, those older than 85 years constitute the most rapidly increasing segment of the population and have a falling mortality rate (Rosenwaike *et al.*, 1980). Overall, approximately 5 to 10 percent of persons over the age of 65 years are demented, and an additional 10 percent have milder intellectual impairment (Besdine *et al.*, 1980; Mortimer *et al.*, 1981). Among nursing home residents, more than 50 percent are intellectually impaired (US Dept of Health, Education and Welfare, 1978).

References

American Psychiatric Association. *Diagnostic and Statistical Manual of Psychiatry* (3rd edition, revised). Washington, DC: American Psychiatric Association Press, 1987.

Benson DF, Cummings JL, Tsai SY. Angular gyrus syndrome simulating Alzheimer's disease. *Arch Neurol* 1982; **39**: 616–20.

Besdine RW, Brody JA, Butler RN, Duncan LE, Jarvik L, Libow L. Senility reconsidered: treatment possibilities for mental impairment in the elderly. *JAMA* 1980; **244**: 259–63.

Creasey H, Schwartz M, Frederickson H, Haxby JV, Rapoport SI. Quantitative computed tomography in dementia of the Alzheimer type. *Neurology* 1986; **36**: 1563–8.

Cummings JL, Benson DF. Dementia of the Alzheimer type: An inventory of diagnostic classical features. *J Am Geriatr Soc* 1986; **34**: 12–19.

Friedland RP, Koss E, Kumar A, Gaine S, Metzler D, Haxby JV, Moore A. Motor vehicle crashes in dementia of the Alzheimer type. *Ann Neurol* 1988; **24**: 782–6.

Gould SJ. *The Mismeasure of Man*. New York: WW Norton and Company, 1981, p. 99.

Mortimer JA, Schuman LM, French LR. Epidemiology of dementing illness. In: *The Epidemiology of Dementia* (Mortimer JA, Schuman LM, eds). New York: Oxford University Press, 1981.

Plum F. Dementia: an approaching epidemic. *Nature* 1979; **279**: 372–3.

Rosenwaike I, Yaffe N, Sagi PC. The recent decline in mortality of the extreme aged: an analysis of statistical data. *Am J Public Hlth* 1980; **70**: 1074–80.

Rubin EH, Kinscherf DA. Psychopathology of very mild dementia of the Alzheimer type. *Am J Psychiat* 1989; **146**: 1017–21.

Soininen H, Puranen M, Riekkinen PJ. Computed tomographic findings in senile dementia and normal aging. *J Neurol Neurosurg Psychiat* 1982; **45**: 50–4.

Terry RD, Katzman R. Senile dementia of the Alzheimer type. *Ann Neurol* 1983; **14**: 497–506.

US Department of Health, Education and Welfare publication No. (PHS) 78–1780, Profile of Chronic Illness in Nursing Homes, 1973–1974, National Center for Health Statistics, series 13, No. 29, 1978.

15. *Extensive complaints of cognitive dysfunction and variable performance on mental status testing suggest depressive pseudodementia*

Kiloh (1961) introduced the term pseudodementia to describe patients in whom the diagnosis of dementia is considered, 'but has to be abandoned because of the subsequent course of the illness'. His patients were ultimately diagnosed as having depression, conversion disorder, malingering, mania, paraphrenia (or psychosis of late life), or Ganser's syndrome (a dissociative disorder in which patients give 'approximate answers' to questions, and amnesia and disorientation are often present). Kiloh recognized that the term pseudodementia is 'purely descriptive and carries no diagnostic weight'.

Pseudodementia has since emerged as a popular and practical descriptor of functional and organic disorders that mimic dementia but are usually non-progressive and treatable. Organic disorders that mimic dementia usually arise from medications and are discussed in Maxims 20 and 21. By far, the most common functional cause of pseudodementia is depression.

Affective disorder has a prevalence of 10 to 15 percent in persons over 65 years of age (Roth, 1976), with depression accounting for the vast majority of cases. Some specialists estimate that as many as 10 percent of patients initially diagnosed with dementia will later be found to have primary depression (Wells, 1977). In people of all ages, depression causes psychic symptoms, such as sadness, helplessness, hopelessness, worthlessness, as well as vegetative symptoms, such as sleep disturbance (especially early morning awakening), diminished appetite, and impaired libido. In the elderly, however, intellectual dysfunction is a prominent feature: 10 to 20 percent of older, depressed patients have serious cognitive deficits (Roth, 1955, 1976; Folstein, 1979; Reifler *et al.*, 1982; Knesevich *et al.*, 1983). Therefore, in some depressed patients, a true dementia coexists.

Although psychometric tests, radiological studies and EEG are useful ancillary tests, clinical assessment is the most powerful tool in recognizing pseudodementia (Kiloh, 1961). Differentiation between depressive pseudodementia and dementia is best made by observing both an improvement in affective and cognitive symptoms with antidepressant therapy and the absence of progressive intellectual decline after at least one year of follow-up.

In addition, Reynolds *et al.* (1988) found additional characteristics that distinguish depressive pseudodementia from dementia, including early morning awakening, increased anxiety and more severe impairment of libido. Demented patients showed significantly more disorientation to time, greater difficulty finding their way about familiar streets or houses, and more impairment in dressing.

When evaluating a patient with possible dementia, it is imperative to inquire about affective and vegetative symptoms. Be specific: 'What time do you awaken in the morning?' 'Are you refreshed?' 'Do you sleep a lot during the day or have trouble falling asleep?' 'Do you ever wish you were dead?' Some patients actively deny depressive feelings and symptoms. It is a grave error to discount the seriousness of patients who complain 'how miserable life is' and ask 'what's the point of living?' The elderly have a high rate of suicide.

Also keep in mind that chronic complainers or 'kvetches' can get depressed, although they are often dismissed by family and physicians as worry-warts and guilt-mongers. Frequently, their complaints are no longer heard, and their apparent behavioral problems may be attributed to dementia.

Table 15.1 shows the clinical features that distinguish depressive pseudodementia from primary degenerative dementias. Although this table suggests that these disorders are easily separable and mutually exclusive,

Table 15.1.   Differential diagnosis of dementia and pseudodementia.

Feature	Dementia	Pseudodementia
Onset	Often insidious	Usually acute or subacute
Progression	Usually slow, early changes often missed	Usually rapid
Symptom duration at presentation	Long	Short
Prior psychiatric history or recent life crisis	Uncommon	Common
Extensive self-report of mental impairment	Uncommon	Common
Mental status/ psychometric testing	Progressive decline	Variable, effort related
Memory impairment	Common, most severe for recent events	Common, often selective amnesia, inconsistent deficits over time
Affective changes	Apathy, shallow emotions	Depression common
Nocturnal exacerbation of symptoms	Common	Uncommon

depressive pseudodementia and degenerative dementia may overlap clinically and coexist in the same patient. Demented patients are often unaware of or offer only modest complaints of cognitive impairment, whereas depressive patients may exaggerate or focus on cognitive problems. Mental status testing reveals stable or progressive deficits in dementia and variable performance in pseudodementia. Although patients with pseudodementia often show mild cognitive deficits on formal testing, the results are inconsistent with the presentation of severe functional disability.

Neuropsychological testing in dementia shows deficits in many cognitive areas, including orientation to time and place, language, memory, calculations and visuospatial functions. On tests such as the Mini Mental State Examination (Folstein et al, 1975) (Table 15.2), demented patients score lower than those with pseudodementia. However, depressive pseudodementia is characterized by slowing of mental processing and impairment of attention, short-term recall, analysis of detail, abstract thinking and ability to follow three-step commands or change pattern (as manifested by mental inflexibility and perseveration when shifting mental sets). In some pseudodementia cases, the attentional deficit or an unwillingness to cooperate on neuropsychological tests may falsely indicate profound cognitive losses. Retesting will often show dramatic fluctuations in certain cognitive functions, reflecting variability in effort.

If depression is diagnosed, an underlying medical or neurological illness must also be considered, because 'the association between somatic disease and psychiatric disorder is particularly close in senescence' (Roth, 1976). Weight loss and depression are an ominous combination in the elderly and may be due to pancreatic or other types of cancer, endocrine disorder or other somatic illness. Depression is quite common after strokes and can magnify cognitive losses. Affective symptoms also occur in 5 to 20 percent of patients with Alzheimer's disease and in a higher percentage of patients with subcortical dementias, such as Parkinson's disease (see Maxim 84). When depression occurs in patients with Alzheimer's disease, psychic symptoms, which include anxiety and feelings of helplessness and hopelessness, predominate over vegetative symptoms. One must recognize treatable disorders in patients with untreatable illnesses.

Major depression should be treated in the elderly, as in any other age group. Both antidepressant medication and psychotherapy can help to reduce symptoms, prevent recurrence and enhance social adjustment (Weissman and Myers, 1974).

Other psychiatric disorders that may present as pseudodementia in the elderly include personality disorders, late-life psychosis, conversion disorder, somatization disorder, dissociative disorders and paranoid disorder. Paranoia is common among the elderly and results from life stresses (including social isolation, loss of loved ones or loss of employment), physical deterioration and sensory deprivation, as well as from psychopathological processes. In many older persons, paranoia is combined with delusions and hallucinations (Miller et al., 1984).

Table 15.2   Mini Mental State Examination.

Maximum score		Test
		Orientation
5	( )*	What is the (year) (season) (date) (day) (month)?
5	( )	Where are we: (state) (county) (town) (hospital) (floor)?
		Registration
3	( )	Name three objects: one second to say each. Then ask the patient all three after you have said them. Give 1 point for each correct answer. Then repeat them until he learns all three. Count trials and record: number of trials.
		Attention and calculation
5	( )	Serial 7's. 1 point for each correct answer. Stop after five answers. Alternatively spell 'world' backwards.
		Recall
3	( )	Ask for the three objects repeated above. Give 1 point for each correct object.
		Language
9	( )	Name a pencil, and watch (two points) Repeat the following 'No ifs, ands or buts'. (1 point)

Follow a three stage command:

'Take a paper in your right hand, fold it in half, and put it on the floor'. (3 points)

Read and obey the following:

'Close your eyes'. (1 point)

Write a sentence (1 point)

Copy design (1 point)

_____ Total score
ASSESS level of consciousness along a continuum _____

Alert Drowsy Stupor Coma

*( ), patient's actual score.
Folstein et al., 1975 (with permission)

References

Folstein MF, Folstein SE, McHugh PR. Mini-mental state. A practical method for grading the cognitive state of patients for the clinician. *J Psychiatric Res* 1975; **12**: 189–198.

Folstein MF, McHugh PR. Dementia syndrome of depression. In: *Aging* (volume 7) *Alzheimer's Disease, Senile Dementia and Related Disorders* (Katzman R, Terry RD, Beck KL, eds). New York: Raven Press, 1979.

Kiloh LG. Pseudodementia. *Acta Psychiatr Scan* 1961; **37**: 336–51.

Knesevich JW, Martin RL, Berg L *et al.* Preliminary report on the affective symptoms in the early stages of senile dementia of the Alzheimer type. *Am J Psychiat* 1983; **140**: 233–5.

Miller BL, Read SL, Mahler ME, Benson DF. Altered mental status in the elderly. *Primary Care* 1984; **11**: 653–65.

Reifler BV, Larson E, Hanley R. Coexistence of cognitive impairment and depression in geriatric outpatients. *Am J Psychiat* 1982; **139**: 623–36.

Reynolds CF, Hoch CC, Kupfer DJ, Buysee DJ, Houck PR, Stack JA, Campbell DW. Bedside differentiation of depressive pseudodementia from dementia. *Am J Psychiat* 1988; **145**: 1099–103.

Roth M. The natural history of mental disorder in old age. *J Ment Sci* 1955; **101**: 281–301.

Roth M. The psychiatric disorders of later life. *Psychiatr Ann* 1976; **6**: 417–44.

Weissmann MM, Myers JK. Affective disorders in a US urban community. *Arch Gen Psychiat* 1974; **30**: 771–8.

Wells CE. Diagnostic evaluation and treatment in dementia. In: *Dementia* (Wells CE, ed.). Philadelphia: FA Davis Company, 1977, pp. 247–73.

16.   *Subcortical dementia is associated with mental slowing, apathy, depression and motor signs*

The term subcortical dementia was introduced by McHugh and Folstein (1973) to describe the intellectual changes in Huntington's disease. They stressed the preservation of language, recognition and ability to learn new material. In contrast, patients with such cortical dementias as the prototypical Alzheimer's disease develop aphasia, alexia, agnosia and amnesia.

In Huntington's disease, the pathological changes that accompany subcortical dementia are most severe in the basal ganglia (caudate and putamen). However, they also affect the cerebral cortex, especially the third, fourth and fifth layers (Hayden, 1981).

The application of the term subcortical dementia expanded after Albert *et al.* (1974) independently identified four characteristic mental changes in patients with progressive supranuclear palsy (PSP): forgetfulness; slowness of thought processes; personality changes, such as apathy or depression; and impaired ability to manipulate acquired knowledge. In PSP, lesions are localized to the upper brainstem, thalamus and striatum; the cerebral cortex is spared (Steele *et al.*, 1964). Subsequently, the expanding umbrella of subcortical dementia has grown to include the intellectual deterioration observed in Parkinson's disease, Wilson's disease, multiple lacunar infarctions, bilateral thalamic or basal ganglia lesions, spinocerebellar degenerations and even depression (Caine, 1981; Benson, 1983; Cummings and Benson, 1984).

The absence of aphasia, amnesia and apraxia is a hallmark of subcortical dementia. Linguistic aspects of speech, comprehension, repetition, naming, reading and writing are relatively spared, although such patients are slow, dysarthric and clumsy. This can also hold true in the early stages of cortical dementia, however, because language is often relatively normal. In cortical dementias, the first language symptom is usually word-finding difficulty resulting from memory impairment.

In fact, impaired short-term memory is often the initial symptom in cortical dementias, while the initial symptoms in subcortical dementia are mental slowing and apathy. Patients with cortical dementia are often brought to medical attention when relatives become concerned over failing memory. At first, patients are unable to learn new information. As cortical dementia progresses, the memory disorder becomes profound, and patients may fail to recognize their spouse or children by sight or voice (Fisher, 1988). The deficit is not due to primary sensory deficit, agnosia or Balint's syndrome (Maxim 48); it is a disintegration of long-term memory. In contrast, patients with subcortical dementia have difficulty retrieving learned materials: they 'forget to remember' (Albert, 1974). Furthermore, memory disorder is fairly mild even when subcortical dementia is advanced.

Motor disorder is a prominent feature of subcortical dementia. The slowness that is characteristic of cognitive functions also affects motor skills, causing delayed initiation and execution of movements. Adventitious movements, including tremor, chorea and dyskinesia, are common in subcortical dementias, whereas myoclonus may occur with such cortical dementias as Alzheimer's and Creutzfeldt–Jackob diseases. One should always test muscle tone in the neck and extremities when subcortical dementia is suspected, since extrapyramidal rigidity (sometimes called 'lead pipe') is often present in appendicular and truncal muscles. Speech is slow, dysarthric and hypophonic (low in volume). Posture is rigid with flexion, and less often, hyperextension. Gait is unsteady, slow, wide-based and short-stepped. Motor findings are often prominent in multi-infarct dementia, a disorder that includes features of cortical and subcortical dementia. Except in the advanced stages of cortical dementias, however, motor findings are absent or present as mild, most often extrapyramidal, signs.

Depression and apathy are common in subcortical dementia, whereas patients with cortical dementias are often unconcerned about their cognitive and behavioral problems, or are disinhibited with irritability, agitation and loss of social graces. However, patients with bilateral prefrontal lesions, as in Pick's disease or trauma, combine elements from both disorders (i.e. apathy and disinhibited behavior). Major depression also complicates cerebral infarction in patients with multi-infarct dementia and may occur in up to 20 percent of Alzheimer patients (Reifler *et al.*, 1982; Reding *et al.*, 1985).

Despite these distinctions, however, the concept of subcortical dementia remains controversial because: (1) subcortical lesions are present in cortical dementias, as in Alzheimer's disease (Maxim 17); (2) cortical lesions are present in some subcortical dementias; (3) the cortex and subcortex are richly interconnected and, therefore, a subcortical lesion can disrupt corti-cal function (Maxims 10 and 11); (4) aphasia and amnesia, which are char-acteristically absent in subcortical dementias, can result from discrete subcortical lesions; and (5) neuropsychological and neuropathological evi-dence is inadequate to support the separation of these groups. In summary, substantial anatomical and clinical heterogeneity causes an overlap between 'cortical' and 'subcortical' dementia.

For example, although Alzheimer's disease is classed as a cortical dementia, degeneration in Alzheimer's involves subcortical regions, including the basal nucleus of Meynert, locus ceruleus and raphe nuclei (Whitehouse, 1986). These nuclei are also involved in Parkinson's disease, a 'subcortical dementia'. But in Huntington's disease, another 'subcortical dementia', they are relatively spared. Thus, one could argue that Alz-heimer's and Parkinson's diseases are closer to each other, anatomically, than either is to Huntington's disease. Similarly, cortical degeneration occurs in both Huntington's and Parkinson's diseases, but not in PSP. Yet in PSP, the 'purest' of the subcortical dementias, positron emission tomography shows a significant reduction in prefrontal metabolic rate, as measured by glucose utilization (D'Antona et al., 1985). To complicate mat-ters even further, the pattern of cortical glucose hypometabolism in Parkin-son's disease is similar to that found in Alzheimer's disease (Mettler et al., 1984).

Attempts to differentiate cortical and subcortical dementias with neuro-psychological test batteries have produced conflicting results as well (Lees and Smith, 1983; Mayeux et al., 1983; Huber et al., 1986). Although simple bedside inventories such as the Mini Mental Status Examination (Maxim 15) (Folstein et al., 1975) do not reliably distinguish between the two groups, more sensitive test batteries directed at specific cognitive and behavioral findings have shown significant differences between patients with cortical and subcortical dementia (Huber et al., 1986).

To lump or to split the dementias, that is the question. Both research and practical, clinical applications of this somewhat artificial division sug-gest that a separation, but not complete segregation, is in order.

References

Albert ML, Feldman RG, Willis AL. The sub-cortical dementia of progressive sup-ranuclear palsy. *J Neurol Neurosurg Psychiat* 1974; **37**: 121–30.

Benson DF. Subcortical dementia: A clinical approach. In: *The Dementias* (Mayeux R, Rosen WG, eds). New York: Raven Press, 1983, pp. 185–93.

Caine ED. Pseudodementia. *Arch Gen Psychiat* 1981; **38**: 1359–64.

Cummings JL, Benson DF. Subcortical dementia: review of an emerging concept. *Arch Neurol* 1984; **41**: 874–9.

D'Antona R, Baron JC, Samson Y, Serdaru M, Viader F, Agid Y, Cambier J. Sub-cortical dementia: frontal cortex hypometabolism detected by positron emission tomography in patients with progressive supranuclear palsy. *Brain* 1985; **108**: 785–99.

Fisher CM. Neurologic fragments. I. Clinical observations in demented patients. *Neurology* 1988; **38**: 1868–73.

Folstein MF, Folstein SE, McHugh PR. 'Mini-mental state': A practical method for grading the cognitive state of patients for the clinician. *J Psychiatr Res* 1975; **12**: 189–98.

Hayden MR. *Huntington's Chorea*. New York: Springer-Verlag, Berlin, 1981, p. 94.

Huber SJ, Shuttleworth EC, Paulson GW, Bellchambers MJG, Clapp LE. Cortical vs subcortical dementia: neuropsychological differences. *Arch Neurol* 1986; **43**: 392–4.

Lees AJ, Smith E. Cognitive deficits in the early stages of Parkinson's disease. *Brain* 1983; **106**: 257–70.

Mayeux R, Stern Y, Rosen J, Benson DF. Is 'subcortical dementia' a recognizable clinical entity? *Ann Neurol* 1983; **14**: 278–83.

Mettler EJ, Reige WH, Benson DF *et al*. Patterns of regional cerebral glucose metabolism in Alzheimer's disease patients. Presented at the Norman Rockwell Conference on Alzheimer's Disease, Lubbock, Texas, October, 1984.

McHugh PR, Folstein MF. Subcortical dementia. Address to the American Academy of Neurology, Boston, April, 1973 (unpublished).

Reding M, Haycox J, Blass J. Depression in patients referred to a dementia clinic: a three-year prospective study. *Arch Neurol* 1985; **42**: 895–6.

Reifler BV, Larson E, Hanley R. Coexistence of cognitive impairment and depression in geriatric outpatients. *Am J Psychiat* 1982; **139**: 623–6.

Steele JC, Richardson JC, Olezewski J. Progressive supranuclear palsy. *Arch Neurol* 1964; **10**: 333–59.

Whitehouse PJ. The concept of subcortical and cortical dementia: another look. *Ann Neurol* 1986; **19**: 1–6.

17. *Alzheimer's disease is the most common cause of dementia*

Approximately 55 percent of dementia in the USA is associated with Alzheimer's Disease (AD). The landmark case report by Alois Alzheimer (1907) described the silver stain neuropathological findings of neurofibrillary tangles and neuritic plaques in a 55-year-old woman with progressive dementia. While the diagnosis of AD was initially restricted to cases of 'presenile dementia' in those less than 65 years old, the clinical and pathological features of degenerative dementia starting before or after the age of 65 years are indistinguishable (Blessed *et al.*, 1968), and AD is now diagnosed without an age limit. The incidence and prevalence of AD increases with age, with rare cases in the fourth decade and a prevalence of approximately 15 percent after 85 years of age (Terry and Katzman, 1983).

Alzheimer's disease usually occurs sporadically, although autosomal dominant inheritance is found in some cases (Goudsmit *et al.*, 1981). It is possible that most cases are hereditary but that delayed clinical expression of the disease until the age of 80 years or later prevents recognition of familial patterns (Fitch *et al.*, 1988). The high incidence of AD-like clinical and pathological features found among patients with Down's syndrome who survive into their fourth decade has led to a vigorous search for an abnormality on chromosome 21 – as yet without success.

Pathologically, AD is characterized by neuronal loss and neuritic plaques and neurofibrillary tangles scattered in the brain's parietal, frontal and temporal association cortices, limbic areas and subcortical regions, including the basal nucleus of Meynert, locus ceruleus, raphe nucleus and hypothalamus. There is relative sparing of primary motor, somatosensory and visual cortices, as well as of the basal ganglia (Terry and Katzman, 1983). Blessed *et al.* (1968) reported a prospective study of demented patients in whom mental deterioration correlated with the abundance of neuritic plaques at *post mortem*. In addition, amyloid angiopathy is a nearly constant accompaniment of AD, although it varies in severity (Bergeron *et al.*, 1987; Joachim, 1988), and there is an increased incidence of AD in patients with amyloid angiopathy and intracerebral lobar hematomas.

The diagnosis of AD during life is primarily one of exclusion. There are no biochemical tests or histological findings in readily accessible tissue that permit a definitive diagnosis. The demonstration of plaques and tangles in the brain is the only absolute criterion for diagnosis. Brain biopsy is not indicated, however, because of its risks and the lack of treatment for AD. Furthermore, the chances of discovering a treatable disorder by brain biopsy are exceeding low, when other diagnostic studies are negative (Maxim 21).

Given these circumstances, it is not surprising that AD is frequently misdiagnosed. Patients with AD may be considered 'normal for an old person' or, at the other extreme, incorrectly diagnosed and treated for such disorders as multi-infarct dementia (Maxim 18) and occult hydrocephalus (Maxim 22). Also, patients with treatable disorders, such as depression or hypothyroidism are incorrectly diagnosed with AD, and therapeutic opportunities are missed (Maxims 15, 20 and 21). Such misdiagnosis also occurs easily in patients with lesions of the dominant angular gyrus, because they often develop alexia, fluent aphasia, constructional disturbances and Gertsmann's syndrome of agraphia, finger agnosia, acalculia and right–left disorientation (Benson *et al.*, 1982). Preservation of memory and visuospatial function help to distinguish the angular gyrus syndrome from AD.

The first step in the diagnosis of AD is to be certain that the patient is demented (Maxim 14). The second step is to exclude dementia's treatable causes of dementia (Maxim 21). Commonly, the dementia work-up reveals equivocal findings such as (1) hydrocephalus that is 'in between' *ex vacuo* (atrophy) and occult (normal pressure); (2) a small area of encephalomalacia or multiple, small unidentified bright objects on imaging studies; or (3) a moderately elevated serum calcium level. Under these circumstances, conservative therapeutic trials, such as a tap-test for hydrocephalus (Maxim 23) or judicious hydration for hypercalcemia, may be helpful.

Alzheimer's disease often coexists with other medical, neurological and psychiatric disorders that are treatable. There is an increased frequency of seizures and myoclonus in AD; seizures occur at any stage, but myoclonus usually occurs late in the course (Hauser *et al.*, 1986). Furthermore, there is an increased incidence of thyroid disease in women with AD (Heyman *et al.*, 1983).

The slow progressive course of intellectual and behavioral deterioration is the most characteristic clinical feature of AD. During the first stage (years 1–4), there is an insidious loss of short-term memory. Patients forget information, misplace objects, annoyingly repeat questions or stories, and commonly get lost in new places; they are often brought to medical attention when relatives become concerned by their memory failure. Difficulty in finding words during spontaneous speech and diminished capacity for abstract thought and planning are among the earliest cognitive problems. In addition, patients in the early stages of disease may realize the brain is failing, responding with irritability, withdrawal and sadness. Occasionally, AD presents as delirium in a patient with a medical illness such as pneumonia. When the pneumonia and delirium resolve, the patient is no longer the same – dementia is finally recognized.

As the disease progresses to the second stage (years 2–10), the cognitive and behavioral symptoms worsen and the spectrum of impaired functions widens. Memory for both recent and remote events is severely impaired. Patients are unable to recall their addresses or telephone numbers. They may misplace the list that compensated for amnesia in the first stage, or worse still, forget to make it. However, even in moderately advanced cases, inappropriate insertions of fragments from a conversation 10 to 30 minutes before can occur, demonstrating that some information does 'get in' (Fisher, 1988). Spatial disorientation causes the patient to get lost in the neighborhood. A dangerous combination of cognitive deficits, slowed reaction time, and impaired vision and hearing makes motor vehicle accidents more likely (Friedland *et al.*, 1988). Fluent aphasia with circumlocution and empty speech, diminished auditory and written comprehension, and difficulty with even simple calculations develop (Cummings *et al.*, 1985; Thal *et al.*, 1988).

During the second stage, personality changes that were annoying during the initial stage can move to the forefront, causing great difficulty for family, friends and support personnel. Apathy, indifference and rigidity may intensify. Premorbid personality traits may be grossly exaggerated or reversed. Patients become fearful, paranoid and delusional. They may accuse their spouses of infidelity, blame nursing aids for losing their misplaced items, or demand police be called to remove imaginary burglars and enemies from their house. Stubborn insistence on their wants and opinions often provokes disagreements and, in some cases, is accompanied by agitated and aggressive behaviors (Fisher, 1988; Petry *et al.*, 1988). Patients often refuse to participate in or allow others to provide basic care. They may become restless, impatient and argumentative. Rude behavior extends from embarrassing comments to undressing, passing flatus and urinating in public. Others remain quiet throughout the illness.

Major depression occurs in 15 to 20 percent of AD patients, most often during the second stage (Reifler *et al.*, 1982; Reding *et al.*, 1985). Such depression has been correlated with significantly more degenerative changes in the locus ceruleus and substantia nigra, lower cortical norepinephrine levels, and relative preservation of choline acetyltransferase activity in subcortical regions relative to that found in AD patients without depression (Zubenko and Moossy, 1988; Zubenko, 1990).

Even at this stage of severe mental disability, the motor and sensory systems and sphincter control are preserved. Primitive reflexes, such as snouting, sucking and grasping, develop during the second or third stages. While mild extrapyramidal signs (e.g. bradykinesia and slight rigidity) are common in AD patients (Molsa *et al.*, 1984), more prominent extrapyramidal symptoms or myoclonus occasionally develop (Kaye *et al.*, 1988a,b). However, focal weakness or atrophy, rigidity, tremor, dysarthria, ataxia, hyperreflexia or Babinski sign are not typical of any stage of AD. If these findings are noted within five years of onset of behavioral change, consider alternative diagnoses, including multi-infarct dementia, Binswanger's encephalopathy, Parkinson's disease or occult hydrocephalus.

The third and terminal stage of AD (years 7–14) is a near-vegetative existence for the patient, as she becomes more akinetic and mute. After 6 to 12 years of illness, intellect and memory deteriorate to the point that patients no longer recognize spouses or children. Personal hygiene and nutrition are ignored. Sphincter control is lost, and a progressive gait disorder with smaller and less certain steps, rigidity and flexed extremities causes the patient to become bedridden. Seizures may occur. Male sex, onset of symptoms before the age of 65 years, and severity of behavioral impairment are all associated with decreased survival (Barclay *et al.*, 1985). Death commonly results from infection and trauma (Chandra *et al.*, 1986).

A syndrome of slowly progressive aphasia without generalized dementia was reported by Mesulam (1982) in six patients with clinical courses lasting 6 to 11 years. Additional cases have been documented (Foster and Chase, 1983; Heath *et al.*, 1983), some with atrophy in the left perisylvian areas on computed tomography (CT) or magnetic resonance imaging (MRI) (Sapin *et al.*, 1989), and others with glucose hypometabolism on positron emission tomographic (PET) scan (Chawluck *et al.*, 1986). The aphasia is most often anomic and is often paired with acalculia. Although Mesulam proposed that this collection of symptoms represent a distinct syndrome, his proposition remains controversial (Foster and Chase, 1983; Gordon and Selnes, 1984; Chawluck *et al.*, 1986; Poeck and Luzzatti, 1988). Do the cases of slowly progressive aphasia represent a specific disorder or merely a more prolonged and focal onset of a generalized cerebral degenerative disorder? Green *et al.* (1990) found that seven of eight patients with progressive aphasia developed mild dementia within five years of presentation, suggesting that this disorder is a precursor of dementia.

Alzheimer's, Pick's and Creutzfeldt–Jackob diseases may also present with anomic aphasia, but other cognitive deficits and behavioral changes usually occur within one year (Progacar and Williams, 1984; Holland *et al.*, 1985; Shuttleworth *et al.*, 1985; Mandell *et al.*, 1989).

Benson *et al.* (1988) reported five patients with progressive dementia presenting as a disorder of higher visual functioning. All developed visual agnosia, alexia, agraphia and components of Balint's, Gertsmann's and transcortical sensory aphasia syndromes. Memory and insight were relatively preserved until late in the course. Two of these patients had atrophy on CT or MRI that was maximal in the parietal and occipital lobes. As with progressive aphasia, the question of pathogenesis and whether this is an atypical form of Alzheimer's disease, a posterior lobar atrophy similar to Pick's except for location, or a new and unique disease remains uncertain. Additional neuropathological, neurochemical and molecular studies are needed to define further the 'focal dementias', as well as the subtypes of AD.

Subtypes of AD have been described based on the presence of associated motor findings (Mayeux *et al.*, 1985). Alzheimer's disease patients with myoclonus or prominent extrapyramidal features of rigidity, bradykinesia and flexed posture have an earlier age of onset and more severe dementia than those without these features (Mayeux *et al.*, 1985; Kaye *et al.*, 1988a,b). Patients with extrapyramidal features have lower CSF levels of homovanillic acid (HVA) and biopterin, while those with myoclonus have lower CSF levels of HVA, biopterin and 5-hydroxyindoleacetic acid. The myoclonus in AD does not differ clinically from Creutzfeldt–Jackob disease and may cause diagnostic problems. The electroencephalogram in AD, however, shows a focal, contralateral central, negative cerebral potential that precedes the myoclonic jerk by 25 to 40 mseconds and lasts 40 to 80 mseconds in AD. In Creutzfeldt–Jackob, the negative potential precedes the jerk by 50 to 85 mseconds and lasts 100 to 160 mseconds (Wilkins *et al.*, 1984).

Pick's disease is a degenerative dementia that affects the frontal and temporal lobes. Patients present with personality changes of the frontal lobe syndrome (Maxims 54): disinhibition, loss of social graces, jocularity and apathy punctuated by irritability. Difficulty with concentration and language dysfunction is common during the early stages, with reduced verbal output and word-finding difficulty (anomic aphasia) (van Mansvelt, 1954; Balajthy, 1964; Lishman, 1987). Temporal involvement may predominate early on, with transcortical or fluent aphasias and memory loss (Balajthy, 1964; Wechsler *et al.*, 1982; Morris *et al.*, 1984).

Pick's disease occurs in adulthood, with a peak between 55 and 65 years. There is a slight female predominance. In most cases, the disease is thought to be inherited as an autosomal dominant trait (Schenk, 1958–59), although the cause is unknown.

The differentiation of Alzheimer's and Pick's diseases has been debated for decades (Davison, 1938; Stengel, 1943). During the initial stages of illness, prototypic cases of Pick's disease, with prominent personality changes but relatively preserved memory, arithmetic and visuospatial skills and praxis, can be recognized as distinct from Alzheimer's disease, in which cognitive disorders predominate. As the diseases progress, however, they become more difficult to distinguish clinically. Because there is approximately one case of Pick's for every 75–100 cases of Alzheimer's disease[1] (Pearce and Miller, 1973; Terry, 1976) and Alzheimer's disease may present with atypical features including personality changes, reliable differentiation can only be made pathologically.

The gross neuropathology of Pick's disease is striking: the frontal and temporal lobes show severe atrophy and gyri appear knife-like. In contrast to Alzheimer's disease, in which the atrophy is mainly cortical, both cortical and white matter are affected in Pick's disease. Mixed frontotemporal atrophy is found in 54 percent of cases, predominantly frontal atrophy occurs in 25 percent, predominantly temporal atrophy occurs in 17 percent and approximately 4 percent have significant parietal or occipital atrophy (Tomlinson and Corsellis, 1984). While this atrophy may be symmetrical, it predominates on one side in more than half of cases. Atrophy may also occur in the basal nucleus of Meynert and the caudate nucleus (van Mansvelt, 1954; Uhl, 1983), but the primary motor area is usually spared. Microscopically, cell loss predominates in the outer cortical layers with intense astrocytic gliosis and abundant Pick's cells. There are enlarged, circular cells with intranuclear inclusions seen best with silver staining (Tomlinson and Corsellis, 1984).

Creutzfeldt–Jakob disease (CJD) is a rare, potentially transmissible form of dementia that is caused by a slow virus. The virus has an average incubation period of two years and the clinical illness usually lasts between 3 and 15 months; 90 percent of patients die within a year of onset (May, 1968; Brown *et al.*, 1986). Approximately 5 percent of cases are familial.

Although rare, the unconventional nature of the virus and the difficult process required to kill it have made CJD a source of great interest and concern (Brown *et al.*, 1983). Creutzfeldt–Jackob disease may be spread with depth electrodes, transplantation of cadaver corneas or dura matter, and cadaver pituitary-derived growth hormone; there is an increased incidence of CJD in patients who have intraocular pressure testing, sustain head trauma or require sutures for physical trauma (Brown *et al.*, 1985; Davanipour *et al.*, 1985; Fross, 1986; Rapaport, 1987).

Clinically, CJD usually presents with vague complaints of aesthenia, anxiety and changes in sleeping and eating patterns. These symptoms are usually followed within a month by neurological symptoms: mental deterioration occurs in two-thirds of cases, while cerebellar symptoms (e.g. gait disorder or clumsiness), diplopia or visual symptoms (e.g. altered color perception, visual loss) are found in the remaining third. Although neurological symptoms usually evolve over weeks or months, Brown *et al.* (1986) report that 20 percent of patients experience a rapid or even sudden onset of these symptoms. As the disease progresses, there is a global deterioration in mentation and behavior, accompanied by myoclonic jerks

---

[1] Outside Sweden, where there is a high incidence of Pick's disease (Sjögren *et al.*, 1952).

(88 percent), extrapyramidal rigidity (67 percent), cerebellar (61 percent) and oculomotor (16 percent) disorders, seizures (8 percent) and lower motor neuron dysfunction (11 percent) (Brown *et al.*, 1986).

The characteristic EEG finding of biphasic and triphasic sharp waves with a repetition rate of 0.5–1.5 per second is found in more than 80 percent of cases. However, during the early stages of illness, the EEG usually shows diffuse slowing that is often asymmetric (Burger *et al.*, 1972; Levy *et al.*, 1986).

The triad of dementia, myoclonus and periodic sharp waves in the EEG strongly suggests CJD, but this triad occurs in only three-quarters of patients and often develops once the disease has progressed. One final note: if CJD is suspected, warn the neuropathologist!

References

Alzheimer A. Uber eine eigenartige Erkrangkung der Hirnrinde. *All Z Psychiatr* 1907; **64**: 146–8.

Balajthy B. Symptomatology of the temporal lobe in Pick's convolutional atrophy. *Acta Med Acad Sci Hug* 1964; **20**: 301–16.

Barclay LL, Zemcov A, Blass JP, McDowell FH. Factors associated with duration of survival in Alzheimer's disease. *Biol Psychiat* 1985; **20**: 86–93.

Benson DF, Cummings JL, Tsai SY. Angular gyrus syndrome simulating Alzheimer's disease. *Arch Neurol* 1982; **39**: 616–20.

Benson DF, Davis RJ, Snyder BD. Posterior cortical atrophy. *Arch Neurol* 1988; **45**: 789–93.

Bergeron C, Ranalli PJ, Miceli PN. Amyloid angiopathy in Alzheimer's disease. *Can J Neurol Sci* 1987; **14**: 564–9.

Blessed G, Tomlinson BE, Roth M. The association between quantitative measures of dementia and of senile change in the cerebral grey matter of elderly subjects. *Br J Psychiat* 1968; **114**: 797–811.

Brown P, Cathala F, Castaigne P, Gajdusek DC. Creutzfeldt–Jakob Disease: Clinical analysis of a consecutive series of 230 neuropathologically verified cases. *Ann Neurol* 1986; **20**: 597–602.

Brown P, Gajdusek DC, Gibbs CJ, Asher DM. Potential epidemic of Creutzfeldt–Jakob disease from human growth hormone therapy. *New Engl J Med* 1985; **313**: 728–30.

Brown P, Gibbs CJ, Amyx HL, Kingsbury KT, Tohwer RG, Sulima MP, Gajdusek DC. Chemical disinfection of Creutfeldt–Jakob disease virus. *New Engl J Med* 1983; **306**: 1279–82.

Burger LJ, Rowan AJ, Goldensohn ES. Creutzfeldt–Jakob disease. An electro-encephalographic study. *Arch Neurol* 1972; **26**: 428–33.

Chawluck JB, Mesulam M-M, Hurtig H, Kushner M, Weintrabu S, Saykin A, Rubin N, Alavi A, Reivich M. Slowly progressive aphasia without generalized dementia: Studies with positron emission tomography. *Ann Neurol* 1986; **19**: 68–74.

Chandra V, Bharucha NE, Schoenberg BS. Conditions associated with Alzheimer's disease at death: Case – control study. *Neurology* 1986; **36**: 209–11.

Cummings JL, Benson DF, Hill MA, Read S. Aphasia in dementia of the Alzheimer type. *Neurology* 1985; **35**: 394–7.

Davanipour Z, Alter M, Sobel E, Asher D, Gajdusek DC. Creutzfeldt–Jakob disease: Possible medical risk factors. *Neurology* 1985; **35**: 1483–6.

Davison C. Circumscribed cortical atrophy in the presenile psychoses. Pick's disease. *Am J Psychiat* 1938; **94**: 801–18.

Fisher CM. Neurologic fragments. I. Clinical observations in demented patients. *Neurology* 1988; **38**: 1868–73.

Fitch N, Becker R, Heller A. The inheritance of Alzheimer's disease: A new interpretation. *Ann Neurol* 1988; **23**: 14–19.

Foster NL, Chase TN. Diffuse involvement in progressive aphasia. *Ann Neurol* 1983; **13**: 224–5.

Friedland RP, Koss E, Kumar A, Gaine S, Metzler D, Haxby JV, Moore A. Motor vehicle crashes in dementia of the Alzheimer type. *Ann Neurol* 1988; **24**: 782–6.

Fross RD. Ophthalmological precautions in Creutzfeldt–Jakob disease. *Ann Neurol* 1986; **20**: 748.

Gordon B, Selnes O. Progressive aphasia 'without dementia': evidence of more widespread involvement. *Neurology* 1984; **34**: 102. (suppl 1).

Goudsmit JAAP, White BJ, Weitkamp LR, Keats BJB, Morrow CH, Gajdusek DC. Familial Alzheimer's disease in two kindreds of the same geographic and ethnic origin: a clincial and genetic study. *J Neurol Sci* 1981; **49**: 79–89.

Green J, Morris JC, Sandson J, McKeel DW, Miller JW. Progressive aphasia: A precursor of global dementia? *Neurology* 1990; **40**: 423–9.

Hauser WA, Morris ML, Heston LL, Anderson VE. Seizures and myoclonus in patients with Alzheimer's disease. *Neurology* 1986; **36**: 1226–30.

Heath PD, Kneedy P, Kapur N. Slowly progressive aphasia without generalized dementia. *Ann Neurol* 1983; **13**: 687–8.

Heyman A, Wilkinson WE, Hurwitz BJ, Schmechel D, Sigmon AH, Weinberg T, Helms MJ, Swift M. Alzheimer's disease: genetic aspects and associated clinical disorders. *Ann Neurol* 1983; **14**: 507–15.

Holland AL, McBurney DH, Moossy J, Reinmuth OM. The dissolution of language in Pick's disease with neurofibrillary tangles: a case study. *Brain Lang* 1985; **24**: 36–58.

Joachim CL, Morris HJ, Selkoe DJ. Clinically diagnosed Alzheimer's disease: autopsy results in 150 cases. *Ann Neurol* 1988; **24**: 50–6.

Kaye JA, May C, Atack JR, Daly E, Sweeney KL, Beal MF, Kaufman S, Milstein S, Friedland RP, Rapoport SI. Cerebrospinal fluid neurochemistry in the myoclonic subtype of Alzheimer's disease. *Ann Neurol* 1988a; **24**: 647–50.

Kaye JA, May C, Daly E, Atack JR, Sweeney BS, Luxenberg JS, Kat AD, Kaufman S, Milstien S, Friedland RP, Rapoport SI. Cerebrospinal fluid monoamine markers are decreased in dementia of the Alzheimer type with extrapyramidal features. *Neurology* 1988b; **38**: 554–7.

Levy SR, Chiappa KH, Burke CJ, Young RR. Early evolution and incidence of electroencephalographic abnormalities in Creutzfeldt–Jakob disease. *J Clin Neurophysiol* 1986; **3**: 1–21.

Lishman WA. *Organic Psychiatry*. Oxford: Blackwell Scientific Publications, 1987, pp. 391–3.

Mandell AM, Alexander MP, Carpenter S. Creutzfeldt–Jackob disease presenting as isolated aphasia. *Neurology* 1989; **39**: 55–8.

May WW. Creutzfeldt–Jakob disease. *Acta Neurol Scand* 1968; **44**: 1–32.

Mayeux R, Stern Y, Spanton S. Heterogeneity in dementia of the Alzheimer type: Evidence of subgroups. *Neurology* 1985; **35**: 453–61.

Mesulam MM. Slowly progressive aphasia without generalized dementia. *Ann Neurol* 1982; **11**: 592–8.

Molsa PK, Marttila RJ, Rinne UK. Extrapyramidal signs in Alzheimer's disease. *Neurology* 1984; **34**: 1114–16.

Morris JC, Cole M, Banker BQ, Wright D. Hereditary dysphasic dementia and the Pick–Alzheimer spectrum. *Ann Neurol* 1984; **16**: 455–66.

Pearce J, Miller E. *Clinical Aspects of Dementia*. London: Bailliere-Tindall, 1973.

Petry S, Cummings JL, Hill MA, Shapira J. Personality alterations in dementia of the Alzheimer type. *Arch Neurol* 1988; **45**: 1187–90.

Poeck K, Luzzatti C. Slowly progressive aphasia in three patients. *Brain* 1988; **111**: 151–68.

Progacar S, Williams RS. Alzheimer's disease presenting as slowly progressive aphasia. *RI Med J* 1984; **67**: 181–5.

Rapaport EB. Iatrogenic Creutzfeldt–Jakob disease. *Neurology* 1987; **37**: 1520–2.

Reding M, Haycox J, Blass J. Depression in patients referred to a dementia clinic: a three-year prospective study. *Arch Neurol* 1985; **42**: 894–6.

Reifler BV, Larson E, Hanley R. Coexistence of cognitive impairment and depression in geriatric outpatients. *Am J Psychiat* 1982; **139**: 623–6.

Sapin LR, Anderson FH, Pulaskki PD. Progressive aphasia without dementia: further documentation. *Ann Neurol* 1989; **25**: 411–13.

Schenk VWD. Re-examination of a family with Pick's disease. *Ann Hum Genet* 1958–59; **23**: 325–33.

Shuttleworth EC, Yates AJ, Paltin-Ortiz JD. Creutzfeldt–Jakob disease presenting as progressive aphasia. *J Natl Med Assoc* 1985; **77**: 649–55.

Sjögren T, Sjögren H, Lindgren AGH. Morbus Alzheimer and morbus Pick: Genetic, clinical and pathoanatomic study. *Acta Psychiatr Neurol Scand*, 1952 (Suppl 82), pp. 1–152.

Stengel E. A study on the symptomatology and differential diagnosis of Alzheimer's disease and Pick's disease. *J Ment Sci* 1943; **89**: 1–21.

Terry RD. Dementia. *Arch Neurol* 1976; **33**: 1–4.

Terry RD, Katzman R. Senile dementia of the Alzheimer type. *Ann Neurol* 1983; **14**: 497–506.

Thal LJ, Grundman M, Klauber MR. Dementia: characteristics of a referral population and factors associated with progression. *Neurology* 1988; **38**: 1083–90.

Tomlinson BE, Corsellis JAN. Aging and the dementias. In: *Greenfield's Neuropathology* (4th edition) (Adams HJ, Corsellis JAN and Duchen LW, eds). New York: Wiley and Sons, 1984, pp. 951–1024.

Uhl GR, Hilt DC, Hedreeen JC, Whitehouse PJ, Price DL. Pick's disease (lobar sclerosis): depletion of neurons in the nucleus basalis of Meynert. *Neurology* 1983; **33**: 1470–3.

van Mansvelt J. *Pick's Disease. A Syndrome of Lobar Cerebral Atrophy*. The Netherlands: Enschede, 1954.

Wechsler AF, Verity MA, Rosenschein S, Fried I, Scheibel A. Pick's disease: a clinical, computed tomographic, and histologic study with golgi impregnation observations. *Arch Neurol* 1982; **39**: 287–90.

Wilkins DE, Hallett M, Beradelli A, Walshe T, Alvarez N. Physiologic analysis of the myoclonus of Alzheimer's disease. *Neurology* 1984; **34**: 898–903.

Zubenko GS. Progression of illness in the differential diagnosis of primary depression. *Am J Psychiatr* 1990; **147**: 435–8.

Zubenko GS, Moossy J. Major depression in primary dementia: clinical and neuropathologic correlates. *Arch Neurol* 1988; **45**: 1182–6.

18.   Multi-infarct dementia is characterized by a stepwise or stuttering course, strokes and focal neurological signs

Vascular lesions are the second most common cause of dementia after Alzheimer's disease (Tomlinson and Henderson, 1976). Hachinski *et al.* (1974) coined the term multi-infarct dementia because the underlying pathology usually consists of multiple small or large infarcts. The distinction between primary degenerative and vascular dementia is usually straight-forward and based on clinical, radiographic, or pathological criteria. However, some patients have mixed forms.

The diagnosis of vascular dementia is strongly suggested by a history of sudden, stepwise deterioration in neurological function. This includes intellectual changes, as well as dysarthria, hemiparesis, reflex asymmetry, and somatosensory and visual field deficits. There is often partial recovery or stabilization of neurological dysfunction followed by another sudden decline. Urinary and gait disturbances are early markers for multi-infarct dementia (Kotsoris *et al.*, 1987). Additional features that suggest vascular dementia include relative preservation of memory function, prominent language disorder and pseudobulbar palsy, which is characterized by bilateral upper motor neuron lesions that cause spastic dysarthria, dysphagia, increased jaw jerk reflex and impaired emotional expression with spontaneous crying and laughing. Finally, a history of hypertension, transient ischemic attacks, cardiac source of emboli and peripheral vascular disease provides weak supportive evidence for the diagnosis of vascular dementia.

Hachinski *et al.* (1975) developed a scale for the diagnosis of vascular dementia based on a combination of clinical features (Table 18.1). Scores of 7 or higher are more likely to be associated with multi-infarct dementia while those below 5 are not.

The diagnosis of vascular dementia must be based on specific clinical and radiological findings. Hypertension, arteriosclerosis and other forms of peripheral vascular disease are common among the elderly. Yet such imprecise, clinicopathologic constructs as hardening of the cerebral arteries, 'arteriosclerotic dementia' and poor cerebral circulation are often used in reference to elderly patients with mental impairment. Similarly, it

Table 18.1 Ischemic score.

Feature	Score
Abrupt onset	2
Stepwise deterioration	1
Fluctuating course	2
Nocturnal confusion	1
Relative preservation of personality	1
Depression	1
Somatic complaints	1
Emotional incontinence	1
History of hypertension	1
History of strokes	2
Evidence of associated atherosclerosis	1
Focal neurological symptoms	2
Focal neurological signs	2

From Hachinski *et al.* 1975 (with permission).

is a mistake to diagnose vascular dementia simply because the patient is hypertensive, or to presume that arteriosclerosis has caused dementia.

Caution should likewise reign when magnetic resonance imaging (MRI) reveals white matter hyperintensities, also known as unidentified bright objects (Hunt et al., 1989), since these MRI signals are of uncertain clinical significance, and a small amount of encephalomalacia is common in non-demented old people (Tomlinson et al., 1968). How much encephalomalacia is pathological? Tomlinson et al. (1970) have related volumes of encephalomalacia from vascular insults to dementia. In non-demented subjects, they observed, the volume of softened tissue rarely exceeded 50 ml and there were no cases in which the volume of destroyed parenchyma was greater than 100 ml. In contrast, nearly 20 percent of demented elderly subjects had volumes of encephalomalacia exceeding 100 ml. Thus, as with degenerative dementia, the severity of pathology correlates with the clinical severity of the dementia.

In vascular dementia, lesion sites are also important in determining the pattern and severity of behavioral abnormality. Cerebral blood flow (CBF) is reduced in a bilateral patchy distribution in patients with vascular dementia, especially in the middle cerebral artery territory (Yamaguchi et al., 1980). Reduction in CBF correlates with severity of dementia (Meyer et al., 1988).

There are several vascular syndromes of dementia. The most obvious and least controversial cause is multiple, moderate-to-large cortical or subcortical strokes. Patients with this stroke pattern usually have a history of strokes causing focal neurological deficits, such as hemiparesis or aphasia. Less often, one or more large strokes involve clinically silent brain areas (e.g. right prefrontal or temporal cortex) or cause a transient confusional state that is attributed to other causes. Multiple large infarcts, on the other hand, are rarely confused with degenerative dementia, because accompanying behavioral changes often differ from those in dementia and prominent focal deficits are also present. Although these patients often have more language disturbance and less memory disorder than patients with degenerative dementia, their requirements for social support are similar to those of other dementias.

The lacunar state is characterized by multiple small areas of subcortical infarction due to lipohyalinotic occlusion of small, penetrating arteries (Fisher, 1969). Following individual lacunar infarcts, no apparent deficit or characteristic syndromes may occur. These syndromes include pure motor hemiparesis, pure sensory stroke, clumsy-hand dyarthria and ataxic hemiparesis. Dementia only results from multiple lacunes. Patients are usually hypertensive and often have other vascular risk factors, such as diabetes or cigarette smoking. Lacunar dementia, which shares many clinical features of the frontal lobe syndrome, is characterized by lack of spontaneity, emotional lability, i.e. pseudobulbar palsy, episodes of confusion, small-stepped gait, dysarthria, urinary incontinence, grasp reflex and pyramidal signs (Ishii et al., 1986).

Personality is relatively preserved in the lacunar state, in contrast with degenerative dementia, in which early personality changes are common. Many patients with multiple subcortical lacunes do not fulfil clinical criteria for dementia, although neuropsychological testing often reveals frontal dysfunction, with deficits in shifting mental set, response inhibition and executive function (Wolfe *et al.*, 1990).

Binswanger's subcortical encephalopathy or Binswanger's disease is a form of vascular dementia characterized by multiple white matter infarcts and lacunes, located in the border zones between penetrating cortical and lenticulostriate arteries. Patients are usually hypertensive and have extensive cerebrovascular atheromatous lesions (Burger *et al.*, 1976; Caplan and Schoene, 1978). Also, these patients often present with a stuttering, stepwise course that includes pseudobulbar palsy, and focal motor and sensory changes.

As Binswanger's disease progresses, some patients follow a fulminant course, while others experience gradual mental deterioration without neurological signs (Loizou *et al.*, 1981; Kinkel *et al.*, 1985). The clinical course may be lengthy, with long plateau periods (Caplan and Schoene, 1978). Behavioral features are similar to those of the lacunar state, with prominent frontal lobe symptoms.

Cerebral microinfarction is an uncommon cause of progressive dementia often accompanied by visual field defects, peripheral vascular disease and signs of motor neuron dysfunction (Kaplan *et al.*, 1985). Patients are usually middle-aged men who present with stroke that is followed by dementia. Valvular or ischemic heart disease is often present.

The existence of a dementia syndrome resulting from chronic cerebral ischemia due to either bilateral carotid stenosis or to diffuse arteriolar narrowing is controversial. If it exists, it is very rare. There is little evidence to support vascular surgical intervention or medications that alter vasomotor tone as a remedy for persistent cognitive and behavioral deficits.

References

Burger PC, Burch JG, Kunze U. Subcortical arteriosclerotic encephalopathy (Binswanger disease). *Stroke* 1976; **7**: 626–31.

Caplan LR, Schoene WC. Clinical features of subcortical arteriosclerotic encephalopathy (Binswanger disease). *Neurology* 1978; **28**: 1206–15.

Fisher CM. The arterial lesions underlying lacunes. *Acta Neuropath* 1969; **12**: 1–15.

Hachinski VC, Iluff LD, Zilhka E, DuBoulay GH, McAllister VL, Marshall J, Ross Russell RW, Symon L. Cerebral blood flow in dementia. *Arch Neurol* 1975; **32**: 632–7.

Hachinski VC, Lassen NA, Marshal J. Multi-infarct dementia: a cause of mental deterioration in the elderly. *Lancet* 1974; **ii**: 207–10.

Hunt AL, Orrison WW, Yeo RA, Haaland KY, Rhyme RL, Garry PJ, Rosenberg GA. Clinical significance of MRI white matter lesions in the elderly. *Neurology* 1989; **39**: 1470–4.

Ishii N, Nishihara Y, Imamura T. Why do frontal lobe symptoms predominate in vascular dementia with lacunes? *Neurology* 1986; **36**: 340–5.

Kaplan JG, Katzman R, Horoupian DS, Fuld PA, Mayeux R, Hays AP. Progressive dementia, visual deficits, amyotrophy, and microinfarcts. *Neurology* 1985; **35**: 789–96.

Kinkel WR, Jacobs L, Polachini I, Bates V, Heffner RR. Subcortical arteriosclerotic encephalopathy (Binswanger's disease) computed tomograpic, nuclear magnetic resonance, and clinical correlations. *Arch Neurol* 1985; **42**: 951–9.

Kotsoris H, Barclay LL, Kheyfets S, Hulyalkar A, Dougherty J. Urinary and gait disturbances as markers for early multi-infarct dementia. *Stroke* 1987; **18**: 138–41.

Loizou LA, Kendall BE, Marshall J. Subcortical arteriosclerotic encephalopathy: A clinical and radiological investigation. *J Neurol Neurosurg Psychiat* 1981; **44**: 294–304.

Meyer JS, Rogers RL, Judd BW, Mortel KF, Sims P. Cognition and cerebral blood flow fluctuate together in multi-infarct dementia. *Stroke* 1988; **19**: 163–9.

Tomlinson BE, Henderson G. Some quantitative cerebral findings in normal and demented old people. In: *Neurobiology of Aging* (Terry RD, Gershon S, eds). New York: Raven Press, 1976 pp. 183–204.

Tomlinson BE, Blessed G, Roth M. Observations on the brains of non-demented old people. *J Neurol Sci* 1968; **7**: 331–56.

Tomlinson BE, Blessed G, Roth M. Observations on the brains of demented old people. *J Neurol Sci* 1970; **11**: 205–42.

Wolfe N, Linn R, Babikian VL, Knoefel JE, Albert ML. Frontal systems impairment following multiple lacunar infarcts. *Arch Neurol* 1990; **47**: 129–32.

Yamaguchi F, Meyer JS, Yamamoto M *et al.* Non-invasive regional cerebral blood flow measurements in dementia. *Arch Neurol* 1980; **37**: 114–19.

19. *Supportive care for the patient and family, avoidance of stressors and judicious use of medication comprise the mainstay of dementia treatment*

The medical and supportive care of patients with dementia is often neglected by physicians who consider their obligation fulfilled once they have made the diagnosis and ruled out curable disorders.

Referring patients and family to self-help groups, day-care and respite centers for relief of the burden of providing care, and sources of management suggestions is part of the physician's charge when caring for patients with Alzheimer's disease. One good resource is the book, *The 36-Hour Day* (Mace and Rabins, 1981), which provides insightful discussions on (1) the nature of dementia; (2) problems of independent living, such as when a patient should give up her job, stop managing her own money, stop driving, or move to a supervised home; (3) problems in daily care, such as nutrition, personal hygeine and smoking; (4) medical problems associated with dementia, such as falls, constipation and seizures; (5) what to do if the patient's caretaker becomes ill; (6) locating resources for the patient and their family; and (7) how the caretaker and family of the patient can learn to cope with the illness. Other books that cover these and related topics include *Alzheimer's: A Caregiver's Guide and Sourcebook* (Gruetzner,

1988), *Alzheimer's Disease: The Long Bereavement* (Forsythe, 1990), *Alzheimer's Disease: The Standard Reference* (Reisberg, 1984), *Caring for the Person with Dementia: A Guide for Families and other Carers* (Alzheimer's Disease Society, 1984) and *Alzheimer's Disease: A Practical Guide for Families and Other Caregivers* (Ronch, 1991). These books provide a wealth of practical information for families and should also be consulted by any physician who cares for affected patients. It may be useful to have a copy of these paperbacks for families to look over at the time of their office visits. The Appendix lists organizations that can be helpful for patients and their families.

Alzheimer's patients are particularly sensitive to medications, and dosages should be lowered or drugs discontinued if possible. The incidence of falls and fractures is increased in Alzheimer's disease (AD), and such incidents are partly due to medication (Buchner and Larson, 1987). However, judicious use of medications can often overcome difficult problems. For example, intermittent, low doses of haloperidol controls agitated or aggressive behavior, and short courses of low doses of benzodiazepines or antihistamines may be used to treat insomnia and reversal of the day–night sleep–wake cycle.

The search for drugs to prevent, reverse or stabilize dementia continues. However, except for drugs to treat hypertension and other cardiovascular risk factors for stroke, no clearly effective agent has been found for the treatment of degenerative, vascular or alcoholic dementias.

There has been a major push to find a drug to rejuvenate the degenerating brain. In AD, the major neurotransmitter change is loss of cholinergic input to the cortex. The cell loss in the basal nucleus, from which cholinergic fibers arise, accounts for a 50 to 90 percent decrease of the biosynthetic enzyme choline acetyltransferase in the cortex of AD patients (Katzman, 1986). This cholinergic deficiency, coupled with the well-known amnesic effects of muscarinic blocking agents, such as scopolamine (previously used during labor so that the mother would not remember the pain), led to great excitement that AD might be the cholinergic analog to Parkinson's disease, a dopamine deficiency disease. Initial clinical trials to test this hypothesis, using with cholinergic precursors (choline and lecithin) and anticholinesterase blockers (physostigmine) have observed no, or limited, benefit (Maxim 21) (Terry and Katzman, 1983). In addition, other neurotransmitters (e.g. norepinephrine, serotonin, dopamine) and neuropeptides (e.g. somatostatin and corticotropin-releasing hormone) are reduced in many AD patients (Katzman, 1986; Zubenko and Moossy, 1988). Theoretical problems with a simple 'chemical cocktail' fix thus include: (1) difficulty achieving a physiological balance, and (2) extensive cortical cell loss, which negates the therapeutic effect of pumping in missing subcortically synthesized compounds since the target site for these transmitters may already be destroyed. In early stages of disease, however, certain drug therapies, such as lecithin, may be beneficial.

Although control of hypertension in the elderly reduces cerebrovascular, myocardial and peripheral vascular insults, reduction of blood pressure in demented hypertensive patients may have either positive or adverse effects on cognition and behavior (Whalley, 1989). The degree of blood pressure reduction, as well as the type of antihypertensive used may be important. For example, beta-blockers may have greater motor, cognitive and behavioral side effects than angiotensin-converting enzymes; the latter may be preferable in patients with depression and dementia (Solomons *et al.*, 1985; Croog *et al.*, 1986; Lichter *et al.*, 1986). Cerebral vasodilators, stimulants and vitamins have also been tried, but have not shown a reproducible, beneficial effect.

Dementia in alcoholics may be due to Korsakoff's syndrome, other neurotoxicity related to alcohol or poor nutrition, hepatic dysfunction, head trauma or vascular disease. Unlike Wernicke's encephalopathy, the memory disorder in Korsakoff's syndrome does not respond to thiamine. Clonidine, an alpha-2 adrenergic agonist, may improve memory in some patients with Korsakoff's syndrome (McEntee and Mair, 1980), but cholinergic as well as noradrenergic deficits may contribute to memory disorders in alcoholics, and clonidine cannot be expected to help all patients (Lishman 1986).

Appendix: Organizations concerned about Alzheimer's disease

Administration on Aging, 330 Independence Ave, SW, Washington, DC 20201

Age Concern England, Astral House, 1268 London Road, London SW16 4ER

Alzheimer's Disease and Related Disorders Association, Inc., 360 N. Michigan Ave, Chicago, IL 60601 (this national office can provide information on local affiliates)

Alzheimer's Disease Society, 158–160 Balham High Road, London SW12 9BN

American Association of Homes for the Aging, 1050 17th St, NW, Washington DC 20036

American Nursing Home Association (American Health Care Association), 1025 Connecticut Ave, NW, Washington DC 20036

Disabled Living Foundation, 380–384 Harrow Road, London W9 2HU

Family Service Association of America, 44 East 23rd St, New York, NY 10010

Gray Panthers, 3700 Chestnut St, Philadelphia, PA 19104.

National Council for Homemakers, Home Health Aide Services, 1790 Broadway, New York, NY 10019

National Council of Senior Citizens, 1511 K St, NW, Washington, DC 20005

National Institute on Aging, Information Office, Bldg 31, Room 5C-36, National Institutes of Health, Bethesda, MD 20205

References

Alzheimer's Disease Society (1984). *Caring for the Person with Dementia: A Guide for Families and Other Carers*. ADS, London.

Buchner DM, Larson EB. Falls and fractures in patients with Alzheimer-type dementia. *JAMA* 1987; **257**: 1492–5.

Croog SH, Levine S, Tests M *et al*. The effects of antihypertensive therapy on the quality of life. *New Engl J Med* 1986; **314**: 1657–64.

Forsythe E. *Alzheimer's Disease: The Long Bereavement*. New York: Faber and Faber, 1990.

Gruetzner H. *Alzheimer's: A Caregiver's Guide and Sourcebook*. New York: J. Wiley and Sons, Inc., 1988.

Katzman R. Alzheimer's disease. *New Engl J Med* 1986; **314**: 964–73.

Lichter I, Richardson P, Wyke M. Differential effects of atenolol and enalapril on memory during treatment for essential hypertension. *Br J Clin Pharm* 1986; **21**: 641–5.

Lishman WA. Alcoholic dementia: a hypothesis. *Lancet* 1986; **i**: 1184–6.

Mace NL, Rabins PV. *The 36-Hour Day: A Family Guide to Caring for Persons with Alzheimer's Disease*. Baltimore: Johns Hopkins Press, 1981.

McEntee WJ, Mair RG. Memory enhancement in Korsakoff's psychosis by clonidine: further evidence for a noradrenergic deficit. *Ann Neurol* 1980; **7**: 466–70.

Reisberg, B. (ed.) *Alzheimer's Disease: The Standard Reference*. London: Free Press/Collier Macmillan, 1984.

Ronch JL. *Alzheimer's Disease: A Practical Guide for Families and Other Caregivers*. New York: Continuum Publishing Company, 1991.

Solomons S, Hotchkiss E, Saravay S *et al*. Impairment of memory function by antihypertensive medication. *Arch Gen Psychiat* 1985; **40**: 1109–12.

Terry RD, Katzman R. Senile dementia of the Alzheimer type. *Ann Neurol* 1983; **14**: 497–506.

Whalley LJ. Drug treatment of dementia. *Br J Psychiat* 1989; **155**: 595–611.

Zubenko GS, Moossy J. Major depression in primary dementia: clinical and neuropathologic correlates. *Arch Neurol* 1988; **45**: 1182–6.

20.   *The elderly are exquisitely sensitive to the effects of medication*

A common and potentially treatable cause of pseudodementia is encephalopathy caused by drugs, toxins and metabolic abnormalities. In the geriatric population, drugs are commonly prescribed and used in combination, with nearly 25 percent of elderly patients taking between four and six medications (Williamson and Chopin, 1980). Adverse drug reactions are approximately two and one-half times more common in patients over the age of 60 years (Editorial, 1978), and adverse reactions to many commonly used drugs include such serious mental symptoms as confusion, agitation, depression, hallucinations, paranoia and psychosis (*Medical Letter*, 1989). Psychiatric symptoms occur as either dose-related or idiosyncratic side effects.

A 75-year-old retired attorney who had been in excellent health developed depression with suicidal ideation and complaints of rapidly progressive loss of short-term memory over a three-month period. Evaluation by a neurologist and psychiatrist confirmed the symptoms; magnetic resonance imaging (MRI) was normal. He was diagnosed with depression and possible Alzheimer's disease and a tricyclic antidepressant was prescribed. This prescription was discontinued one month later because of agitation. It was then discovered that, a year earlier, a physician friend of the patient had prescribed 0.25 mg triazolam at night for sleep. Six months previously the patient found that the prescribed dose was ineffective and doubled the dose. Within three months following taper and discontinuation of triazolam, his behavioral symptoms resolved.

In addition, withdrawal of either alcohol or sedative–hypnotic and anti-anxiety agents often provokes prominent behavioral reactions, including psychosis. Withdrawal symptoms are common after hospital admission; their occurrence may be delayed with long-acting drugs such as clorazepate (Tranxene) or diazepam (Valium).

Increased sensitivity to medications among the elderly is related to a combination of factors. The endogenous factors include (1) decreased hepatic detoxification and renal excretion; (2) decreased serum albumin and therefore protein binding (resulting in increased free drug levels); (3) decreased volume of distribution (decreased total body water); and (4) defective homeostatic mechanisms. The exogenous factors include polypharmacy and drug interactions (Vestal, 1978). Furthermore, it is not uncommon for even very low doses of medication to cause disabling mental side effects in old people.

Any elderly patient with mental impairment should have all prescription and non-prescription medications carefully reviewed. Low doses that are not toxic to younger patients may be responsible for unexpected and severe side effects. Include all drugs, ranging from antibiotics to antiepileptics to antihypertensives, in this review.

Table 20.1 lists the principal medications which cause neurobehavioral disorders in the elderly. Diuretics, the most commonly prescribed drugs in the elderly, can cause metabolic derangements (e.g. hyponatremia, hypokalemia, hyperkalemia, hypercalcemia), dehydration and hypotension, which contribute to cognitive and psychomotor retardation as well as delirium. Cardiovascular drugs are also a frequent cause of behavioral change among the elderly. Beta-adrenergic blockers and antihypertensives can cause depression, delirium, hallucinations, paranoia and delusions. Antiarrhythmic agents can cause delirium, panic and terror, agitation, depression and psychosis.

Anticholinergic agents commonly cause confusion, agitation, delirium, memory impairment, hallucinations and paranoia. Histamine H2-receptor blockers (cimetidine and ranitidine) can cause confusion, depression, hallucinations and paranoia.

Non-steroidal anti-inflammatory drugs may cause a wide range of mental

Table 20.1 Medications that commonly cause neurobehavioral disorders in the elderly.

Diuretics	*Non-steroidal anti-inflammatory drugs*
Hydrochlorthiazide	*Histamine H_2-receptor blockers*
Furosemide	Cimetidine
Cardiovascular drugs	Ranitidine
Non-selective beta-blockers	*Glucocorticoids*
Propranolol	*Narcotics*
Antihypertensives	*Antiepileptic drugs*
Prazosin	Carbamazepine
Clonidine	Phenobarbital
Methyldopa	Primidone
Nifedipine	Phenytoin
Captopril	Valproic acid
Antiarrhythmias	*Antiparkinsonism drugs*
Lidocaine	Levodopa
Procainamide	Amantadine
Digitalis	Bromocriptine
Disopyramide	Lergotrile
Anticholinergics	*Psychotropic drugs*
Scopolamine (oral, transdermal)	Benzodiazepines
Atropine (oral, ocular)	Antidepressants
Antibiotics	Antipsychotic drugs
Isoniazid	Lithium
Gentamycin	
Tobramycin	

side effects, including delirium, depression and hallucinations. Glucocorticoids can cause mania, psychosis, depression, paranoia, hallucinations and catatonia. Elderly patients are very sensitive to narcotics.

Antiepileptic and antiparkinsonism drugs can cause delirium, depression, psychosis, hallucinations, agitation and aggression.

Psychotropic drugs are frequently prescribed for the elderly and are among the most common causes of confusion and other behavioral problems (Prien, 1980). Benzodiazepines with long half-lives (e.g. diazepam, flurazepam and chlordiazepoxide) should not be prescribed for elderly patients for extended periods because decreased hepatic metabolism leads to frequent toxicity. However, benzodiazepines with shorter half-lives, such as temazepam and oxazepam, also produce behavioral disorders. In elderly patients tricyclic and newer antidepressants, antipsychotic drugs and lithium are likely to cause behavioral side-effects, especially at routine or high doses.

References

Editorial. Medication in the elderly. *J Irish Med Assoc* 1978; **71**: 136–7.

Medical Letter. Drugs that cause psychiatric symptoms. 1989; **31**: 113–18.

Prien RF. Problems and practices in geriatric psychopharmacology. *Psychosomatics* 1980; **21**: 213–23.

Vestal RE. Drug use in the elderly: A review of problems and special considerations. *Drugs* 1978; **16**: 358–82.

Williamson J, Chopin JM. Adverse reactions to prescribed drugs in the elderly: A multicentre investigation. *Age and Ageing* 1980; **9**: 73–80.

21.   *There are many treatable causes of dementia, but these affect only a minority of dementia patients*

All patients should be thoroughly evaluated for treatable causes of global cognitive dysfunction. Approximately 15 percent of demented patients have fully or partially reversible disorders (Marsden and Harrison, 1972; Wells, 1978). However, because the potentially treatable causes of dementia include such a vast spectrum of disorders (Table 21.1), it is impractical to pursue clinical and laboratory tests to explore each one. A minimum workup is summarized in Table 21.2.

Within this extensive differential diagnosis, the medical history and physical examination often provide the most important clues. In addition, a complementary medical history from at least one close relative or friend and a thorough review of the patient's past medical records are essential because of the limited mnemonic and communicative skills of many patients. For example, a history of previous radioiodine treatment for hyperthyroidism, depression, tuberculosis, or subarachnoid hemorrhage suggests a specific, treatable cause of dementia.

Therapeutic drug intoxication is the most common cause of reversible intellectual dysfunction in the elderly (Maxim 20), so investigate current use of both prescribed and over-the-counter medications. If possible, a family member should be instructed to search the medicine cabinet and supervise all medication use for one week to ensure that the patient is not taking too much or incorrect medication. Check serum levels of certain drugs (e.g. phenytoin, phenobarbital and digoxin), bearing in mind that elderly patients are often exquisitely drug sensitive and frequently develop toxic reactions in the low therapeutic or subtherapeutic dosage range. The patient's medications should be re-evaluated, as many can often be gradually tapered or discontinued safely. Medical or psychiatric consultation is often required before certain medications are reduced.

Serial examinations are often helpful to identify a fluctuating course, and can uncover additional historical or physical findings. The mental status

Table 21.1   Potentially reversible causes of dementia.

Chemical intoxication
Alcohol (ethyl or methyl)
Aniline dyes
Arsenic
Carbon monoxide
Lead
Mercury
Organophosphates
Nitrobenzenes

Deficiency states
B_{12} (subacute combined degeneration)
Folate
Marchiafava–Bignami (primary degeneration of the corpus callosum)
Niacin (pellagra)
Thiamine

Drug intoxication
Anticholinergics (e.g. atropine, scopolamine)
Antidepressants (e.g. imipramine, amitryptiline)
Barbiturates
Benzodiazepines (e.g. diazepam, Iorazepam)
Beta-adrenergic blockers (e.g. propranolol)
Bromides
Cardiac glycosides (e.g. digoxin)
Clonidine
Disulfarim
Histamine H2 receptor antagonists (e.g. cimetidine)
Levodopa
Lithium
Metoclopramide
Neuroleptics (e.g. haloperidol, chlorpromazine)
Non-steroidal anti-inflammatory agents
Opiates
Phenytoin
Prazosin
Quinidine

Systemic disorders

Cardiovascular
  Arrhythmia
  Congestive heart failure
  Endocarditis
  Hypertensive encephalopathy
  Left-ventricular outflow obstruction (e.g. aortic stenosis)

Collagen–vascular
  Sarcoidosis
  Systemic lupus erythematosus
  Systemic necrotizing vasculitis
  Temporal arteritis

Hematological
  Polycythemia
  Severe anemia

Infectious
  Aquired immunodeficiency syndrome
  Cryptococcus
  Cystercicosis
  Tuberculosis
  Whipple's disease

Metabolic and endocrine disorders
  Addison's disease
  Cushing's syndrome
  Dialysis
  Hepatic insufficiency
  Hypercalcemia
  Hyperlipidemia
  Hyperthyroidism
  Hypoglycemia
  Hyponatremia
  Hypothyroidism
  Hypopituitarism
  Pheochromocytoma

Pulmonary
  Emphysema
  Pneumonia
  Sleep apnea

Neurologic disorders
Epilepsy (repeated bouts of status epilepticus)
Demyelination (multiple sclerosis)
Hydrocephalus (occult, obstructive)
Infections (AIDS, herpes encephalitis, chronic meningitis, neurosyphilis, subdural empyema, abscess)
Parkinson's disease
Trauma (intracerebral, subdural, epidural hematoma)
Tumor (primary or metastatic)

Psychiatric
Conversion disorder
Depression
Dissociative disorder
Malingering

Miscellaneous
Fat embolism
Fecal impaction
Hospitalization
Paraneoplastic
Porphyria
Sensory deprivation
Surgery–Anesthesia
Wilson's disease

Table 21.2   History, physical, and laboratory examinations in dementia.

History
Nature of onset and pace of progression
Description of behavioral changes
  Cognitive problems (memory, language, calculation, judgment,
    geographic disorientation (getting lost))
  Personality change (irritability, apathy, agitation)
  Psychiatric symptoms (anxiety, depression, hallucinations, delusions,
    paranoia)
Sleep disorder
Life stresses (loss of loved ones, jobs, etc.)
Previous medical, neurological and psychiatric disorders
Alcohol and other drug use
Prescription and over-the-counter medications
Toxic exposure
Family history

Physical examination
Appearance – posture, facial expression, hygiene, dress
Vital signs – orthostatic blood pressure changes
Head – trauma, exophthalmos, Kayser–Fleischer ring
Neck – bruit, thyromegaly
Lymph nodes – adenopathy
Pulmonary
Cardiovascular
Abdomen – ascites, mass
Extremities – vascular insufficiency, edema

Neurological examination
Must be thorough; always test smell, eye movements, tone and gait

Psychiatric examination

Laboratory examination
Hematological tests: electrolytes (Na, K, CO_2, Cl, Ca, Phos), glucose,
  complete blood cell count, thyroid and liver function tests, blood urea
  nitrogen, and creatinine, vitamin B_{12} and folate levels, VDRL,
  erythrocyte sedimentation rate
Urinalysis (glucose, albumin and ketone levels, microscopic examination)
Stool examination for occult blood
Chest X-ray
Electrocardiogram
Electroencephalogram
Computed tomography or magnetic resonance imaging of the brain
Lumbar puncture

examination is particularly important, because focal neurological, disorders (e.g. aphasia, amnesia, left-sided neglect) may be misdiagnosed as dementia.

Depression must be considered in all demented patients. Affective disorders are common in the elderly and cause psychic symptoms, including anxiety, hopelessness, helplessness and worthlessness, as well as vegetative symptoms, such as decreased sleep, appetite and libido. Not all depressed patients have a sad face and slowed mentation, some are agitated or may appear 'normal'. Also, treatable affective disorders may coexist with, or present as, dementia (Maxim 15).

Paranoia, delusions, hallucinations and illusions are common in patients who have degenerative dementing illnesses, medication intoxication, other organic mental disorders and primary psychiatric disorders. These symptoms should be specifically sought from patients and observers. For all these reasons, it is prudent to have any patient with these symptoms examined by a psychiatrist before diagnosing a degenerative, incurable dementia.

Computed tomography (CT) or magnetic resonance imaging (MRI) of the brain are invaluable in detailing intracranial lesions such as tumor, hemorrhage, abscess and empyema, infarction and hydrocephalus. Generalized or restricted cerebral atrophy can also be identified on these imaging studies. Computed tomography of the brain should also be obtained with contrast dye if there are no contraindications. Gadolinium is not required for routine MRI scanning in dementia, although it may be helpful in certain situations (e.g. multiple small metastases or meningeal carcinomatosis). Radionuclide scanning, single photon emission computed tomography (SPECT), and cerebral angiography are helpful in occasional cases (e.g. obese patients too large for CT or MRI).

Lumbar puncture should be performed if there are no contraindications, such as bleeding diathesis or an intracranial mass with potential for herniation. Laboratory studies of the cerebrospinal fluid (CSF) should include cell count, glucose and protein analysis, culture, Indian ink stain, Venereal Disease Research Laboratories (VDRL) and cytology. In selected cases CSF lyme antibody titres should be obtained. The low yield in seeking a treatable cause of dementia, when the workup has so far yielded negative findings, has dissuaded many from performing lumbar puncture routinely. However, the risks of lumbar puncture are extremely small if there are no contraindications, and despite the low yield, the benefits of identifying a treatable cause of dementia are enormous. Furthermore, if clinical findings are suggestive of central nervous system infection (e.g. fever, headache, stiff neck, previous history of syphilis, tuberculosis or cryptococcus), it is essential to examine the CSF. An elevated protein level without any structural brain abnormality in a demented patient with hydrocephalus may rarely result from a spinal cord tumor secreting protein that obstructs CSF reabsorption (Feldmann et al., 1986).

The diagnostic workup outlined above should be performed *early* in the course of mental decline. Most of dementia's treatable causes become more refractory with time.

References

Feldmann E, Bromfield E, Navia B, Pasternak GW, Posner JB. Hydrocephalic dementia and spinal cord tumor. *Arch Neurol* 1986; **43**: 714–18.
Marsden CD, Harrison MJG. Outcome of investigation in patients with presenile dementia. *Br Med J* 1972; **2**: 249–52.
Wells CE. Chronic brain disease: An overview. *Am J Psychiat* 1978; **135**: 1–12.

22. Occult hydrocephalus was first described in adults as the triad of gait disturbance, dementia and incontinence

Occult (normal pressure) hydrocephalus is a chronic condition in which the cerebrospinal fluid (CSF) pressure is less than 180 mm H_2O but there is a slight pressure gradient between the ventricles and brain or intermittent increases in intracranial pressure. Often, the pressure gradient causes progressive ventricular enlargement and compression of adjacent white matter, triggering progressive cerebral dysfunction. In milder cases, the pressure gradient sustains the overinflated ventricular system (most likely inflated from previous increased CSF pressure) and results in static cerebral dysfunction. The symptoms may be reversed with removal of cerebrospinal fluid by lumbar puncture or shunting (Adams *et al.*, 1965).

Gait disturbance is the principal symptom; it usually develops first and is the sole problem in most patients (Fisher, 1982). Patients often describe imbalance, unsteadiness, slowness, falling, and difficulty traversing stairs and curbs. Complaints of tiredness and weakness when walking or standing are also common. The gait disorder's onset is usually insidious, and its severity fluctuates widely in many patients. Following falls, patients may be unable to get up and walk for several hours (Fisher, 1977), although subsequent examination reveals no weakness. As the course progresses, the shorter, shuffled steps occur on a wider base and are less certain; the feet become 'glued to the ground'in this 'magnetic gait disorder' (Fisher, 1977). Turning and rapid postural changes become more difficult, and smooth movements degenerate into slow, disarticulated, clumsy sequences. Other movements may also be quite slow and delayed.

Some specialists have described this gait disorder as an apraxia, but this concept is controversial (Knutsson and Lying-Tunell, 1985; Sudarsky and Simon, 1987). Denny-Brown (1958) introduced the term gait apraxia to characterize the effects of frontal lesions. The observation that some patients with occult hydrocephalus can imitate walking movements while supine, but are glued to the floor when they stand, has been used to support the designation of apraxia (Fisher, 1982). However, many patients cannot imitate walking movements while supine. Furthermore, the imitation of walking while supine is a far cry from the actual, complex motor act. Therefore, the fundamental gait problem is not apraxia, or inability to carry out a movement on command (Maxim 43). It is instead a disorder of motor integration and execution.

Patients with occult hydrocephalus may also have parkinsonian symptoms such as stooped posture, slow movements and short-stepped gait. On motor and reflex examination, patients may have Gegenhalten or paratonic rigidity, slowing of fine or serial hand movements, poor handwriting, brisk reflexes, extensor plantar reflexes and grasp reflexes (Estanol, 1981; Fisher, 1982).

Eventually, most patients develop mental symptoms, which rarely occur without a pre-existing gait disorder. The form and severity of mental changes vary. Deficiencies of attention, initiative, spontaneity and drive, slowing of thought and memory impairment are common. Some patients also become disoriented, irritable, aggressive or manic.

Bladder dysfunction, usually the last triad component to develop, occurs in about half of patients. Early symptoms include urgency and frequency, while incontinence complicates later stages. Unnecessary prostate surgery for urinary complaints is not uncommon. Some incontinent patients show no embarrassment or concern, as may also be seen in those with frontal lobe lesions (Maxim 54). Cystometrograms may reveal bladder hyperactivity and detrusor instability (Ahlberg *et al.*, 1988).

The diagnosis of occult hydrocephalus is based on a combination of clinical and radiological findings. Signs of increased intracranial pressure such as papilledema are absent. Computed tomography (CT) and magnetic resonance imaging (MRI) of the brain show enlargement of the ventricular system with variable gyral atrophy. Prominent ventriculomegaly without convolutional atrophy strongly supports occult hydrocephalus, but sulcal enlargement neither refutes the diagnosis nor predicts shunt failure. On MRI, increased periventricular density and white matter signal on T2-weighted images, CSF flow void sign (or loss of signal in flowing CSF relative to more stationary CSF) seen in the cerebral aqueduct, and corpus callosum thinning are found in occult hydrocephalus, as well as in other dementing illnesses (Jack *et al.*, 1987).

The 'tap-test' is a simple and useful test for evaluating patients with possible occult hydrocephalus (Maxim 23) (Wikkelso *et al.*, 1982). Bedside quantitative tests of psychometric and motor capacities are performed before and after removal of 35 to 45 ml CSF. Definite, albeit transient, improvement supports the diagnosis of occult hydrocephalus. Additional tests for establishing the diagnosis include radioisotope cisternography (Le May and New, 1970), saline infusion into the lumbar subarachnoid space with pressure measurements (Katzman and Hussey, 1970) and measurement of conductance to CSF outflow (Borgesen and Gjerris, 1982). However, the value of these additional tests is uncertain (Maxim 23).

The differential diagnosis of adult occult hydrocephalus includes hydrocephalus with increased pressure, Alzheimer's disease and multi-infarct dementia, Parkinson's disease, progressive supranuclear palsy, frontal lobe lesions and cervical myelopathy.

Occult hydrocephalus also occurs in children, in whom the onset may be insidious and the symptoms may be subtle. Some patients are incorrectly diagnosed with 'arrested hydrocephalus' and therapeutic opportunities are missed. The pediatric form of occult hydrocephalus is characterized by an enlarged head, mild spastic paraparesis and a history of delayed psychomotor and cognitive development, in which the deficit in perfomance IQ exceeds the deficit in verbal IQ (Milhorat, 1984). The differential diagnosis includes arrested or compensated hydrocephalus, in which there is no pressure gradient between the ventricles and brain, atrophy, porencephaly and aqueductal stenosis and other forms of obstructive hydrocephalus.

A slight obstruction of CSF outflow is believed to cause the gradual ventricular distention in occult hydrocephalus. The etiology of the obstruction includes subarachnoid hemorrhage, head trauma, chronic meningitis or other central nervous system infections, basilar artery ectasia and craniotomy. However, many cases are idiopathic.

References

Adams RD, Fisher CM, Hakim S, Ojemann RG, Sweet WH. Symptomatic occult hydrocephalus with 'normal' cerebrospinal fluid pressure. A treatable syndrome. *New Engl J Med* 1965; **273**: 117–26.

Ahlberg J, Norlen L, Blomstrand C, Wikkelso C. Outcome of shunt operation on urinary incontinence in normal pressure hydrocephalus predicted by lumbar puncture. *J Neurol Neurosurg Psychiat* 1988; **51**: 105–8.

Borgesen SE, Gjerris F. The predictive value of conductance to outflow of CSF in normal pressure hydrocephalus. *Brain* 1982; **105**: 65–86.

Denny-Brown D. The nature of apraxia. *J Nerv Ment Dis* 1958; **126**: 9–32.

Estanol BV. Gait apraxia in communicating hydrocephalus. *J Neurol Neurosurg Psychiat* 1981; **44**: 305–8.

Fisher CM. The clinical picture of occult hydrocephalus. *Clin Neurosurg* 1977; **24**: 270–84.

Fisher CM. Hydrocephalus as a cause of disturbances of gait in the elderly. *Neurology* 1982; **32**: 1358–63.

Jack CR, Mokri B, Laws ER, Houser OW, Baker HL, Petersen RC. MR findings in normal-pressure hydrocephalus: Significance and comparison with other forms of dementia. *J Comp Assist Tomogr* 1987; **11**: 923–31.

Katzman R, Hussey F. A simple constant-infusion manometric test for measurement of CSF absorption: I. Rationale and method. *Neurology* 1970; **20**: 534–44.

Knutsson E, Lying-Tunell U. Gait apraxia in normal-pressure hydrocephalus. *Neurology* 1985; **35**: 155–60.

Le May M, New PFJ. Pneumoencephalography and isotope cisternography in the diagnosis of occult normal pressure hydrocephalus. *Radiology* 1970; **96**: 347–58.

Milhorat TH. Hydrocephalus: Historical Notes, Etiology, and Clinical diagnosis. In: *Pediatric Neurosurgery*, (McLaurin RL, ed.). New York: Grune and Stratton, 1984, pp. 197–210.

Sudarsky L, Simon S. Gait disorder in late-life hydrocephalus. *Arch Neurol* 1987; **44**: 263–7.

Wikkelso C, Andersson H, Blomstrand C, Lindqvist G. The clinical effect of lumbar puncture in normal pressure hydrocephalus. *J Neurol Neurosurg Psychiat* 1982; **45**: 64–9.

23.   *A known cause, a short duration of symptoms and a positive tap-test predict a good response to cerebrospinal fluid shunting in patients with occult hydrocephalus*

The recognition that occult hydrocephalus is a reversible disorder led to an enthusiastic surge of support for shunting procedures. This enthusiasm has been subsequently tempered because improvement is variable and shunt complications occur in about one-third of patients. The critical element in successful treatment of occult hydrocephalus is identification of patients likely to benefit from shunting.

The diagnosis of occult hydrocephalus must be established before therapy is considered. When mental changes or urinary symptoms are present without gait impairment, the diagnosis of occult hydrocephalus is unlikely. When characteristic clinical findings are accompanied by hydrocephalus, the diagnosis should be strongly considered. The best clinical predictors of response to shunting are (1) clinical onset with gait disorder; (2) a known cause (e.g. subarachnoid hemorrhage, head trauma, meningitis); (3) a short duration of symptoms, especially dementia (i.e. less than 1–2 years); (4) the absence of structural lesions (e.g. stroke) that could explain symptoms; and (5) resting cerebrospinal fluid (CSF) pressure greater than 100 mm H$_2$O (Fisher, 1977; Thomsen *et al.*, 1986; Petersen *et al.*, 1985; Graff-Radford *et al.*, 1989).

Computed tomography (CT) and magnetic resonance imaging (MRI) are important aids in evaluating patients with occult hydrocephalus. A practical CT or MRI definition of hydrocephalus is a greater than 5:1 ratio of the transverse inner skull diameter, measured at the level of Monro's foramina, to the lateral ventricular width at the same level (Vassilouthis, 1984). Alternatively, a lateral ventricular span of greater than 50 mm at the level of the anterior horns is consistent with hydrocephalus (Adams and Victor, 1989). Obliteration of cerebral sulci on high CT or MRI cuts and areas of periventricular low density on CT or an increased signal on T2-weighted MRI support the diagnosis of occult hydrocephalus. The periventricular white matter changes represent transependymal displacement of CSF due to the ventricular–brain pressure gradient. This radiographic sign predicts a good response to shunting.

The tap-test is a simple and useful bedside procedure for assessing clinical change following removal of CSF. Several psychometric parameters (e.g. short-term memory, reaction time and visuospatial function) and gait (e.g. number of steps needed to walk 50 feet) are measured at the same hour on two consecutive days. On the second day, a lumbar puncture with removal of 35 to 45 ml of CSF is performed two hours prior to testing. Improvements of 25 percent on memory and visuospatial testing, and 5 percent on reaction time and gait testing are meaningful (Wikkelso *et al.*, 1986). There is a highly significant correlation between improvement following the lumbar puncture and subsequent shunt.

In difficult cases, or when the tap-test is equivocal, ancillary studies to predict responsiveness to shunting are often done, but their clinical usefulness is limited. They include (1) radionuclide cisternography demonstrating reflux into the ventricles and delayed pericerebral diffusion (Bannister *et al.*, 1967; Le May and New, 1970); (2) lumbar infusion test (Katzman and Hussey, 1970); (3) conductance to outflow of CSF (Borgesen and Gjerris, 1982); and (4) 24-hour CSF pressure monitoring to determine the percentage of time B-waves are present and the CSF pressure exceeds 15 mm Hg (Graff-Radford *et al.*, 1989). Radionuclide cisternography may show reflux into the ventricles and delayed pericerebral diffusion in patients with hydrocephalus *ex vacuo*, for example, in Alzheimer's disease. The infusion test (Katzman and Hussey, 1970), which measures lumbar subarachnoid pressure in response to a constant infusion of 0.76 ml/min of saline for 30 to 60 minutes, produces inconsistent results. Measurement of CSF outflow conductance has not found widespread use in the USA. This technique requires monitoring of intraventricular pressure and was a poor predictor of surgical outcome in studies by Graff-Radford *et al.* (1989).

In many cases, a problem remains in differentiating between such degenerative processes as Alzheimer's disease and occult hydrocephalus because patients have a mild gait disorder, dementia and hydrocephalus. This problem is especially severe in those patients with idiopathic hydrocephalus, convolutional atrophy and no periventricular white matter changes. In such problematic cases, the tap-test can be useful, but unfortunately, there is only one way to find out truly if the shunt will help: to shunt the patient.

Ventriculoperitoneal shunts with low or medium pressure valves are the most common treatments for occult hydrocephalus. Some improvement is seen in 75 to 90 percent of carefully selected patients, but is sustained for two years in only 50 percent (Petersen *et al.*, 1985). Complications develop in one-third of patients (Petersen *et al.*, 1985; Hughes *et al.*, 1978). They include subdural hematoma, cerebral infarction, intracerebral hemorrhage, seizures, infections and shunt malfunctions. Symptomatic low intracranial pressure is an important complication in shunted adults. In the upright position, patients complain of headache, nausea, lethargy and diplopia (Foltz and Blanks, 1988). Measurement of intracranial pressure via shunt reservoir reveals normal findings in the supine position but extremely low pressures with standing.

These rates of success and complication are from excellent centers operating on highly selected cases. Clearly then, the decision to shunt is often difficult. The following factors must be taken in to consideration: (1) the severity of clinical symptoms; (2) evidence of clinical progression; (3) clinical and radiographic predictors of shunt success; and (4) recognition that complications are not rare. Finally, the patient and family must be involved in the decision process.

References

Adams RD, Victor M. *Principles of Neurology*. New York: McGraw-Hill, Inc., 1989, p. 508.

Bannister R, Gilford E, Koen R. Isotope encephalography in the diagnosis of demential due to communicating hydrocephalus. *Lancet* 1967; **ii**: 1014–17.

Borgesen SE, Gjerris F. The predictive value of conductance to outflow of CSF in normal pressure hydrocephalus. *Brain* 1982; **105**: 65–86.

Fisher CM. The clinical picture of occult hydrocephalus. *Clin Neurosurg* 1977; **24**: 270–84.

Foltz EL, Blanks JP. Symptomatic low intracranial pressure in shunted hydrocephalus. *J Neurosurg* 1988; **68**: 401–8.

Graff-Radford NR, Godersky JC, Jones MP. Variables predicting surgical outcome in symptomatic hydrocephalus in the elderly. *Neurology* 1989; **39**: 1601–4.

Hughes CP, Seigel BA, Coxe WS, Gado MH, Grubb RL, Coleman RE, Berg L. Adult idiopathic communicating hydrocephalus with and without shunting. *J Neurol Neurosurg Psychiat* 1978; **41**: 961–71.

Katzman R, Hussey F. A simple constant-infusion menometric test for measurement of CSF absorption: I. Rationale and method. *Neurology* 1970; **20**: 534–44.

Le May M, New PFJ. Radiological diagnosis of occult normal-pressure hydrocephalus. *Radiology* 1970; **96**: 347–58.

Petersen RC, Mokri B, Laus ET. Surgical treatment of idiopathic hydrocephalus in elderly patients. *Neurology* 1985; **35**: 307–11.

Thomsen AM, Borgesen SE, Bruhn P, Gjerris F. Prognosis of dementia in normal-pressure hydrocephalus after a shunt operation. *Ann Neurol* 1986; **20**: 304–10.

Vassilouthis J. The syndrome of normal-pressure hydrocephalus. *J Neurosurg* 1984; **61**: 501–9.

Wikkelso C, Andersson H, Blomstrand C, Lindqvist G, Svedsen P. Normal pressure hydrocephalus: Predictive value of the cerebrospinal fluid tap-test. *Acta Neurol Scand* 1986; **73**: 566–73.

3
Aphasia

24. Assessment of handedness is essential in the diagnosis and localization of language disorders

The two cerebral hemispheres in humans are not created equal. Language was the first behavior whose distribution was found to be asymmetrical (Broca, 1861). Left hemisphere language dominance has been recognized for more than a century and has been confirmed by repeated observations in right-handed people. For example, perisylvian and other left hemisphere lesions cause aphasia, while identical right-sided lesions do not.

Right-handedness is predominant in all human races, comprising 90 to 92 percent of the population (Coren and Porac, 1977; Hardyck and Petrinovich, 1977). However, handedness is not a homogeneous trait. Rather, handedness ranges along a spectrum from strongly right-handed to ambidextrous to strongly left-handed. In general, 'lefties' are less strongly left-handed than 'righties' are right-handed.

Handedness is determined by genetic, developmental and environmental factors. Left-handed people should be asked about a family history of left-handedness. If the patient's family is large, and no other members are left-handed, then the patient is more likely to be strongly left-handed. In contrast, people with a strong family history of left-handedness tend to be ambidextrous (Hecaen and de Ajuriaguerra, 1964). Indeed, some scientists have theorized that the absence of a family history of left-handedness is associated with early-life injury to the left hemisphere (Orsini and Satz, 1986). This theory of 'pathological left-handedness' may explain why individuals without a family history of left-handedness are strongly left-handed: left hemisphere damage impairs control of the right hand. Furthermore, a high incidence of left-handedness exists among patients with epilepsy, mental retardation and developmental dyslexia. Many of these patients with neurological disorders probably have pathological left-handedness.

In some cultures and families, left-handedness is treated as a disorder, and children are taught to be right-handed. A history of conversion from left- to right-handedness is important, because the language dominance pattern does not necessarily join this conversion process.

Clinically, handedness is most often assessed by asking the patient which hand he uses to write. Some individuals perform all fine and skilled motor functions (e.g. writing, sewing, using a knife, cutting with scissors, or throwing and kicking a ball) with the right hand and foot, while others write with their right hand but perform many other skilled tasks with their left hand or foot. These ambidextrous individuals may have different patterns of hemispheric specialization from strongly right-handed subjects. Because handedness predicts cerebral dominance for speech and language, the physician should inquire about the writing hand, the hand used for other dextrous functions, a history of natural left-handedness with subsequent conversion to right-handedness and family handedness. Detailed handedness questionnaires are available, but are mainly used as a research tool (Annett, 1967; Oldfield, 1971).

The left hemisphere is dominant for language in 99 percent of right-handed and about 60 percent of left-handed persons. Aphasia is rare following right hemisphere lesions in right-handers, but does occur (Archibald and Wepman, 1968; Kinsbourne, 1971; Searleman, 1977; Habib et al., 1983; Brust et al., 1986). Left-handedness and ambidexterity are associated with greater right-hemisphere language capabilities (Naeser and Borod, 1986). Approximately 30 percent of left-handed persons have right hemisphere language dominance and 10% have mixed dominance. In left-handed and ambidextrous subjects, there is a tendency towards bilateral representation of language and visuospatial functions. Hemispheric specialization in left-handers may be dissociated for handedness, speech output and language comprehension. For example, left-handers may have left hemisphere dominance for language comprehension and right hemisphere dominance for skilled manual functions and speech output. Aphasia tends to be milder and shorter among left-handers after either left or right hemisphere insults than among right-handers after left hemisphere insults (Brown and Hecaen, 1976).

References

Annett M. The binominal distribution of right, mixed and left handed. *Q J Exp Psychol* 1967; **19**: 327–33.

Archibald YM, Wepman JR. Language disturbance and nonverbal cognitive performance in either patients following injury to the right hemisphere. *Brain* 1968; **91**: 117–30.

Broca P. Perte de la parole, ramollissement chronique et destruction partielle du lobe ant erieur gauche du cerveau. *Bull Soc Anthropol Paris* 1861; **2**: 235–8.

Brown JW, Hecaen H. Lateralization and language representation. *Neurology* 1976; **26**: 183–9.

Brust JCM, Plank C, Burke A, Goudadia MMI, Healton EB. Language disorder in a right-hander after occlusion of the right anterior cerebral artery. *Neurology* 1982; **32**: 492–7.

Coren S, Porac C. Fifty centuries of right-handedness: the historical record. *Science* 1977; **198**: 631–2.

Habib M, Joanette Y, Ali-Cherif A, Poncet M. Crossed aphasia in dextrals. *Neuropsychologia* 1983; **21**: 413–18.

Hardyck C, Petrinovich LF. Left-handedness. *Psychol Bull* 1977; **84**: 385–404.

Hecaen H, de Ajuriaguerra J. *Left Handedness: Manual Superiority and Cerebral Dominance*. New York: Grune and Stratton, 1964.

Kinsbourne M. The minor cerebral hemisphere as a source of aphasic speech. *Arch Neurol* 1971; **25**: 302–6.

Naeser MA, Borod JC. Aphasia in left-handers: Lesion site, lesion side, and hemispheric asymmetries on CT. *Neurology* 1986; **36**: 471–88.

Oldfield RC. The assessment and analysis of handedness: the Edinburgh Inventory. *Neuropsychologia* 1971; **9**: 97–113.

Orsini DL, Satz P. A syndrome of pathological left-handedness: correlates of early left hemisphere injury. *Arch Neurol* 1986; **43**: 333–7.

Searleman A. A review of right hemisphere linguistic capabilities. *Psychol Bull* 1977; **84**: 503–28.

25.   Most aphasias are easily, although imprecisely, diagnosed and localized

The lack of a systematic approach and framework for organizing observations perpetuates the mystique surrounding language disorders. The clinical findings in an aphasic syndrome are variable. Language disorders do not strictly obey anatomical landmarks. However, language examination uncovers recognizable and reproducible clinical patterns. By analysing these patterns in the light of behavioral and neurological signs and symptoms, one can often localize aphasia with reasonable accuracy.

There are eight principal forms of aphasia, which result from cortical lesions (Table 25.1). Four of these forms – Broca's aphasia, mixed transcortical, transcortical motor and global aphasia – have non-fluent spontaneous speech. The remaining four – Wernicke's aphasia, conduction, transcortical sensory and anomic aphasia – have fluent speech. Two-thirds of patients with aphasia can be classified into one of these forms. The remaining cases are mixed forms or subcortical aphasias.

In many patients, one aphasic disorder evolves or resolves into another. For example, Broca's aphasia can evolve into global aphasia, global aphasia can resolve into Broca's aphasia, or Broca's aphasia can resolve into transcortical motor aphasia. Specific cortical and subcortical aphasias are discussed in greater detail in Maxims 28–34.

Aphasia screening requires testing of the patient's *spontaneous speech, comprehension of spoken language, repetition of speech, confrontational naming ability, reading and writing.*

Language assessment begins by listening to *spontaneous speech.* Two critical questions can usually be answered while the patient gives the chief complaint: Does the patient speak spontaneously? Is speech fluent? For example, when you enter the room, does the patient greet you, return your greeting, only speak in response to questions or speak in one or two-word answers? It is critical to hear the patient speak in sentences, so

Table 25.1 Clinical features of cortical aphasias.

Aphasia	Language findings						Associated neurolopsychiatric findings				
	Para-phasias	Compre-hension	Repetition	Naming	Reading	Writing	Motor	Somato-sensory	Visual field	Apraxia	Behavior
Non-fluent											
Broca's	−	+	−	±	±	−	HP	±HS	N	±left limbs	Depression
Mixed transcortical	−	−	+	−	-	−	HP	HS	HA		
Transcortical motor	−	+	+	±	+	−	±HP	N	N	±left limbs	
Global	−	−	−	−	−	−	HS	HS	HA		Depression
Fluent											
Wernicke's	+	−	−	−	−	−	N	±HS	±superior QA		Agitation confusion, violence
Conduction	+	+	−	±	+	−	N	±HS	±HA	±bilateral	
Transcortical sensory	+	−	+	−	−	−	±HS	±HS	HA		
Anomic	−	+	+	−	+	+	N	N	N		

−Impaired/absent. + Normal/present. QA, quadrantanopsia. HP, hemiparesis. HS, hemisensory loss. N, normal. HA, hemianopsia.

ask open-ended questions such as 'Why have you come to the hospital?', 'What is your typical weekday like?' Some patients conceal major language disorders with 'yes' and 'no' answers.

Spontaneity is an important concept in behavioral neurology. The absence of motor and speech spontaneity can be the most prominent manifestation of lesions in the frontal lobe or of the reticular activating system, located in the upper midbrain or diencephalic reticular formation. Patients with aspontaneous speech often go unnoticed because they are unaware of the problem, offer no complaints and 'make no trouble'. Broca's aphasia and transcortical motor aphasia are characterized by hesitating, effortful speech produced only in response to questioning.

Verbal fluency is the ability to produce flowing, smooth speech without word-finding pauses. Non-fluent speech is slow, with a rate that is usually less than 40 words per minute, sparse, or often consisting of single words, effortful, dysarthric, dysprosodic (see below) and agrammatical. Patients with non-fluent aphasias omit grammatical, syntactical words such as prepositions, articles and adverbs as well as word endings such as plurals and tense (Goodglass and Berko, 1960). Fluent aphasics typically speak effortlessly with normal articulation and prosody, and their phrase length or number of words between pauses, is also normal. In some fluent aphasics, verbal output is excessive (logorrhea or verborrhea). The most prominent feature of fluent aphasia is 'empty' speech that contains grammatical words but lacks substantive, lexical words, such as in, 'Yes, you know, of course, and well yes, as a matter of fact, if you did, yes'.

The differentiation of fluent from non-fluent speech is critical in distinguishing anterior from posterior aphasias. Fluency is severely disrupted by lesions anterior to the Rolandic fissure (central sulcus), while most patients with fluent, paraphasic speech have lesions posterior to this landmark (Benson, 1967; Poeck et al., 1972; Naeser et al., 1989). Anatomical localization is less reliable during the early stages of aphasia because many patients with posteriorly situated lesions are acutely non-fluent. Aphasic children with both anterior and posterior lesions are usually non-fluent, although dysarthria and agrammatism (the inability to speak or write grammatically due to brain injury) are usually found only with anterior lesions (Benson and Geschwind, 1985).

Spontaneous speech should also be assessed for articulation (Maxim 26), prosody and paraphasias. Prosody refers to the distribution of stress and melody of speech, and includes both affective and non-affective components (Maxim 51). Prosody is the chief affective component of speech and introduces subtle shades of meaning or completely changes the impact of a statement (Ross, 1981; Weintraub et al., 1981). The right hemisphere is dominant for affective prosody, and both hemispheres contribute to non-affective, propositional prosody (Heilman et al., 1984). Affective prosody is the emotional tone that flavors our speech and allows our children and pets to 'understand' what we are saying even though they cannot comprehend the words. Non-affective prosody is the alteration in pitch and stress that conveys different messages with the same words. For example, one can change the statement 'Let's have pizza' to the question 'Let's have pizza?' by raising the pitch as ones says 'pizza'. Ross (1981) proposed a clinical –anatomical correlation of prosody: anterior right hemisphere lesions (analog of Broca's area) impair spontaneous prosody, causing monotonous speech that lacks emotion and intonation, while posterior right hemisphere lesions (analog of Wernicke's area) impair comprehension of prosody, leaving patients unable to distinguish subtle shades of meaning in others' speech. Prosody is more fully discussed in Maxim 51.

Paraphasias are syllable or word-substitution errors and are most common in fluent aphasia. Literal, or phonemic, paraphasia is replacement of letters or syllables in otherwise correct word usages, as in, 'John drove my *di*cycle', 'Jane *st*ew the ball'. Verbal, or semantic, paraphasias are word substitutions, as in, 'John drove my apple', or 'Jane threw the house'. Neologisms are word creations, for example, 'Shoua Mousante, the *clamorific* Martian queen'. These creations are sometimes considered a form of paraphasia.

Comprehension is assessed after spontaneous speech. If the patient constructs well-formulated answers to questions, comprehension is usually normal. There are four common pitfalls in assessing comprehension: (1) being lulled into assuming that comprehension is normal because the patient is verbose and fluent (Wernicke's aphasia); (2) incorrectly diagnosing a comprehension deficit because the patient cannot verbally respond to a question or command; (3) asking the patient to perform a learned motor command, such as 'Show me how you salute', which also assesses praxis (Maxim 43); and (4) overestimating language comprehension because the examiner provides meaningful non-verbal cues, such as inflection, tone and facial expression.

Comprehension deficits should be suspected if the patient talks but makes little sense, appears confused, or moves from one topic to another without completing a thought. Comprehension can be tested in a mute or aphasic patient by asking the patient to point to objects in the room. In quadriplegic patients, comprehension can be tested by asking the patient to make eye movements or blinks. It is also useful to ask yes – no questions. For example, ask 'Are you lying in bed?' or 'Do two pounds of flour weigh more than one?' A slightly more difficult question: 'Is it true that in South America helicopters eat their young?' If the patient responds no, then ask 'Do helicopters eat their young in Europe?' If the patient again responds no, ask if that was a silly question, and observe for hesitation or uncertainty in the answer. Because a normal person does not have to ponder long about any of these questions, undue hesitation is often a sign of impaired comprehension. Also, since the patient has a 50 percent chance of guessing the correct answer to each yes or no question, ask at least three or four questions when you suspect a comprehension deficit. Finally, a good tool for quantifying comprehension disturbance is the Token Test, which measures the patient's ability to follow simple commands in manipulating colored tokens (DeRenzi and Vignolo, 1962).

Repetition is tested by asking the patient to repeat words, phrases and sentences. 'There are no ifs, ands, or buts about it' or 'The phantom soared across the foggy heath' are difficult sentences, and if either is repeated correctly, then repetition is normal. Listen carefully for omissions (e.g. plural endings), additions, perseverations or repetitions, paraphasias and grammatical errors. Accurate repetition is usually impaired by lesions in the anterior or posterior perisylvian language areas. Preserved repetition in mild aphasia has little localizing value. In contrast, normal repetition in moderate to severe aphasia is indicative of transcortical aphasia with lesions outside the perisylvian language areas.

Confrontational naming is tested by pointing to objects and asking the patient to name them. Various categories (e.g. body parts, clothing, appliances, colors) and various levels of difficulty (e.g. commonly used words such as nose, belt, television, red and uncommonly used words such as eyebrow, shin, watch crystal, second hand, tie knot, belt buckle) should be tested. Patients most often have difficulty naming object parts, especially those names that are not commonly used in everyday speech. One must be careful to avoid cultural or sexual bias in selecting items (someone who never wears a tie may have never heard the name for the 'knot' of a tie). If the patient fails to name an indicated object but selects the correct word from a short list, then comprehension is normal, but naming is not. Naming errors occur with most aphasias and have limited localizing value (Maxim 32). Also, non-aphasic misnaming occurs with diffuse central nervous system insults, the frontal lobe syndrome with facetiousness known as Witzelsucht, conversion disorder and malingering (Weinstein and Keller, 1964; Geschwind, 1967).

Naming and word finding can be formally tested with the Boston Naming and Animal Naming Tests, respectively (Kaplan *et al.*, 1982; Goodglass and Kaplan, 1983). The Boston Naming Test (Maxim 5; Table 5.2) is the most widely used test of naming, and healthy elderly subjects perform as well as young adults (Labarge *et al.*, 1986). The Animal Naming Test assesses both word finding and fluency. In this test, the patient is given 90 seconds to name as many animals as possible and the score is derived from the most productive 60 seconds. A word-finding disorder is suggested by a score of less than 13 animals and confirmed by a score of less than 10 animals, as long as potentially complicating factors are excluded (e.g. motor speech disorder, severe educational handicap).

Reading can be assessed by asking the patient to read a few sentences aloud. Many patients with aphasia cannot read aloud but can comprehend written material. In these patients, comprehension must be tested with questions that can be answered by nodding the head yes or no. Alexia, the failure to comprehend written material, is usually accompanied by errors with oral reading and is acquired through brain damage (Maxim 42).

Writing is tested with a series of tasks of increasing difficulty. Tasks begin with signing one's name, then require writing single words by dictation before moving on to composition of descriptive passages, which are often about such topics as work, favorite foods or the weather. When spoken language is aphasic, writing is invariably aphasic. Therefore, writing is an excellent screen of language function; if the patient writes a short paragraph normally, he is probably not aphasic. Writing impairment due to an acquired brain lesion, called agraphia, can result from disruption of motor or language systems (Maxim 41).

References

Benson DF. Fluency in aphasia: Correlation with radioactive scan localization. *Cortex* 1967; **3**: 257–67.

Benson DF, Geschwind N. Aphasia and related disorders: A clinical approach. In: *Principles of Neurology* (Mesulam MM, ed.). Philadelphia: Davis Company, 1985.

DeRenzi E, Vignolo L. The token test: A sensitive test to detect receptive disturbances in aphasics. *Brain* 1962; **85**: 665–78.

Geschwind N. The varieties of naming errors. *Cortex* 1967; **3**: 97–112.

Goodglass H, Berko J. Agrammatism and inflectional morphology in English. *J Speech Hear Res* 1960; **3**: 257–67.

Goodglass H, Kaplan E. *The Assessment of Aphasia and Related Disorders* (2nd edition). Philadelphia: Lea and Febiger, 1983.

Heilman KM, Bowers D, Speedie L, Coslett HB. Comprehension of affective and nonaffective prosody. *Neurology* 1984; **34**: 917–21.

Kaplan E, Goodglass H, Weintraub S. *The Boston Naming Test (Experimental Edition)*: Boston: Lea and Febiger, 1982.

Labarge E, Edwards D, Knesevich JWM. Performance of normal elderly on the Boston Naming Test. *Brain Lang* 1986; **27**: 380–4.

Naeser MA, Palumbo CL, Helm-Estabrooks N, Stiassny-Eder D, Albert ML. Severe nonfluency in aphasia. *Brain* 1989; **112**: 1–38.

Poeck K, Kerschensteiner M, Hartje W. A quantitative study on language understanding in fluent and nonfluent aphasia. *Cortex* 1972; **8**: 299–305.

Ross ED. The aprosodias: Functional-anatomic organization of the affective components of language in the right hemisphere. *Arch Neurol* 1981; **38**: 561–9.

Weinstein EA, Keller NJS. Linguistic patterns of misnaming in brain injury. *Neuropsychologia* 1964; **1**: 79–90.

Weintraub S, Mesulam MM, Kramer L. Disturbances in prosody: A right-hemisphere contribution to language. *Arch Neurol* 1981; **38**: 742–4.

26.   *Acquired speech impairment results from aphasic and non-aphasic disorders*

In cases of acquired speech impairment, the possibility of a non-aphasic disorder must be considered. The first step in evaluating a language or communicative disorder is to determine whether or not the patient is aphasic. Aphasia is acquired language dysfunction caused by brain injury and it is not congenital or developmental.

Disorders of mechanical sound production are commonly misdiagnosed as aphasia. Speech requires the coordinated functions of the pyramidal and extrapyramidal motor systems, the cerebellum, lower motor neurons, the neuromuscular junction and muscles. Lesions of these neural systems impair speech spontaneity, fluency, articulation, volume, resonance, phonation and prosody. Structural lesions of the larynx, oropharynx, soft palate, tongue and lips also impair speech. In contrast with aphasia, however, these motor speech disorders are not associated with language errors, for example, the patient can use written language normally.

Dysarthria, in its strictest sense, refers to abnormal articulation. Used most broadly, the term connotes any non-linguistic speech disorder. Dysarthria is common in anterior non-fluent aphasia, such as Broca's aphasia, and rare in posterior fluent aphasia, such as Wernicke's aphasia. It also often occurs without aphasia.

Dysarthria is classified into five types, according to its qualitative features and which neuroanatomical systems are affected.

Paretic (flaccid) dysarthria results from weakness of articulatory muscles. The vocal cord adductors are most commonly paretic. Weakness in other muscles, including the laryngeal and pharyngeal, diaphragm, tongue, orbicularis oris, masseter and pterygoid muscles may also contribute to impaired oral communication (Tepperman and Thacker, 1980). The lesion may be in lower motor neurons (e.g. progressive bulbar palsy, idiopathic polyneuritis, recurrent laryngeal nerve), the neuromuscular junction (e.g. myasthenia) or the muscle (e.g. myositis). The voice is typically soft or barely audible, low-pitched and nasal. Patients with laryngeal weakness have difficulty with prolonged phonation of vowel sounds, such as 'ee'. Articulation is also impaired by weakness of the (1) soft palate, resulting most often from bilateral vagal lesions or myasthenia gravis and causing nasal voice, especially when the head is tilted forward; (2) tongue, as a result of hypoglossal palsy and myopathies, causing lisping or muffled speech; and (3) lip musculature, caused by facial palsy. Asking the patient to imitate sounds, for example, 'Ga Ga' to test the soft palate, 'Ta Ta' to check the tongue, 'Ba Ba' for the lips and 'ee' for the larynx, helps to distinguish the affected muscles. For example, a patient who cannot repeat the sounds 'ga ga' or 'ee' most probably has weakness in the soft palate and larynx.

Spastic (hypertonic, pseudobulbar) dysarthria results from upper motor neuron (corticobulbar) lesions, usually due to multiple, bilateral small lacunar infarcts. Speech is slow, strained, thick and monopitched. Articulation is imprecise, especially for consonants, and volume may be explosive (Darley *et al.*, 1969). On neurological examination, the jaw jerk is usually increased and the tongue is unable to make rapid, alternating movements.

Ataxic (cerebellar) dysarthria results from lesions of the cerebellum or its connections, and it is most common in patients with cerebellar degeneration and multiple sclerosis. The slurred speech is dysarticulated into jerky, irregular components. Speech rhythm, volume and pitch are variable, and speech may be explosive with poorly regulated expiration. In 'scanning' cerebellar speech, the hallmark is staccato sentences in a sing-song, mono- tonous meter that lacks the normal stress on syllables and words. In some cases, a voice tremor occurs as part of a more generalized cerebellar tremor, and further disrupts the phonatory rhythm. Scanning speech is rarely due to a pure cerebellar lesion. Most often, patients have cerebellar, pyramidal and extrapyramidal lesions (Kremer *et al.*, 1947).

Extrapyramidal dysarthria takes many forms. Patients with caudate- putamen infarcts have slow, dysarthric speech and may have hemiplegia (Naeser *et al.*, 1982; Caplan *et al.*, 1990). Parkinsonism is associated with hypokinetic dysarthria, a disorder characterized by slow, monotonous speech with decreased pitch and variable loudness, low volume, inappro- priate silences and imprecise consonants (Tepperman and Thacker, 1980). Huntington's chorea victims may have erratic breathing with explosive speech; in severe cases, all utterances are unintelligible (Wilson, 1940). Choreic dysarthria is caused by involuntary respiratory, tongue and facial movements and results in hesitant speech with irregular speed, loudness and articulation.

Aphemia or cortical dysarthria is a rare disorder resulting from lesions that affect the left (dominant) inferior frontal motor cortex and adjacent white matter but that spare Broca's area. Infarction is the most common pathol- ogy (Schiff *et al.*, 1983). In aphemia, preserved language function must be demonstrated by normal writing, because true aphemia patients have effective written communication (Benson, 1979). Many patients with aphemia also have oral–buccal–lingual apraxia (Maxim 43), which can be demonstrated by asking them to suck, blow or whistle. In the acute stage, patients often have mutism and right hemiparesis. Over time, however, these deficits often resolve, with near-normal recovery of both limb strength and speech, which is frequently slow, hypophonic and difficult to understand during early recovery. Primary laryngeal lesions causing mutism or dysarthria are occasionally misdiagnosed as aphemia.

Patients whose impaired speech primarily results from laryngeal dis- orders are said to be *dysphonic*. If their speech is entirely absent from these causes, they are *aphonic*. Dysphonia can be distinguished from the aphasias by preservation of comprehension, fluency and use of written language. Although dysphonic speech may be mistakenly considered dys- fluent, tests of fluency such as the Animal Naming Test (Maxim 25) are normal. However, dysphonia may coexist with aphasia.

Spastic (spasmodic) dysphonia is a gradually progressive focal dystonia involving laryngeal speech musculature. Onset is usually in adulthood. Although the dystonia is almost always isolated to laryngeal musculature, in some cases, the dystonia extends to other muscles, such as the orbicu- laris oculi (blepharospasm) and hand. Simultaneous contraction of all speech muscles produces loud, strained and dysfluent speech, which has been likened to the speech of a person being strangled (Adams and Victor, 1989). While patients are unable to speak in a soft and rhythmic manner, they are typically able to sing, shout, whisper and swallow. This dissociation of actions that involve the same muscles has led some to suggest a psychogenic etiology. Rather, spastic dysphonia is an extrapyramidal disorder, a focal dystonia similar to writer's cramp. Relaxation techniques and psychotherapy are not helpful. Destruction of one recurrent laryngeal nerve or injection of botulinus toxin into one vocal cord may be beneficial (Dedo, 1976).

The following disorders are acquired speech impairments that must also be distinguished from aphasia.

Stuttering is usually a developmental childhood disorder but may also begin after brain injury in adulthood. Acquired stuttering usually occurs acutely and is characterized by involuntary repetitions, prolongations and blocks that are not restricted to initial syllables or substantive words. For example, grammatical words such as 'and' and 'if' are affected (Helm *et al.*, 1978). Most patients with acquired stuttering have left hemisphere lesions and aphasia, most often Broca's aphasia, although the exact lesion site and even lateralization varies (Caplan, 1972; Benson, 1979; Ardila and Lopez, 1986). Acquired stuttering is often transient, but can persist in patients with bilateral lesions (Benson, 1979). Antiepileptic drugs have been reported to improve acquired stuttering (Baratz and Mesulam, 1981).

Palilalia is involuntary repetition of words, phrases and less often, syllables. In most patients, speech rate increases and volume decreases with repetition (Lapointe and Horner, 1981). Post encephalitic parkinsonism was once the most common cause (Critchley, 1927). Currently, most cases of this uncommon disorder result from idiopathic parkinsonism, progressive supranuclear palsy and other diseases with bilateral upper brainstem, thalamic, or basal ganglia lesions, such as pseudobulbar palsy (Brain, 1961; Boller *et al.*, 1973; Yasuda *et al.*, 1990). Rarely, palilalia is associated with seizures originating in the left parasagittal region (Alajouanine *et al.*, 1959).

Echolalia is the parrot-like repetition of words and phrases heard from others. In the most severe cases, i.e. combined anterior and posterior transcortical aphasia, patients have no comprehension of what is said, although they faithfully repeat what they hear (Maxim 31) (Geschwind *et al.*, 1968). Echolalia and palilalia may coexist (Schneider, 1938). Echolalia also occurs in infantile autism, schizophrenia, Alzheimer's disease and Tourette's syndrome.

Functional, or psychogenic, voice disorders occur in patients presenting with prominent complaints of impaired phonation despite normal mucosa, full vocal cord movement and complete closure on phonation (Bridger and Epstein, 1983). Excessive voice use does not appear to play a role. Increased tension in laryngeal muscles during speech and psychogenic factors are important. When such patients present, complaining of complete inability to speak, bear in mind that functional voice impairment is ten times more common than functional loss of voice (Bridger and Epstein, 1983).

References

Adams RD, Victor M. *Principles of Neurology*. New York: McGraw-Hill Company, 1989, p. 392.

Alajouanine T, Castaigne P, Sabouraud O *et al*. Palilalie paroxystique et vocalisations iteratives au cours de crises epileptiques par lesion interessant l'aire motrice supplementaire. *Rev Neurol* 1959; **101**: 685–97.

Ardila A, Lopez MV. Severe stuttering associated with right hemisphere lesion. *Brain Lang* 1986; **27**: 239–46.

Baratz R, Mesulam M-M. Adult-onset stuttering treated with anticonvulsants. *Arch Neurol* 1981; **38**: 132.

Benson DF. *Aphasia, Alexia, and Agraphia*. Edinburgh, New York: Churchill Livingstone, 1979, pp. 129–31.

Boller F, Boller M, Denes G *et al*. Familial palilalia. *Neurology* 1973; **23**: 1117–25.

Brain R. *Speech Disorders–Aphasia, Apraxia, and Agnosia*. Oxford: Butterworths, 1961.

Bridger MWM, Epstein R. Functional voice disorders: A review of 109 patients. *J Laryngol Otol* 1983; **97**: 1145–8.

Caplan LR. An investigation of some aspects of stuttering-like speech in adult dysphasic patients. *J S Afr Speech Hear Assoc* 1972; **19**: 52–66.

Caplan LR, Schahmann JD, Kase CS, Feldmann E, Baquis G, Greenberg JP, Gorelick PB, Helgason C, Hier DB. Caudate infarcts. *Arch Neurol* 1990; **47**: 133–43.

Critchley M. On palilalia. *J Neurol Neurosurg Psychiat* 1927; **8**: 23–32.

Darley FL, Aronson EA, Brown JR. Differential diagnostic patterns of dysarthria. *J Speech Hear Res* 1969; **12**: 246–69.

Dedo HH. Recurrent laryngeal nerve section for spastic dysphonia. *Ann Otol* 1976; **85**: 451–9.

Geschwind N, Quadfasel FA, Segarra JM. Isolation of the speech area. *Neuropsychologia* 1968; **6**: 327–40.

Helm NA, Butler RB, Benson DF. Acquired stuttering. *Neurology* 1978; **18**: 1159–65.

Kremer M, Russell WR, Smyth GE. A mid-brain syndrome following head injury. *J Neurol Neurosurg Psychiat* 1947; **10**: 49–60.

Lapointe LL, Horner J. Palilalia: A descriptive study of pathological reiterative utterances. *J Speech Hear Dis* 1981; **46**: 34–8.

Naeser MA, Alexander MP, Helm-Estabrooks N, Levine HL, Laughlin SA, Geschwind N. Aphasia with predominantly subcortical lesion sites. *Arch Neurol* 1982; **39**: 2–14.

Schiff HB, Alexander MR, Naeser MA, Galaburda AM. Aphemia: clinical-anatomic correlations. *Arch Neurol* 1983; **40**: 720–7.

Schneider DE. The clinical syndromes of echolalia, echopraxia, grasping and sucking. *J Nerv Ment Disord* 1938; **88**: 18–35.

Tepperman PS, Thacker RC. Motor speech disorders. *Postgrad Med* 1980; **68**: 86–97.

Wilson SAK. *Neurology*. Baltimore, MA: Williams and Wilkins Company, 1940, p. 849.

Yasuda Y, Akiguchi I, Ino M, Nabatabe H, Kameyama M. Paramedian thalamic and midbrain infarcts associated with palilalia. *J Neurol Neurosurg Psychiat* 1990; **53**: 797–9.

27. *Mutism often occurs in non-aphasic disorders*

Mutism, the inability or refusal to speak, has an extensive differential diagnosis (Table 27.1)

Initially, patients with Broca's or global aphasia may be unable to even attempt speaking. Associated symptoms usually include right facial weakness or hemiparesis in both Broca's and global aphasia, as well as right hemisensory loss and hemianopsia in global aphasia. As mute aphasic patients recover, aspontaneous and non-fluent speech emerges. Aphasic patients with mutism make linguistic writing errors (Maxims 28 and 33). These include word substitutions or paralexias, such as 'pair' instead of 'chair'; telegraphic writing in which connecting grammatical words are deleted, such as, 'I store rice' for 'I want to go to the store to buy rice'; and non-sensical fluent writing, as in, 'The only thing that I wish well you must know that the other thing yes that thing of course'. These errors help distinguish such patients from those with non-aphasic mutism.

However, mutism is most often associated with non-aphasic disorders, which can be neurological or functional.

In *aphemia* (Maxim 26), muteness often precedes a characteristic pattern of slow, hypophonic and dysarthric speech. Aphemia results from lesions that affect the left inferior frontal motor cortex and underlying white matter but spare Broca's area. Stroke is the most common cause, and such patients often have right hemiparesis following the ictus (Schiff *et al.*, 1983).

Lesions in the supplementary motor area (SMA) of the dominant hemisphere can cause muteness during the first several weeks. Recovery of spontaneous speech and repetition follows, but an impairment of writing per-

Table 27.1 Differential diagnosis of mutism.

Aphasic syndromes
  Global aphasia
  Broca's aphasia
Aphemia (pure word mutism)
Supplementary motor area lesion
Pseudobulbar palsy
Abulia
Akinetic mutism
Locked-in syndrome
Chronic vegetative state
Cerebellar lesions
Lower motor neuron lesions
  Idiopathic polyneuritis
  Bulbar poliomyelitis
Laryngeal disorders
Psychiatric–psychogenic disorders

sists (Masdeu, 1978). Dominant SMA lesions rarely cause aphasia (Laplane *et al.*, 1977; Masdeu, 1978). Laplane *et al.* (1977) described three stages that follow selective SMA ablations. The acute stage is associated with a global akinesia that is more prominent contralaterally and causes arrest of speech. The second, subacute stage is characterized by reduced spontaneous motor activity contralaterally, facial weakness for emotional expression and reduced spontaneous speech. In the third, chronic stage, patients display slowing of rapid, alternating hand movements and normal speech. In experimental studies, electrical stimulation and spontaneous focal seizure discharges from the dominant SMA have been observed to cause speech arrest (Guidetti, 1957; Penfield and Roberts, 1959).

Pseudobulbar palsy results from bilateral lesions in the pyramidal (and often extrapyramidal) motor pathways that supply musculature innervated by cranial nerves (Tilney and Morrison, 1912). Spastic weakness with minimal atrophy of muscles supplied by cranial nerves V, VII and IX–XIII occurs. Although dysarthria is the most common motor speech complication in pseudobulbar palsy, mutism can occur, especially when lesions are located in limbic–brainstem motor pathways (Cummings *et al.*, 1983). The pseudobulbar state is often accompanied by pathological laughing, crying and grimacing; these prominent emotional displays often follow little or no stimulation. Drugs that modulate biogenic amine activity including levodopa, methylphenidate, amantadine, amitriptyline, imipramine and fluoxetine may ameliorate these paroxysmal affective attacks (Lawson and Macleod, 1969; Udaka *et al.*, 1984; Jankovic, 1985; Schiffer *et al.*, 1985; Seliger and Hornstein, 1989).

Abulia may cause mutism. It is a general behavioral slowing and lowered activity which results from a variety of pathological processes (Table 27. 2). Abulic patients show little spontaneous motor or speech activity and may intermittently fail to respond to questions or commands for minutes (Fisher, 1968). When responses do occur, they are slow and apathetic.

Table 27.2   Pathological processes and lesion sites associated with abulia and akinetic mutism.

Focal processes
Unilateral or bilateral prefrontal lesions (medial or lateral)
Thalamic lesions
Cerebellar lesions
Midbrain lesions

Diffuse or non-focal processes
Head trauma
Hydrocephalus
Metabolic disorders (hypoxia, hypoglycemia, hepatic encephalopathy)
Postictal state
Fat embolism
Catatonic depression or schizophrenia

Akinetic mutism represents the most intense form of abulia (Fisher, 1983). Cairns *et al.* (1941) originally described akinetic mutism as a condition in which the patient appears awake and may follow the examiner with his eyes but lacks spontaneous motor and verbal responses. In addition, he is doubly incontinent and responds incompletely to noxious stimuli. Akinetic mutism has been reported with bilateral lesions in the frontal lobes, including cingulate and orbital gyri and the septal area (Nielsen and Jacobs, 1951; Freemon, 1971), and with bilateral lesions of the paramedian reticular formation, which includes the diencephalon and midbrain (Cravioto *et al.*, 1960; Kemper and Romanul, 1967). In patients with subcortical lesions, akinesia and muteness may be improved by treatment with dopamine agonists, such as lergotrile or bromocriptine (Ross and Stewart, 1981).

The *locked-in syndrome* results from de-efferentation of central motor fibers supplying facial and body musculature (Plum and Posner, 1966). Lesions are located usually in the ventral pons or occasionally in the ventral midbrain. Pathological processes include infarction, hemorrhage, central pontine myelinolysis, tumor and encephalitis (Patterson and Grabois, 1986). Patients are fully alert and conscious but can only communicate by blinking or moving the eyes. The EEG reveals normal or mildly slowed background activity. Any patient who is mute should be asked to blink or move the eyes on command; otherwise, this diagnosis may be missed.

Patients with the *chronic vegetative state* emerge from coma and resume relatively normal sleep–wake cycles in which the eyes open during 'wakefulness', but intellectual activity is minimal or absent. Unlike patients with locked-in syndrome, those in the chronic vegetative state do not produce any clear-cut, high-level response to verbal stimuli. This disorder usually follows severe, diffuse brain insults such as hypoxia, ischemia, hypoglycemia or head trauma. The EEG usually reveals background slowing with decreased voltage. The prognosis for a meaningful recovery is dismal.

Acute bilateral cerebellar lesions that damage hemispheric and deep dentate nuclei can cause temporary speech loss (Rekate *et al.*, 1985). These patients have little or no cognitive impairment, and cranial nerve signs may be absent. Muteness lasts less than three months, but patients are usually severely dysarthric during recovery.

Lower motor neuron lesions involving both vagus nerves paralyze laryngeal speech muscles. In addition, there may be associated weakness of other muscles needed for speech production, such as those in the soft palate and tongue. Idiopathic polyneuritis is the most common cause of muteness in patients with lower motor neuron deficits. Idiopathic vocal cord paralysis usually results from viral neuronitis.

Viral and, less often, bacterial *laryngitis* often causes hoarseness and may produce acute muteness or 'aphonia'. Other laryngeal disorders, such as tumors, produce voice loss more insidiously. Laryngeal disorders should be considered in all patients with speech disorders who can write normally; vocal cords should be examined and imaging studies obtained when indicated.

Psychiatric causes of mutism are not rare (Bridger and Epstein, 1983). Catatonic depression, schizophrenia and psychogenic illness may mimic structural brain or laryngeal disease.

Elective mutism is a disorder in which a child refuses to talk in specific social situations, such as school, but can comprehend spoken language and speaks in other settings (Wilkins, 1985; Furst, 1989). Predisposing factors to elective mutism are social isolation, parental overprotection (usually by the mother), shyness and withdrawal of one parent (usually the father), language and speech disorders, mental retardation and immigration before the age of 3 years (Pustrom and Speers, 1964; Wright, 1968; Meijer, 1979).

References

Bridger M, Epstein R. Functional voice disorders. *J Laryng Otol* 1983; **97**: 1145–8.

Cairns H, Oldfield RC, Pennybacker JB *et al.* Akinetic mutism with an epidermoid cyst of the third ventricle. *Brain* 1941; **64**: 273–90.

Cravioto H, Silberman J, Feigin I. A clinical and pathologic study of akinetic mutism. *Neurology* 1960; **10**: 10–21.

Cummings JL, Benson DF, Houlihan JP, Gosenfeld LF. Mutism: Loss of neocortical and limbic vocalization. *J Nerv Ment Dis* 1983; **17**: 255–9.

Fisher CM. Intermittent interruption of behavior. *Trans Am Neurol Assoc* 1968; **93**: 209–10.

Fisher CM. Abulia minor vs agitated behavior. *Clin Neurosurg* 1983; **31**: 9–31.

Freemon FR. Akinetic mutism and bilateral anterior cerebral artery occlusion. *J Neurol Neurosurg Psychiat* 1971; **34**: 693–8.

Furst AL. Elective mutism: Report of a case successfully treated by a family doctor. *Isr J Psychiat Relat Sci* 1989; **26**: 96–102.

Guidetti B. Desordres de la parole associes a des lesions de la surface interhemispherique frontale posterieure. *Rev Neurol* 1957; **97**: 121–31.

Jankovic J. Amitriptyline in amyotrophic lateral sclerosis. *N Engl J Med* 1985; **313**: 1478–9.

Kemper TL, Romanul FCA. State resembling akinetic mutism in basilar artery occlusion. *Neurology* 1967; **17**: 74–80.

Laplane D, Talairach D, Meninger V, Bancard J, Bouchareine A. Motor consequences of motor area ablations in men. *J Neurol Sci* 1977; **31**: 29–49.

Lawson IR, MacLeod RDM. The use of imipramine ('Tofranil') and other drugs in organic emotionalism. *Br J Psychiat* 1969; **115**: 281–5.

Masdeu JC, Schoene WC, Funkenstein H. Aphasia following infarction of the left supplementary motor area. *Neurology* 1978; **28**: 1220–3.

Meijer A. Elective mutism in children. *Isr Ann Psychiat* 1979; **17**: 93–100.

Nielsen JM, Jacobs LL. Bilateral lesions of the anterior cingulate gyri. *Bull Los Angeles Neurol Soc* 1951; **16**: 231–4.

Patterson JR, Grabois M. Locked-in syndrome: A review of 139 cases. *Stroke* 1986; **17**: 758–64.

Penfield W, Roberts L. Speech and brain mechanisms. Princeton, NJ: Princeton University Press, 1959.

Plum F, Posner JB. *The Diagnosis of Stupor and Coma.* Philadelphia: FA Davis Company, 1966.

Pustrom E, Speers RW. Elective mutism in children. *J Am Acad Child Psychiat* 1964; **3**: 287–97.

Rekate HL, Grubb RL, Aram DM, Hahn JF, Ratcheson RA. Muteness of cerebellar origin. *Arch Neurol* 1985; **42**: 697–8.

Ross ED, Stewart RM. Akinetic mutism following hypothalamic damage: Successful treatment with dopamine agonists. *Neurology* 1981; **31**: 1435–9.

Schiff HB, Alexander MR, Naeser MA, Galaburda AM. Aphemia: clinical–anatomic correlations. *Arch Neurol* 1983; **40**: 720–7.

Schiffer RB, Herndon RM, Rudick RA. Treatment of pathologic laughing and weeping with amitryptiline. *New Engl J Med* 1985; **312**: 1480–2.

Seliger GM, Hornstein A. Serotonin, fluoxetine, and pseudobulbar affect. *Neurology* 1989; **39**: 1400.

Tilney F, Morrison JF. Pseudobulbar palsy, clinically and pathologically considered, with the clinical report of five cases. *J Nerv Ment Dis* 1912; **39**: 505.

Udaka T, Yamao ZS, Nagata H, Nakamura S, Kameyama M. Pathological laughing and crying treated with levodopa. *Arch Neurol* 1984; **41**: 1095–6.

Wilkins R. A comparison of elective mutism and emotional disorders in children. *Br J Psychiat* 1985; **146**: 198–203.

Wright HL. A clinical study of children who refuse to talk in school. *J Am Acad Child Psychiat* 1968; **7**: 603–17.

28.   Broca's aphasia consists of non-fluent, effortful speech with relatively preserved comprehension following left frontal lesions

The clinical features of Broca's aphasia are summarized in Table 28.1. Mutism may occur at the onset of the aphasia, or patients may produce only single syllables or words. Speech is aspontaneous, sparse and slow; its rate is fewer than a dozen words per minute. Verbal output is agrammatic, even 'telegraphic', because patients utter substantive nouns and verbs that carry sentence meaning but omit grammatical 'connecting' words, including prepositions, articles, conjunctions and adverbs. An example is 'go . . . store . . . me', for 'Do you want to go to the store with me?'. The writing of patients with Broca's aphasia also contains grammatical errors.

Auditory and written comprehension are relatively normal in Broca's aphasia. However, deficits that parallel those found in spoken expression commonly affect linguistic comprehension. Linguistic comprehension requires interpretation of both lexical and grammatical, or syntactic, components. Lexical items are nouns, verbs and adjectives that relate the sentence to the physical world, e.g. mother, brother, sister, female. The grammatical components include word order, articles, and inflection and provide specific meaning. Thus 'mother's sister's brother' and 'mother's brother's sister' are different people and sexes. Broca's aphasia impairs grammatical comprehension, resulting in subtle comprehension deficits that can be elicited by testing the patient's understanding of complex grammatical relationships. For example, those with Broca's aphasia often have difficulties with such questions as 'Is it true that my mother's brother's sister is a female?'.

Table 28.1   Clinical features of Broca's aphasia.

Feature	Observations
Speech	Not spontaneous, non-fluent, dysprodic, telegraphic, effortful, some literal paraphasias
Comprehension (auditory and written)	Good; deficit with complex grammatical structures
Repetition	Impaired
Naming	Impaired, but improved with cues
Reading aloud	Impaired, similar to speech
Writing	Impaired, poorly formed letters; right hemiparesis forces many to write with their left hand
Elementary neurological findings	Right hemiparesis; variable right hemisensory loss
Behavioral findings	Depression; Apraxia of left limbs
Localization	Left posterior–inferior frontal cortex and underlying white matter
Pathology (typical)	Stroke (upper division of left MCA), hemorrhage, tumor, trauma

The 'tip-of-the-tongue' phenomenon, in which patients utter the initial letter or syllable of a word but cannot complete it, is common in Broca's aphasia (Goodglass et al., 1976). Also, confrontational naming is usually impaired. Often, such difficulties with word finding can be offset by cueing the patient with clues to the correct answer (Love and Webb, 1977). Both phonetic cues, such as giving the patient the first sound or syllable, and contextual cues, as in 'I take my coffee with cream and ____', are helpful.

Other clinical features of Broca's aphasia include severe disruption of articulation and prosody (melody and inflection), impairment of repetition that is less severe than impairment of spontaneous speech, and frequent phonemic paraphasias, which consist of sound or syllable substitutions.

Broca's aphasia must be distinguished from aphemia, a syndrome of dysarthria without aphasia caused by small lesions of the motor system that controls articulation (pars opercularis, inferior prerolandic gyrus or white matter underlying those regions) (Schiff et al., 1983). Aphemic patients have normal, non-aphasic writing and naming.

Motor or expressive aphasia should not be used as a synonym for Broca's aphasia. This terminology fosters confusion because spoken expression is altered in all aphasic and many non-aphasic disorders.

The most common cause of Broca's aphasia is embolic or thrombotic infarction in the distribution of the superior branch of the middle cerebral artery. Other causes include tumor, head trauma and infections.

In the acute stage of stroke-induced Broca's aphasia, patients commonly display right hemisensory loss and usually have right hemiparesis that affects the face and arm more than the leg. When patients do not have hemiparesis, Broca's aphasia is often transient (Masdeu and O'Hara, 1983; Henderson, 1985). In addition, patients with stroke-induced Broca's aphasia frequently have ideomotor apraxia of the left arm and leg (sympathetic apraxia) and orofacial muscles (Maxim 43). For example, when a verbal command is given to use the left arm, e.g. 'Show me how you salute with your left hand', patients with sympathetic apraxia are unable to perform the act, although they comprehend the question and can often imitate the movement when it is performed first by the examiner.

Broca's area is the posterior portion of the left inferior frontal gyrus (Brodmann area 44; Figures 7.1, 31.1a) (Broca, 1977). Strokes restricted to Broca's area may cause mutism followed by transient, effortful dysarthria, but no persistent aphasic disorder (Mohr *et al.*, 1978; Tonkonogy and Goodglass, 1981). The classic syndrome of Broca's aphasia results from more extensive left frontal lesions, reaching back to the Rolandic fissure and involving underlying white matter (Mohr *et al.*, 1978; Knopman *et al.*, 1983; Naeser *et al.*, 1989). Persistent, severe non-fluency is associated with white matter lesions in both the rostral portion of the medial subcallosal fasciculus (connecting the cingulate gyrus and supplementary motor area with the caudate) and in the areas adjacent to the lateral ventricle body (underlying the sensorimotor cortex for the mouth). The medial subcallosal fasciculus is important for preparation, initiation and limbic aspects of speech; the periventricular white matter is critical for motor execution and sensory feedback in spontaneous speech (Naeser *et al.*, 1989).

Depression occurs in many aphasic patients with anterior lesions (Robinson *et al.*, 1983). Goldstein (1948) first described the 'catastrophic reaction' to left frontal injuries, in which non-fluent aphasia is associated with profound depression, anxiety and withdrawal. Depression in patients with brain injuries is discussed in Maxims 75, 84 and 95.

References

Broca P. Remarks on the seat of the faculty of articulate speech, followed by the report of a case of aphemia (loss of speech). In (Rottenberg DA, Hochberg FH, eds) *Neurologic Classics in Modern Translation.* New York: Hafner Press, 1977, pp 136–49.

Goldstein K. *Language and Language Disturbances.* New York: Grune and Stratton, 1948.

Goodglass H, Kaplan E, Weintraub S, Ackerman N. The 'tip-of-the-tongue' phenomenon in aphasia. *Cortex* 1976; **12**: 258–65.

Henderson VM. Lesion localization in Broca's aphasia: Implications from Broca's aphasia without hemiparesis. *Arch Neurol* 1985; **42**: 1210–12.

Knopman DS, Selnes OA, Niccum N, Rubens AB, Yock D, Larson D. A longitudinal study of speech fluency in aphasia: CT correlates of recovery and persistent nonfluency. *Neurology* 1983; **33**: 1170–8.

Love RJ, Webb WG. The efficiency of cueing techniques in Broca's aphasia. *J Speech Hear Disord* 1977; **42**: 170–8.

Masdeu JC, O'Hara RJ. Motor aphasia unaccompanied by faciobrachial weakness. *Neurology* 1983; **33**: 519–21.

Mohr JP, Pessin MS, Finkelstein S, Funkenstein HH, Duncan GW, Davis KR. Broca aphasia: Pathologic and clinical. *Neurology* 1978; **28**: 311–24.

Naeser MA, Palumbo CL, Helm-Estabrooks N, Stiassny-Eder D, Albert ML. Severe nonfluency in aphasia. *Brain* 1989; **112**: 1–38.

Robinson RG, Starr LB, Kubos KL, Price TR. A two-year longitudinal study of post-stroke mood disorders: Findings during the initial evaluation. *Stroke* 1983; **14**: 736–41.

Schiff HB, Alexander MP, Naeser MA, Galaburda AM. Aphemia: Clinical–anatomic correlations. *Arch Neurol* 1983; **40**: 720–7.

Tonkonogy J, Goodglass H. Language function, foot of the third frontal gyrus, and rolandic operculum. *Arch Neurol* 1981; **38**: 486–90.

29.   *Wernicke's aphasia is often misdiagnosed as a psychiatric disorder*

When evaluating any patient with a sudden change in behavior – beware – and assess mental status, especially comprehension, carefully. Some patients will have Wernicke's aphasia, but others will have treatable disorders such as herpes encephalitis. The following case report demonstrates the misdiagnosis of Wernicke's aphasia:

> A neurological consultation was requested on a 64-year-old man because psychological testing raised the question of 'organicity'. Family members had brought him to the emergency room because of confusion and irritability. The man had no prior psychiatric history and was well until several hours before admission. Prior to neurological consultation, he was hospitalized for a month on a psychiatric ward with the diagnosis of atypical psychosis. When asked by the neurologist why he was in the hospital, he replied 'I don't think that's fair, no, not that thing'. He spoke fluently with slightly pressured speech and paraphasias. When asked if helicopters in South America eat their young, he replied 'I should hope so'. Head computed tomography showed a left posterior, superior temporal lucency consistent with infarction.

Wernicke's aphasia is one of the most dramatic and distinctive neurological syndromes. Behavioral and linguistic features predominate, while such elementary neurological signs and symptoms as hemiparesis or sensory loss are often absent, although right superior quadrantanopia may occur (Table 29.1). Acutely, there is often prominent alteration of mood and affect. The most characteristic behavioral feature is lack of awareness and concern for the condition. While many patients are euphoric, others act irritable, angry and paranoid, and they may become violent (Benson, 1973). These behavioral changes probably result from disruption of limbic functions when the lesion extends to the medial temporal lobe. Alternatively, some patients may 'emotionally comprehend' that something is very wrong and become frustrated and upset.

Linguistically, Wernicke's aphasia is the antithesis of Broca's aphasia.

Table 29.1   Clinical features of Wernicke's aphasia.

Feature	Observations
Speech	Fluent, normal prosody, frequent paraphasias
Comprehension (auditory and written)	Impaired
Repetition	Impaired
Naming	Impaired, paraphasic errors
Reading aloud	Impaired
Writing	Well-formed letters, but meaningless content
Elementary neurological findings	Right hemianopsia, right superior quadrantanopsia, or normal fields
Behavioral findings	Unconcern, euphoria, confusion, agitation, irritability, suspiciousness
Pathology	Stroke (lower division of MCA), hemorrhage, tumor, trauma

Patients with Wernicke's aphasia are fluent with normal prosody, often speak excessively (logorrhea, verborrhea), create paraphasias and neologisms, and have impaired comprehension (Benson, 1979).

Wernicke's aphasia is sometimes confused with psychiatric illness because of the absence of obvious neurological signs. The behavior is clearly 'different', but the patient is unconcerned and unaware; mood changes and suspiciousness occur, and speech is vague with loose associations and 'confusion' (Gerson *et al*, 1977). Fluent aphasia can usually be distinguished from psychiatric disorders on historical grounds. The behavioral change usually develops suddenly without prior personality or mood disorders; precipitating events, such as death of a spouse, are absent; and patients are usually old. Although stroke is the most common cause and produces an acute disorder, tumors can trigger presentation with a more insidious onset of symptoms. The language examination is diagnostic.

Several features distinguish the speech of patients with 'loose' schizophrenia ('word salad') and Wernicke's (or conduction) aphasia. Responses to open-ended questions are shorter in aphasia; paraphasias are common in aphasia and rare in schizophrenia; vague responses occur in both disorders, but are due to word-finding problems in aphasia and to circumstantiality in psychosis; and bizarre and delusional themes occur in psychosis (Benson *et al.*, 1977).

Language disorder in Wernicke's aphasia is always present but varies among patients. Acutely, patients may be mute before the characteristic fluent, overflowing speech filled with empty phrases, circumlocutions and paraphasias. Indeed, a foreigner with Wernicke's aphasia – speaking an unknown language – would sound almost identical to one with normal speech. Paraphasias and the lack of meaningful substantive words, such as nouns and verbs, are most apparent in spontaneous speech. Paraphasias are usually verbal rather than literal; that is, they are more likely to consist of word substitutions than substitutions of phonemes or sounds. Jargon speech contains abundant neologisms, or new words, such as 'thintoke'. Children with Wernicke's aphasia tend to speak less fluently than adults, but recover more fully (Woods and Tueber, 1978).

Verbal comprehension deficit is the central linguistic component of Wernicke's aphasia. However, it is usually overlooked if not specifically tested, because patients perceive non-verbal cues, such as speech tone, facial expression, and hand and body gestures, that obscure their lack of verbal comprehension. The best test of comprehension is a series of nonsense questions asked in a serious, inquisitive manner (Maxim 25). Simple questions, such as 'Do two pounds of flour weigh more than one?' and 'Are you lying in bed?', can also reveal prominent impairment of comprehension.

If the patient is unable to respond verbally, one should assess comprehension with non-verbal responses, such as 'Show me your hand'. However, it is important to distinguish comprehension and praxis (Maxim 43). Some apraxic patients are able to follow commands involving the axial musculature, as in 'Blink' or 'Turn your head to the right', but not those commands involving the extremities, such as 'Flip a coin'.

Auditory and reading comprehension are usually impaired to a similar degree. In occasional cases, either of these two abilities (more often reading comprehension) may be relatively spared (Heilman *et al.*, 1979; Kirshner *et al.*, 1981; Sevush *et al.*, 1983). It is imperative to test auditory and reading comprehension separately, because preservation of one modality may open a therapeutic window. For example, patients who comprehend written material may learn to communicate effectively with sign language (Kirshner and Webb, 1981).

Patients with Wernicke's aphasia also have impaired naming and repetition. Word-finding deficiency is severe during both spontaneous speech and confrontation testing, and patients may happily produce bizarre, paraphasic, naming errors. Reading aloud is also commonly impaired, although it may be relatively intact, with or without some preservation of reading comprehension. Writing is legible but incomprehensible, with the same emptiness, circumlocution and paraphasic errors that contaminate speech.

Wernicke's area is situated in the posterior third of the left superior temporal gyrus (Brodmann area 22; Figures 7.1, 31.1a). Lesions confined to Wernicke's area usually produce persistent aphasia, but occasionally cause no language deficits (Selnes *et al.*, 1983, 1985). However, when the characteristic features of Wernicke's aphasia occur, lesions are reliably found in this area (Benson, 1988). Comprehension of spoken language is more severely affected by medial temporal extension of the lesion, while comprehension of written language is more severely affected by extension posteriorly into the parietal lobe (Hecaen, 1969). Involvement of the posteriorly contiguous infrasylvian parietal lobe, or supramarginal gyrus, is common in Wernicke's aphasia patients and contributes to aphasia and alexia (Mohr *et al.*, 1978). The most common etiology of Wernicke's aphasia is stroke, usually an embolus to the inferior division of the left middle cerebral artery. Other causes include tumor, abscess and hemorrhage, especially posterior putaminal hemorrhages that extend into the temporal lobe isthmus. Occasionally, epileptic discharges produce symptoms of this aphasic syndrome (Serafetinides and Falconer, 1963; Gabr *et al.*, 1989). Rarely, partial status epilepticus presents as Wernicke's aphasia (Knight and Cooper, 1986).

Patients with Wernicke's aphasia usually recover some auditory comprehension, although a favorable prognosis is less likely than in Broca's aphasia. Slow presentation of auditory material may improve comprehension (Albert and Bear, 1974). As patients improve, they often develop insight into their language deficits and, as a result, may become depressed. Paranoia may also emerge as a late sequela.

Pure word deafness is a rare syndrome that is theoretically distinct from Wernicke's aphasia. In reality, however, they often overlap. In patients with pure word deafness, comprehension deficit is restricted to words (Buchman *et al.*, 1986). Pure tone audiometric hearing tests are normal, as is comprehension of such non-verbal sounds as music, animal vocalizations and sirens. In pure word deafness, spontaneous speech, writing, reading and naming are intact; only auditory verbal comprehension and repetition are impaired. However, the separation between word deafness and aphasia is often incomplete because many patients with the former have mild paraphasic errors in speech or naming (Goldstein, 1974). In its pure form, word deafness is not an aphasic disorder, but a form of auditory agnosia in which input from primary auditory cortex (Heschl's gyrus) is unable to reach Wernicke's area. Anatomical lesions in pure word deafness conform to this model, occurring unilaterally in the left temporal or bilaterally in the deep temporal regions (Geschwind, 1970; Coslett *et al.*, 1984; Buchman *et al.*, 1986).

References

Albert ML, Bear D. Time to understand. A case study of word deafness with reference to the role of time in auditory comprehension. *Brain* 1974; **97**: 383–94.
Benson DF. Psychiatric aspects of aphasia. *Br J Psychiat* 1973; **123**: 555–66.
Benson DF. *Aphasia, Alexia, and Agraphia.* Edinburgh, New York: Churchill Livingstone, 1979.
Benson DF. Classical syndromes of aphasia. In: *Handbook of Neuropsychology* (volume 1) (Boller F, Grafman J, eds). Amsterdam: Elsevier Science Publishers, 1988, pp. 267–80.
Buchman AS, Garron DC, Trust-Cardamone JE, Wichter MD, Schwartz M. Word deafness: One hundred years later. *J Neurol Neurosurg Psychiat* 1986; **49**: 489–99.
Coslett HB, Brashear HR, Heilman KM. Pure word deafness after bilateral primary auditory cortex infarcts. *Neurology* 1984; **34**: 347–52.
Gabr M, Luders H, Dinner D, Morris H, Wyllie E. Speech manifestations in lateralization of temporal lobe seizures. *Ann Neurol* 1989; **25**: 82–7.

Gerson SN, Benson DF, Frazier SH. Diagnosis: Schizophrenia versus posterior aphasia. *Am J Psychiat* 1977; **134**: 966–9.

Geschwind N. The organization of language and the brain. *Science* 1970; **170**: 940–4.

Goldstein M. Auditory agnosia for speech (pure word deafness): a historical review with current implications. *Brain Lang* 1974; **1**: 195–204.

Hecaen H. Essai de dissociation du syndrome de l'aphasie sensorielle. *Rev Neurol* 1969; **120**; 229–31.

Heilman K, Rothi L, Campanella D, Wolfson S. Wernicke's and global aphasia without alexia. *Arch Neurol* 1979; **36**: 129–33.

Kirshner HS, Webb WG. Selective involvement of the auditory-verbal modality in an acquired communication disorder: benefit from sign language therapy. *Brain Lang* 1981; **13**: 161–70.

Kirshner HS, Webb W, Duncan G. Word deafness in Wernicke's aphasia. *J Neurol Neurosurg Psychiat* 1981; **41**: 564–8.

Knight RT, Cooper J. Status epilepticus manifesting as reversible Wernicke's aphasia. *Epilepsia* 1986; **27**: 301–4.

Mohr J, Hier D, Kirshner H. Modality bias in Wernicke's aphasia. *Neurology* 1978; **28**: 395.

Selnes OA, Knopman DS, Niccum N *et al.* Computed tomographic scan correlates of auditory comprehension deficits in aphasia: a prospective recovery study. *Ann Neurol* 1983; **13**: 558–66.

Selnes OA, Knopman DS, Niccum N, Rubens AB. The critical role of Wernicke's area in sentence repetition. *Ann Neurol* 1985; **17**: 549–57.

Serafetinides EA, Falconer MA. Speech disturbances in temporal lobe seizures. *Brain* 1963; **86**: 333–46.

Sevush S, Roeltgen DP, Campanella DJ, Heilman KM. Preserved oral reading in Wernicke's aphasia. *Neurology* 1983; **33**: 916–20.

Woods B, Teuber HL. Changing patterns of childhood aphasia. *Ann Neurol* 1978; **3**: 273–80.

30.   *Conduction aphasia, marked by disproportionate impairment in repeating spoken language, results from lesions in the temporoparietal operculum and subjacent white matter*

Wernicke (1874) postulated that difficulty with repetition would result from lesions near the insula which would disconnect fibers connecting the anterior (Broca's) and posterior (Wernicke's) language areas. However, available anatomical data documented only one connection between anterior and posterior language areas, the arcuate fasciculus (Dejerine, 1901). This fiber bundle originates in the auditory association area and passes posteriorly and superiorly, making a 'U turn' at the rear margin of the Sylvian fissure, and then traveling beneath the supramarginal and somatosensory areas in the parietal operculum to reach Broca's area. Wernicke later revised his disconnection model, localizing the lesion in conduction aphasia to the arcuate fasciculus. However, there are two pathways connecting anterior and posterior language areas – the arcuate fasciculus and the more direct route through the extreme capsule (passing just beneath the insular cortex) – and lesions in either pathway can cause conduction aphasia (Damasio and Damasio, 1983). Furthermore, cortical lesions as well as disconnection of cortical areas may cause the syndrome of conduction aphasia.

Table 30.1 shows the clinical characteristics of conduction aphasia. Spontaneous speech is usually fluent with frequent literal, phonemic paraphasias, but patients may also have word-finding pauses. In some patients with conduction aphasia, decreased fluency characterized by hesitation, broken melody (dysprosody) and phonemic paraphasias suggests Broca's aphasia. However, preserved articulation, abundant literal paraphasias and the absence of hemiparesis distinguish conduction aphasia from Broca's aphasia in such cases.

Good comprehension of spoken language is a prerequisite for diagnosis of conduction aphasia. As in Broca's aphasia, comprehension may be entirely normal or impaired only for grammatical components, e.g. understanding active versus passive sentences or sentences with indirect objects and embedded clauses (Heilman and Scholes, 1976; Linebarger et al., 1983). However, patients with conduction aphasia have no difficulties comprehending normal conversation. Moderate comprehension impairment with fluent speech supports the diagnosis of Wernicke's aphasia.

Marked impairment of repetition that is accompanied by preserved comprehension constitutes the essence of conduction aphasia. The difficulty in repeating spoken language stands out against the background of fluent, or nearly fluent, conversational speech. Some patients have difficulty repeating single words. Others successfully repeat simple phrases like 'the boy ran', but fail miserably with 'There are no ifs, ands, or buts about it',

Table 30.1 Clinical features of conduction aphasia.

Feature	Observation
Speech	Fluent, frequent paraphasias, ± hesitations
Comprehension (auditory and written)	Normal or mildly impaired
Repetition	Impaired
Naming	Mild-to-moderate impairment
Reading aloud	Impaired
Writing	Impaired
Elementary neurological findings	Right hemisensory loss and hemianopsia may occur; right hemiparesis is uncommon
Behavioral findings	Apraxia
Localization	Left temporoparietal area
Pathology	Stroke (either upper or lower divisions of MCA or their border zones), tumor

'The spy fled to Greece', or 'The phantom soared across the foggy heath'. Impairment of repetition is limited primarily to the auditory–verbal modality, as repetition in visual–verbal and auditory–manual modalities is usually well preserved (Kinsbourne, 1972). Patients with conduction aphasia are unable to recall auditory sequences, which suggests that impaired memory for auditory sequences contributes to their repetition deficit (Tzortzis and Albert, 1974).

Confrontation naming is usually impaired. Errors may be due to phonemic (literal; syllabic substitutions) and, occasionally, verbal (semantic; word substitutions) paraphasias, as well as anomic word-finding difficulties. Reading aloud is usually abnormal with paraphasias and hesitation, while reading comprehension is quite good. Significant impairment of reading comprehension suggests that the conduction aphasia is accompanied by posterior extension of the lesion to produce alexia or by involvement of Wernicke's area to impair comprehension. Writing is typically impaired, with paraphasias, misspellings and word-order errors (Benson et al., 1973).

In patients with stroke, conduction aphasia often emerges one to two weeks after the ictus. Patients may demonstrate Wernicke's aphasia on presentation and, when tested one week later, show improved comprehension without improved repetition. As patients with conduction aphasia recover, repetition improves and may leave only anomia in its wake. In contrast, patients with lesions in Wernicke's area are more likely to have persistent repetition deficits (Selnes et al., 1985).

Conduction aphasia usually results from lesions in the posterior perisylvian cortex or subjacent white matter (Benson et al., 1973; Mazzochi and Vignolo, 1979; Damasio and Damasio, 1980; Selnes et al., 1985; Kempler et al., 1988). Many patients have temporal lesions in the insula, primary auditory cortex or Wernicke's area. The remainder have inferior parietal lesions, usually involving supramarginal gyrus and subjacent white matter (arcuate fasciculus).

In addition, positron emission tomography studies performed in conduction aphasia patients demonstrate widespread glucose hypometabolism in temporal and parietal regions (Levine and Calvanio, 1982) suggesting that both cortical and white matter lesions are important. Thus, either cortical destruction or disconnection may be the relevant mechanism for conduction aphasia (Levine and Calvanio, 1982; Mendez and Benson, 1985). Disconnection is probably the most important mechanism in the pathogenesis of conduction aphasia. Disconnection may result from lesions in the arcuate fasciculus or in the area of the insula and extreme capsule (Damasio and Damasio, 1983).

The most common etiology of conduction aphasia is stroke, although other structural lesions in these locations can produce the characteristic, clinical picture.

References

Benson DF, Sheremata WA, Bouchard R, Segarra JM, Price D, Geschwind N. Conduction aphasia: a clinicopathological study. *Arch Neurol* 1973; **28**: 339–46.

Damasio H, Damasio AR. The anatomical basis of conduction aphasia. *Brain* 1980; **103**: 337–50.

Damasio H, Damasio AR. The localization of lesions in conduction aphasia. In: *Localization in Neuropsychology*. Orlando, FL: Academic Press, Inc., 1983, pp. 231–43.

Dejerine J. *Anatomie des Centres Nerveux*. Paris: Reuff, 1901.

Heilman KM, Scholes RJ. The nature of the comprehension errors in Broca's, conduction, and Wernicke's aphasics. *Cortex* 1976; **12**: 258–65.

Kempler D, Metter J, Jackson CA, Hanson WR, Riege WH, Mazziotta JA, Phelps ME. Disconnection and cerebral metabolism: The case of conduction aphasia. *Arch Neurol* 1988; **45**: 275–9.

Kinsbourne M. Behavioral analysis of the repetition deficit in conduction aphasia. *Neurology* 1972; **22**: 1126–32.

Levine DN, Calvanio R. Conduction aphasia. In: *The Neurology of Aphasia: Neurolinguistics* (volume 12) (Kirshner HS, Freeman FR, eds). Amsterdam: Swets and Zeitlinger, 1982, pp. 79–112.

Linebarger MC, Schwartz MF, Saffran EM. Sensitivity to grammatical structure in so-called agrammatic aphasics. *Cognition* 1983; **13**: 361–92.

Mazzochi F, Vignolo LA. Localization of lesions in aphasia: clinical CT scan correlates in stroke patients. *Cortex* 1979; **15**: 627–54.

Mendez MF, Benson DF. Atypical conduction aphasia: A disconnection syndrome. *Arch Neurol* 1985; **42**: 886–91.

Selnes OA, Knopman DS, Niccum N, Rubens AB. The critical role of Wernicke's area in sentence repetition. *Ann Neurol* 1985; **17**: 549–57.

Tzortzis C, Albert ML. Impairment of memory for sequences in conduction aphasia. *Neuropsychologia* 1974; **12**: 355–66.

Wernicke C. *Der Aphasische Symptomenkomplex*. Breslau, Poland: Cohn and Wigert, 1874.

31.   *Transcortical aphasia results from isolation, not destruction, of the language cortex*

The transcortical aphasias disconnect, and thereby isolate, speech areas from other cortical regions. In contrast with such classic syndromes as Broca's and Wernicke's aphasias, the speech cortices are spared. There are three varieties of transcortical aphasia: anterior, called *transcortical motor aphasia* (TCMA); posterior, called *transcortical sensory aphasia* (TCSA); and the combined anterior and posterior form, known as *mixed transcortical aphasia* (MTCA) or *isolation of the speech cortex* (Table 25.1).

Isolation of the speech cortex or *MTCA* is a rare syndrome with striking features. Patients cannot understand or speak fluently during conversation, but they repeat beautifully. Therefore, on a simplistic level, it is helpful to think of MTCA as the opposite of conduction aphasia: in transcortical aphasia, repetition is better than expected; in conduction aphasia, it is worse.

In addition, MTCA patients are non-fluent and aspontaneous, with impaired naming, auditory and reading comprehension, and writing. In occasional cases, naming is intact (Heilman *et al.*, 1976). Repetition stands alone as an island of preserved language function. Indeed, some patients echolalically repeat everything that is heard, whether spoken or sung (Geschwind *et al.*, 1968). Many patients speak only when spoken to. In milder MTCA cases, comprehension and spontaneous speech are less impaired.

The lesion in MTCA spares Broca's, Wernicke's and the inferior parietal language (supramarginal and angular gyri) areas and their white matter interconnections, but it affects the cortical rim surrounding these perisylvian language areas (Fig.31.1). As a result, the lesion functionally disconnects language areas from other association areas, including frontal, parietal and temporal association cortices that are essential for other cognitive functions. Primary motor and sensory areas are often involved, giving rise to motor, somatosensory and visual field deficits that may be bilateral. Anatomically, MTCA is caused by lesions in the border zone located between the anterior and middle cerebral arteries and between the middle and posterior cerebral arteries.

Hypoxic–ischemic brain insults from cardiac arrest, shock, hypotension and carbon monoxide poisoning produce bilateral border zone infarcts and are the most common causes of severe MTCA. Milder MTCA may result from such lesions as high-grade stenosis or occlusion of the left internal carotid artery, with filling of the left posterior cerebral artery off the carotid. In these cases, hypotension or stenosis of the right internal carotid may cause ischemia in the left border zone. Rarely, MTCA results from large strokes in the left anterior cerebral artery with infarction extending posteromedially into the parietal lobe (Ross, 1980) or from left thalamic strokes (McFarling *et al.*, 1982; Tuszynski and Petito, 1988).

Transcortical motor aphasia is very similar to Broca's aphasia, but is distinguished by preserved repetition, during which patients may even correct syntactic errors in the original sentence (Davis *et al.*, 1978). Mutism may occur with acute onset, for example, following left anterior cerebral artery infarction. Speech, and often motor activity, is characterized by a lack of spontaneity. Verbal output resembles that in Broca's aphasia because it is non-fluent, dysarthric, and agrammatically telegraphic, but in TCMA stuttering and repetition of the same syllable or word are more common.

Patients with TCMA are often facile in answering yes and no questions. They correctly answer simple comprehension questions such as 'Are you in bed?' and 'Do 3 pounds of candy weigh more than 2?', but do poorly with open-ended questions such as 'Why are you in the hospital?' or 'What do you like to do on your day off?' Their response to these open-ended questions is often a single word. If the examiner is not careful, it is easy to mistake these terse answers for the much more common scenario of a patient who is not very interested in answering a lot of questions.

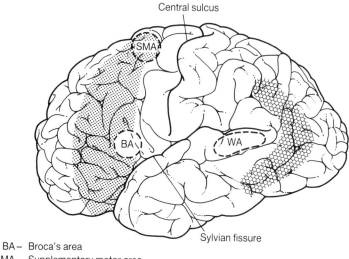

BA – Broca's area
SMA – Supplementary motor area
WA – Wernicke's area

Fig. 31.1(a)   Lateral view of the left hemisphere. Transcortical aphasias.

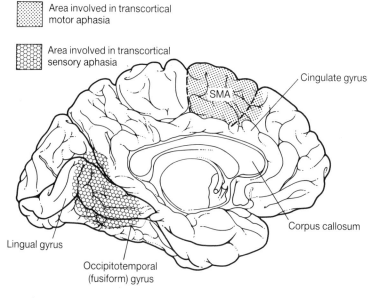

Fig. 31.1(b)   Medial view of the left hemisphere. Transcortical aphasias.

When asked to count to 10, they may have difficulty initiating the sequence. However, if the examiner provides the first few numbers, they can often complete the series. Confrontation naming is usually mildly impaired and can be improved by cues. For example, if the patient cannot name 'watch', providing a contextual cue, such as 'One uses this to tell time', or a phonemic cue, as in 'It starts with WA', may be helpful.

Writing is impaired in TCMA, with poor spelling, a telegraphic lack of grammatical words, and oversized, poorly formed letters. As in spontaneous speech, reading aloud is usually clumsy with dysarthria and repetition of syllables. However, comprehension for both spoken and written language is intact.

Neurological symptoms often associated with TCMA include hemiparesis that affects the leg and shoulder more than the arm or face and is nearly always right-sided, as well as apraxia of the left arm and leg (Maxim 43). Sensory loss is absent or mild and parallels the distribution of motor loss. In addition, right-sided grasp reflexes of the foot and hand, increased muscle tone in the leg and arm, snout reflex and lack of initiative (abulia) may accompany TCMA. However, these signs are usually subtle and result from involvement of frontal cortex. When frontal involvement is extensive or bilateral, TCMA is usually not diagnosed, as the neurobehavioral syndrome is far more prominent (Maxim 54).

The lesion in TCMA is almost always located in the dominant frontal lobe, positioned either anterior and superior to Broca's area or in the supplementary motor area (Luria and Tsvetkova, 1968; Masdeu et al., 1978; Naesser and Hayward, 1978; Jonas, 1981; Freedman et al., 1984). Destruction of the dominant supplementary motor area or its disconnection from Broca's area appears to be the common pathogenic mechanism. However, elective resection of the dominant supplementary motor area for control of epilepsy only causes transient TCMA (Laplane et al., 1977; personal observation). Causes of TCMA lesions include: hemorrhage, acute internal carotid artery occlusion causing infarction in the border zone between the anterior and middle cerebral arteries, thrombotic and embolic infarcts in the anterior cerebral artery distribution, tumor (often following resection) and trauma. Rare cases of TCMA occur with left thalamic lesions (McFarling et al., 1982).

The majority of patients with TCMA improve, but recovery is often incomplete, taking place mostly in the first few weeks after an acute presentation. Occasionally, symptoms completely resolve (Rubens, 1976; Kertesz and McCabe, 1977; Benson, 1979). Bromocriptine may improve speech hesitancy and naming in selected patients (Albert et al., 1988).

Transcortical sensory aphasia is very similar to Wernicke's aphasia, but is distinguished by preserved repetition. Speech is fluent with neologistic and semantic paraphasias. Naming, reading, writing, and auditory and written language comprehension are impaired, although naming is relatively spared in occasional patients (Heilman et al., 1981). Echolalia is often a prominent feature. The examiner's question may be repeated in an automatic, involuntary manner. As with Wernicke's aphasia, these patients are frequently misdiagnosed with schizophrenia or atypical psychosis (Benson, 1973).

The most commonly associated neurological sign in TCSA is visual field loss, most often a right superior quandrantanopia or right hemianopia. Lesions are in the temporoparietooccipital lobes, either in the middle cerebral artery territory, posterior cerebral artery territory (more often medial, inferior and posterior), or in the watershed between the middle and posterior cerebral arteries (more often lateral, superior and anterior) (Damasio, 1981; Kertesz et al., 1982; Alexander et al., 1989). The prognosis in TCSA is variable.

References

Albert ML, Bachman DL, Morgan A, Helm-Estabrooks N. Pharmacotherapy for aphasia. *Neurology* 1988; **38**: 877–9.

Alexander MP, Hillbrunner B, Fischer RS. Distributed anatomy of transcortical sensory aphasia. *Arch Neurol* 1989; **46**: 885–92.

Benson DF. Psychiatric aspects of aphasia. *Br J Psychiat* 1973; **123**: 555–66.

Benson DF. *Aphasia, Alexia, and Agraphia*. Ebinburgh, New York: Churchill Livingstone, 1979.

Damasio H. Cerebral localization of the aphasias. In: *Acquired Aphasia* (Sarno MT, ed.). Orlando, Fl: Academic Press, 1981, pp. 27–50.

Davis L, Foldi NS, Gardner H, Zurif EB. Repetition in transcortical aphasias. *Brain Lang* 1978; **6**: 226–38.

Freedman M, Alexander MP, Naeser MA. Anatomical basis of transcortical motor aphasia. *Neurology* 1984; **34**: 409–17.

Geschwind N, Quadfasel F, Segarra J. Isolation of the speech area. *Neuropsychologia* 1968; **6**: 327–40.

Heilman KM, Tucker DM, Valenstein E. A case of transcortical aphasia with intact naming. *Brain* 1976; **99**: 415–26.

Heilman KM, Rothi L, McFarling D, Rottmann AL. Transcortical sensory aphasia with relatively spared spontaneous speech and naming. *Arch Neurol* 1981; **38**: 236–9.

Jonas S. The supplementary motor region and speech emission. *J Commun Disord* 1981; **14**: 349–73.

Kertesz A, McCabe P. Recovery patterns and prognosis in aphasia. *Brain* 1977; **100**: 1–18.

Kertesz A, Sheppard A, MacKenzie R. Localization in transcortical sensory aphasia. *Arch Neurol* 1982; **39**: 475–8.

Laplane D, Talairach D, Meninger V, Bancard J, Bouchareine A. Motor consequences of motor area ablations in men. *J Neurol Sci* 1977; **31**: 29–49.

Luria A, Tsvetkova LS. The mechanisms of 'Dynamic aphasia'. *Found Lang* 1968; **4**: 296–307.

Masdeu JC, Schoene WC, Funkenstein H. Aphasia following infarction of the left supplementary motor area: A clinicopathological study. *Neurology* 1978; **28**: 1220–3.

McFarling O, Rothi LJ, Heilman KM. Transcortical aphasia from ischemic infarcts of the thalamus: a report of two cases. *J Neurol Neurosurg Psychiat* 1982; **45**: 107–12.

Naesser MA, Hayward RW. Lesion localization in aphasia with cranial computerized tomography and the Boston Diagnostic Aphasia Exam. *Neurology* 1978; **28**: 545–51.

Ross ED. Left medial parietal lobe and receptive language functions: mixed trans-cortical aphasia after left anterior cerebral artery infarction. *Neurology* 1980; **30**: 144–51.

Rubens AB. Transcortical motor aphasia. In: *Studies in Neurolinguistics* (volume I) (Whitaker H, Whitaker HA, eds). Orlando FL: Academic Press, 1976.

Tuszynski MH, Petito CK. Ischemic thalamic aphasia with pathologic confirmation. *Neurology* 1988; **38**: 800–2.

32. *Lesions in any language area can cause anomic aphasia*

Anomia, or naming disorder, results from lesions in any language area, as well as from lesions outside language cortex. Therefore, isolated anomia is of limited localizing value, occurring with lesions in anterior or posterior regions, cortical or subcortical regions, and dominant or non-dominant hemispheres. Like headache, however, anomia is often one of the earliest clues of a brain disorder, such as primary and metastatic tumors.

Anomia is the most common abnormality in aphasia (Goodglass and Geschwind, 1976) and when aphasia is posterior, as in Wernicke's, trans-cortical sensory and conduction aphasias, it can be the only sequela.

Anomic aphasia is characterized by spontaneous, fluent speech that is interrupted by word-finding pauses. The lack of substantive words (e.g. bookshelf and wristband) and the high frequency of non-specific nouns and verbs (e.g. thing, this, do) produces so-called 'empty speech', which is the hallmark of anomic aphasia. Some patients, unable to find the correct substantive word, weave a circuitous, rambling path around the missing target word. This meandering verbiage is referred to as circumlocution. For example, when trying to name 'cat', the patient may respond, 'you know that thing that likes to, uh, that white stuff and it makes those sounds, you know, meow'. In addition to word-finding difficulties in spon-taneous speech, these patients do poorly with confrontation naming and word production tests (Maxim 25), such as 'Name all the farm animals' or 'Name words that begin with the letter S'.

Benson and Geschwind (1985) described four varieties of anomic aphasia: *word production anomia, word selection anomia, semantic anomia* and *disconnec-tion anomias*. The key features that distinguish among these anomias are knowledge of the desired name, understanding of what the object actually is and how it is used, ability to point correctly to the object when the name is presented, and modality-specific or unilateral (e.g. right visual field only) naming deficits.

In *word production anomia*, the patient knows the desired name but is unable to produce it accurately (Benson, 1979). This anomia occurs with both anterior and posterior aphasias. When it accompanies posterior aphasias, literal and verbal paraphasias adulterate speech and prevent correct naming. In anterior (Broca's and transcortical motor) aphasias, word production anomia results from a defect in the articulatory initiation process. Phonetic cues, which give the initial word sound, or such contextual cues as 'you catch a baseball with a _____', are most helpful to anomic patients with anterior lesions.

Word selection anomia is characterized by knowledge of how to use an object and ability to choose the correct object from a group once given the name, but difficulty in naming the object when it is presented in any sensory modality. This uncommon anomia results from lesions in the dominant temporo-occipital junctional cortex (Brodmann area 37).

In *semantic anomia*, the symbolic meaning of words is lost. Such patients are not only unable to name objects, they are also unable to choose the correct object from a group when given the name (Warrington *et al.*, 1975). Semantic anomia often occurs in posterior (transcortical sensory and Wernicke's) aphasia and, paradoxically, can be an early finding in the frontal lobe dementia, Pick's disease (Maxim 17). Semantic anomia classically results from lesions within the angular gyrus (located in the inferior parietal lobe) of the dominant hemisphere. Lesions in this area also produce alexia, impaired interpretation of proverbs and similarities-differences, constructional disturbances, and the components of Gertsmann syndrome as agraphia, acalculia, right–left disorientation and finger agnosia (Benson *et al.*, 1982).

The *disconnection anomias* are divided into modality-specific, category-specific and callosal forms. These anomias result from lesions that sever connections between sensory and language cortices (Geschwind, 1967).

In *modality-specific anomia*, defective naming is limited to one sensory modality. For example, patients with visual anomia are unable to name objects they see but have no difficulty naming the same object when they palpate, hear or smell it – assuming it has a characteristic shape, sound and smell. The distinction is often blurred between such modality-specific anomia and agnosia, which is defined as inability to recognize objects in a sensory modality despite normal attention, language and sensory perception. In this case, inability to name results from inability to recognize. In contrast, with modality-specific anomia, patients can recognize but cannot name an object. In modality-specific anomia, the lesion is usually located in the posterior white matter tracts, functionally disconnecting language and sensory-association cortices.

Category-specific anomia is characterized by naming deficits that are restricted to a specific group of nouns, such as colors or body parts (Geschwind and Fusillo, 1966; Warrington and Shallice, 1984; Hart and Caramazza, 1985). This uncommon anomia is caused by lesions in the posterior white matter.

Callosal anomia results from lesions in the corpus callosum that isolate intact sensory areas of the non-dominant hemisphere from dominant hemisphere language areas (Maxim 52). Such patients can palpate an object in the left hand and accurately assess its size and shape using right hemisphere somatosensory areas. However, they cannot transmit that information to left hemisphere language areas and are therefore unable to name the object. However, these patients can correctly use the object or select it from a group of pictures (Gazzaniga and Sperry, 1967).

In all of the above forms of anomic aphasia, other language functions, including auditory comprehension, repetition, reading and writing, are normal or only mildly impaired. In some patients, defective comprehension with preserved repetition creates a continuum between the syndromes of anomic aphasia and transcortical sensory aphasia. Elementary neurological findings in anomic aphasia are quite variable, as expected from the diverse localization of lesions.

Weinstein and Keller (1964) identified a group of diffuse central nervous system insults, especially those with rapid onset, that result in *non-aphasic naming errors*. They included head injury, subarachnoid hemorrhage, sudden increase in intracranial pressure, and systemic illness. In addition, some patients with frontal lesions and the classic Witzelsucht – moria, jocularity and deliberate facetiousness – may give the appearance of anomia. If the examiner asks 'What is my profession?', the patient may respond 'Someone who asks a lot of questions' (Geschwind, 1967). Perseverative errors, in which the patient repeats prior responses, must also be distinguished from anomic aphasia. Finally, anomia is common in dementia.

Anomia is one of the most common, but least specific, behavioral findings. Regardless of the cause and duration of anomia, treatment can be beneficial. Both phonological therapy, which provides information on the sounds of the unnamed words, and semantic therapy, which gives information on the meaning of the unnamed words, produce small but significant improvements (Howard et al., 1985).

References

Benson DF. Neurologic correlates of anomia. In: *Studies in Neurolinguistics* (volume 4) (Whitaker H, Whitaker HA, eds.). Orlando, FL: Academic Press 1979, pp. 293–328.

Benson DF, Cummings JL, Tsai SY. Angular gyrus syndrome simulating Alzheimer's disease. *Arch Neurol* 1982; **39**: 616–20.

Benson DF, Geschwind N. Aphasia and related disorders: A clinical approach. In: *Principles of Behavioral Neurology* (Mesulam M-M, ed.). Philadelphia: FA Davis Company, 1985, 193–238.

Gazzaniga MS, Sperry RW. Language after section of the cerebral commissures. *Brain* 1967; **90**: 131–48.

Geschwind N. The varieties of naming errors. *Cortex* 1967; **3**: 97–112.

Geschwind N, Fusillo M. Color naming defects in association with alexia. *Arch Neurol* 1966; **15**: 137–46.

Goodglass H, Geschwind N. Language disturbance (aphasia). In: *Handbook of Perception* (volume 7) (Carterette EC, Friedman MP, eds). Orlando, FL: Academic Press 1976, pp. 389–428.

Hart J, Berndt RS, Caramazza A. Category-specific naming deficit following cerebral infarction. *Nature* 1985; **316**: 439–40.

Howard D, Patterson K, Franklin S, Orchard-Lisle V, Morton J. Treatment of work retrieval deficits in aphasia. *Brain* 1985; **108**: 817–29.

Warrington EK. The selective impairment of semantic memory. *Q J Exp Psychol* 1975; **27**: 635–57.

Warrington EK, Shallice T. Category specific semantic impairments. *Brain* 1984; **107**: 829–54.

Weinstein EA, Keller NJS. Linguistic patterns of misnaming in brain injury. *Neuropsychologia* 1964; **1**: 79–90.

33.   Global aphasia usually results from large strokes in the left, middle cerebral artery territory

Global aphasia is moderate-to-severe impairment of all language functions. This common syndrome, accounting for roughly a quarter of all aphasias, represents a combination of anterior and posterior aphasic disorders (Table 33.1) (Brust *et al.*, 1976; Kertesz and McCabe, 1977; Boller, 1981).

Acutely, mutism or only groaning may occur. Non-fluent, effortful, sparse speech is characteristic, and severe impairment of comprehension prevents testing of praxis and other higher cognitive functions. Patients with global aphasia are unable to read, write or name. This syndrome often evolves into Broca's aphasia.

Most often, global aphasia is caused by a large stroke involving the

Table 33.1   Clinical features of global aphasia.

Feature	Observations
Speech	Mute or non-fluent-telegraphic
Comprehension (auditory and written)	Impaired
Repetition	Impaired
Naming	Impaired
Reading aloud	Impaired
Writing	Impaired
Elementary neurological findings	Right hemiparesis, hemisensory loss and hemianopsia*
Behavioral findings	Lethargy, decreased attention
Localization	Left frontotemporoparietal*
Pathology	Stroke (internal carotid or proximal MCA), hemorrhage, tumor

*Global aphasia is almost never seen with unilateral right hemisphere lesions since patients with right hemisphere language function usually have incomplete dominance.

territory of the entire dominant middle cerebral artery, following occlusion of the internal carotid artery or the proximal middle cerebral artery. Global aphasia is usually accompanied by dense right-sided hemiparesis, hemisensory loss, and often hemianopsia. Patients may be lethargic during the acute stage, and patients with progressive edema can lapse into coma after 24 to 96 hours. A single lesion encompassing the frontal, parietal and temporal lobes is usually responsible (Kertesz *et al.*, 1979; Mazzocchi and Vignolo, 1979; Naeser and Hayward, 1978; Damasio, 1981).

Large dominant hemisphere tumors also cause global aphasia, especially when they are accompanied by edema. Occasionally, global aphasia results from discrete, non-contiguous anterior and posterior lesions, or large putaminal hemorrhages (Van Horn and Hawes, 1982; Tranel *et al.*, 1986; Legatt *et al.*, 1987).

In some cases, global aphasia is not accompanied by hemiparesis although right-sided hyperreflexia, Babinski sign and upper extremity drift are usually present. Global aphasia without hemiparesis results from multiple lesions or single large lesions that spare the precentral gyrus and descending pyramidal pathways. Most commonly, lesions are present in both Broca's and Wernicke's areas, or a single lesion is present anterior to the primary motor cortex and often involves the insula (Van Horn and Hawes, 1982; Ferro, 1983; Legatt *et al.*, 1987; Tranel *et al.*, 1987; Deleval *et al.*, 1989). With single anterior lesions, it is postulated that the comprehension deficit results from secondary dysfunction in parietotemporal language areas, which have been disconnected from Broca's and other association areas; i.e. diaschisis (Maxim 10). Lesions causing global aphasia without hemiparesis are usually due to embolic stroke, but also occur with tumor and hemorrhage (Legatt *et al.*, 1987). Recovery is usually rapid, as patients are able to communicate verbally within several weeks, although anterior aphasia usually persists (Deleval *et al.*, 1989).

References

Boller F. Strokes and behavior: disorders of higher cortical functions following cerebral disease. Disorders of language and related functions. *Stroke* 1981; **12**: 532–4.

Brust JCM, Shafer SQ, Richter RW, Bruun B. Aphasia in acute stroke. *Stroke* 1976; 7: 167–74.

Damasio H. Cerebral localization of the aphasias. In: *Acquired Aphasia* (Sarno MT, ed.). Orlando, FL: Academic Press, 1981, pp. 27–50.

Deleval J, Leonard A, Mavroudakis N, Rodesch G. Global aphasia without hemiparesis following prerolandic infarction. *Neurology* 1989; **39**: 1532–5.

Ferro JM. Global aphasia without hemiparesis. *Neurology* 1983; **33**: 1106.

Kertesz A, Harlock W, Coates R. Computer tomographic localization, lesion size, and prognosis in aphasia and nonverbal impairment. *Brain Lang* 1979; **8**: 34–50.

Kertesz A, McCabe P. Recovery patterns and prognosis in aphasia. *Brain* 1977; **100**: 1–18.

Legatt AD, Rubin MJ, Kaplan LR, Healton EB, Brust JCM. Global aphasia without hemiparesis: Multiple etiologies. *Neurology* 1987; **37**: 201–5.

Mazzocchi F, Vignolo LA. Localization of lesions in aphasia: clinical CT scan correlations in stroke patients. *Cortex* 1979; **15**: 627–54.

Naeser MA, Hayward RW. Lesion localization in aphasia with cranial computed
tomography and the Boston Diagnostic Aphasia Exam. *Neurology* 1978: **28**: 545–
51.

Tranel D, Biller J, Damasio H, Adams H. Global aphasia without hemiparesis.
Neurology 1986; **36**: 318 (Suppl).

Tranel D, Biller J, Damasio H, Adams HP, Cornell SH. Global aphasia without
hemiparesis. *Arch Neurol* 1987; **44**: 304–8.

Van Horn G, Hawes A. Global aphasia without hemiparesis: A sign of encephalopathy. *Neurology* 1982; **32**: 403–6.

34.   *Aphasia can result from subcortical lesions*

Human language has been seen as a phylogenetic pinnacle, reflecting the
advanced evolutionary status of association cortex. The finding that subcortical lesions can cause language dysfunction was surprising and paradoxical, since these areas are present in even lower vertebrates, albeit in a
much more primitive form. Subcortical aphasia has provoked a re-examination of how the human brain functions. Rather than refuting the concept
of cortical language areas, the observation that subcortical lesions can
impair language has emphasized the complex interrelations of cortex and
subcortex.

Lesions producing subcortical aphasias usually result from: (1) infarction
in the territory of the lateral lenticulostriate branches of the middle cerebral
artery that supply the basal ganglia and internal capsule; (2) infarction in
the territory of the thalamoperforant, especially the tuberothalamic,
arteries; (3) hemorrhage; and (4) tumor (Damasio *et al.*, 1982; Naeser *et al.*,
1982; Bogousslavsky *et al.*, 1988).

Subcortical areas affected in aphasia include the left putamen, caudate,
anterior limb of the internal capsule and thalamus. Subcortical aphasias
are heterogeneous, correspond imperfectly with classic cortical aphasic
syndromes, and tend to have a good prognosis. The affect of patients
with subcortical aphasia can be normal or range from indifference and
unconcern to mild depression, but the severe depression often present
with cortical aphasias is rare (Alexander and LoVerme, 1980; Watson and
Heilman, 1982).

Naeser *et al.* (1982) reported three aphasic syndromes resulting from
lesions in the *putamen and anterior limb of the internal capsule* and associated
with persistent right-sided hemiplegia. When the putaminal–capsular
lesion extended to anterior–superior white matter, patients had effortful,
slow, dysarthric speech, but normal comprehension and grammar. When
the lesion extended into the posterior white matter to involve the auditory
radiations and temporal isthmus, patients had fluent paraphasic speech

and impaired comprehension. Patients with lesions encompassing both anterior–superior and posterior white matter were globally aphasic.

Lesions involving the *head of the caudate and anterior limb of the internal capsule* often combine features of anterior and posterior cortical aphasias, with prominent stuttering and stammering (Damasio et al., 1982; Caplan et al., 1990). Acutely, speech is non-fluent and contaminated with semantic and phonemic paraphasias. In addition, patients usually have right-sided hemiparesis, dysarthria and dysprosodia. Comprehension and reading are usually normal. However, even if these functions are moderately impaired, improvement in all language symptoms is usually rapid and nearly complete.

When small and discrete lesions affect the anterior limb of the internal capsule, the adjacent corona radiata, or the head of the caudate, pure dysarthria without limb weakness can result (Ozaki et al., 1986; Caplan et al., 1990). Lacunar infarction is the most common etiology. Aphasia is not present in these patients, who usually recover from their dysarthria within two to four weeks.

In addition, subcortical lesions in the basal ganglia and thalamus of the right hemisphere can cause dysprosody (Maxim 51) (Ross, 1981; Wolfe and Ross, 1987). However, the clinical, neuroradiological and pathological data on dysprosody with subcortical lesions are limited.

Thalamic aphasia is characterized by fluctuations in language performance, low speech volume, fading or 'withering' of speech and preserved repetition. Acutely, patients are often mute with right-sided weakness and sensory loss, especially after cerebral hemorrhage. In addition, patients in the acute stage commonly display hypophonia, or low-volume speech, fluctuations in level of consciousness and variable language functions. For example, patients may alternate between an alert state with fairly normal speech and a lethargic condition with dysarthria, paraphasias, perseverations and progressive loss of speech volume (Mohr et al., 1975; McFarling et al., 1982). The aphasia closely resembles transcortical sensory aphasia, because repetition is well preserved and not contaminated by the paraphasias found in spontaneous speech. Speech is fluent or nearly so in most cases; mixed transcortical aphasia may rarely result from a thalamic lesion (McFarling et al., 1982; Tuszynski and Petito, 1988). Comprehension, naming and reading are often mildly impaired. In addition, the language disorder and hypophonia are often most evident as the patient's spontaneous speech fatigues or 'withers'. Thalamic aphasia often resolves or improves markedly with time.

Thalamic aphasia results from left-sided lesions that involve some combination of the ventral anterior, ventral lateral and dorsomedial nuclei (Bogousslavsky et al., 1986, 1988; Tuszynski and Petito, 1988). Right thalamic strokes in right-handed patients do not cause aphasia, but may cause left-sided neglect (Heilman and Valenstein, 1981). However, aphasia has been reported in a left-handed person after a right thalamic stroke (Kirshner and Kistler, 1982). Causes of lesions producing thalamic aphasia include infarction, cerebral hemorrhage, brain tumor and stereotactic surgery (Cheek and Taveras, 1966; Bell, 1968; Riklan *et al.*, 1969; Cappa and Vignolo, 1979; Alexander and LoVerme, 1980; Bogousslavsky *et al.*, 1988).

The mechanism for language impairment following left thalamic lesions is uncertain. Although secondary effects on other subcortical or cortical areas from edema and pressure may contribute in some cases, especially in those with severe hemorrhage, lesions restricted to the left thalamus can produce language dysfunction. Further evidence supporting a thalamic role in language function includes the observation that electrical stimulation of the ventral lateral nucleus and pulvinar produces naming errors (Ojemann *et al.*, 1968; Ojemann, 1975), and the existence of neural connections between these thalamic areas and frontal and parietotemporal language areas.

On the other hand, positron emission tomography and cerebral blood flow studies in patients with subcortical aphasia suggest that secondary effects on cortical function may cause language dysfunction (Olsen *et al.*, 1986; Perani *et al.*, 1987; Metter *et al.*, 1988). In these cases cortical hypometabolism and hypoperfusion may result from independent cortical lesions or diaschisis (Maxim 10).

References

Alexander MP, LoVerme SR. Aphasia after left hemispheric intracerebral hemorrhage. *Neurology* 1980; **30**: 1193–202.

Bell DS. Speech functions of the thalamus inferred from the effects of thalamotomy. *Brain* 1968; **91**: 619–38.

Bogousslavsky J, Miklossy J, Deruaz JP, Regli F, Assal G. Unilateral left paramedian infarction of the thalamus and midbrain: a clinico-pathologic study. *J Neurol Neurosurg Psychiat* 1986; **49**: 686–94.

Bogousslavsky J, Regli F, Uske A. Thalamic infarcts: clinical syndromes, etiology, and prognosis. *Neurology* 1988; **38**: 837–48.

Caplan LR, Schmahmann JD, Kase CS, Feldmann E, Baquis G, Greenberg JP, Gorelick PB, Helgason C, Hier DB. Caudate infarcts. *Arch Neurol* 1990; **47**: 133–43.

Cappa SF, Vignolo LA. 'Transcortical' features of aphasia following left thalamic hemorrhage. *Cortex* 1979; **15**: 121–30.

Cheek WR, Taveras JM. Thalamic tumors. *J Neurosurg* 1966; **24**: 505–13.

Damasio AR, Damasio H, Rizzo M, Varney N, Gersh F. Aphasia with non-hemorrhagic lesions in the basal ganglia and internal capsule. *Arch Neurol* 1982; **39**: 501–6.

Heilman KM, Valenstein E. Thalamic neglect: possible role of the medial thalamus and nucleus reticularis in behavior. *Arch Neurol* 1981; **38**: 501–6.

Kirshner HS, Kistler KH. Aphasia after right thalamic hemorrhage. *Arch Neurol* 1982; **39**: 667–9.

McFarling D, Rothi LJ, Heilman KM. Transcortical aphasia from ischaemic infarcts of the thalamus: a report of two cases. *J Neurol Neurosurg Psychiat* 1982; **45**: 107–12.

Metter EJ, Riege WH, Hanson WR, Jackson CA, Kempler D, van Lancker D. Subcortical structures in aphasia: An analysis based on (F-18)-fluorodeoxyglucose,

positron emission tomography, and computed tomography. *Arch Neurol* 1988;
45: 1229–34.

Mohr JP, Watters WC, Duncan GW. Thalamic hemorrhage and aphasia. *Brain Lang*
1975; **2**: 3–17.

Naeser MA, Alexander MP, Helm-Estabrooks N, Levine HL, Laughlin SA, Geschwind N. Aphasia with predominantly subcortical lesion sites. *Arch Neurol* 1982;
39: 2–14.

Ojemann G. Language and the thalamus: object naming and recall during and after
thalamic stimulation. *Brain Lang* 1975; **2**: 101–20.

Ojemann G, Fedio P, Van Buren J. Anomia from pulvinar and subcortical parietal
stimulation. *Brain* 1968; **91**: 99–116.

Olsen TS, Bruhn P, Oberg RGE. Cortical hypoperfusion as a possbile cause of
'subcortical aphasia'. *Brain* 1986; **109**: 393–410.

Ozaki I, Baba M, Narita S, Matsunaga M, Takebe K. Pure dysarthria due to anterior
internal capsule and/or corona radiata infarction: a report of five cases. *J Neurol
Neurosurg Psychiat* 1986; **49**: 1435–7.

Perani D, Vallar G, Cappa S, Messa C, Fazio F. Aphasia and neglect after subcortical
stroke. *Brain* 1987; **110**: 1211–29.

Riklan M, Levita E, Zimmerman J *et al.* Thalamic correlates of language and speech.
J Neurol Sci 1969; **8**: 307–28.

Ross ED. The aprosodias: Functional anatomic organization of the affective
components of language in the right hemisphere. *Arch Neurol* 1981; **38**: 561–9.

Tuszynski MH, Petito CK. Ischemic thalamic aphasia with pathologic confirmation.
Neurology 1988; **38**: 800–2.

Watson RT, Heilman KM. Affect in subcortical aphasia. *Neurology* 1982; **32**: 102–3.

Wolfe GI, Ross ED. Sensory aprosodia with left hemiparesis from subcortical infarction: Right hemisphere analogue of sensory-type aphasia with right hemiparesis?
Arch Neurol 1987; **44**: 668–71.

35.   *Aphasia therapy is controversial but may help some patients*

The controversy over the efficacy of aphasia therapy endures. The majority
of studies support the role of speech therapy for aphasia (Albert *et al.*,
1973; Hagen, 1973; Darley, 1975; Basso *et al.*, 1979; Wertz *et al.*, 1986)
but several controlled studies have found no benefit from speech therapy
compared with no treatment or therapy by trained volunteers (David *et al.*,
1982; Lincoln *et al.*, 1984).

Spontaneous recovery of language function does occur and is greater in
patients with traumatic than with cerebrovascular lesions (Kertesz and
McCabe, 1977). Among the various types of aphasia, the greatest recovery
is seen in Broca's and conduction aphasias. Anomic aphasia is often a
common end-stage for other acute aphasic syndromes. Long-term follow-
up shows that the prognosis is poor for patients with global aphasia, intermediate in Broca's and Wernicke's aphasias, and good in conduction,
anomic and transcortical aphasias (Kertesz and McCabe, 1977).

Numerous factors influence both spontaneous improvement and

response to speech therapy. Positive prognostic factors include young age at onset and left-handedness. Negative prognostic factors include large lesion, destruction of parietal and temporal language areas, severe comprehension deficit or apraxia, progressive lesions like tumors, limited education, low socioeconomic background, lack of family support and such neurobehavioral problems as depression, neglect and inattention.

The first step in patient assessment is determining whether speech therapy is likely to be beneficial or feasible. Acute medical problems, such as myocardial infarction or sepsis, depressed level of consciousness, delirium, dementia and severe global aphasia are all indications to defer therapy. A large Veterans Administration cooperative study demonstrated that delaying speech therapy for 12 weeks does not compromise ultimate improvement (Wertz *et al.*, 1986).

If the patient is capable of undergoing therapy, the speech pathologist or neuropsychologist then performs detailed analyses of language skills and neurobehavioral functions, such as attention, memory, praxis and visuospatial function. Strengths and weaknesses are identified to plan the treatment approach, which begins by concentrating on relatively preserved language functions, so that patients feel positive about their performance.

Treatment can be successful in either the home, clinic or inpatient setting. For patients with multiple physical, language and behavioral problems, an inpatient rehabilitation service may be most effective. An integrated, multidisciplinary approach involving the neurologist, speech pathologist, occupational and physical therapists, psychologist, social worker and family members is ideal. In many cases, consultation with a psychiatrist is necessary for treatment of depression.

Speech therapies vary with the individual pathologist and according to the different forms of aphasia. Table 35.1 shows some of the more common forms of speech therapy (Skelly *et al.*, 1975; Helm-Estabrooks *et al.*, 1982; Howard *et al.*, 1985). In general, speech therapy is conducted for 30 to 60 minutes daily for two to three months. It is beneficial to enlist family or friends to conduct additional homework sessions on language skills.

If formal speech therapy is not possible, patients may be helped by trained volunteers (David *et al.*, 1982). The volunteers, supervised by speech pathologists, can improve both motivation and communication skills.

Because lack of motivation and depression impair acquisition of language skills, helping the patient maintain a positive frame of mind and offering encouragement and emotional support during therapy are critical. The American Heart Association, American Stroke Association, the British Chest, Heart and Stroke Association, American-Speech-Hearing-Language Association, Easter Seal Foundation, local United Way and speech pathologists are often helpful in identifying community resources.

Table 35.1 Speech therapies.

Therapeutic Technique	Methodology	Aphasic group
Stimulation approach (Basso, 1979)	Use of facilitating stimuli; eliciting a response in an automatic way and then in a more voluntary way by withdrawing facilitory stimuli	All
Language comprehension training (Holland, 1979)	Reteaching meaning with use of verbal and non-verbal materials	Wernicke's; transcortical sensory; global
Amerind (American Indian Sign Language) (Skelly, 1975)	Non-verbal, hand signs to communicate language	Broca's; transcortical motor
Communication Boards	Pointing towards letters, words or pictures	Broca's; transcortical motor
Melodic intonation (Sparks, 1974)	Imbedding short phrases in simple melody; later, the melodic aspect is withdrawn	Broca's; transcortical motor
Visual action therapy (Helm-Estabrooks, 1982)	Facilitate gestural communication	Global
Word retrieval therapy (Howard, 1985)	Semantic (cues on word meaning) and phonologic (cues on word sounds)	All aphasias with anomia

References

Albert ML, Sparks RW, Helm NA. Melodic intonation therapy for aphasia. *Arch Neurol* 1973; **29**: 130–1.

Basso A, Capitani, Vignolo LA. Influence of rehabilitation on language skills in aphasic patients: A controlled study. *Arch Neurol* 1979; **36**: 190–6.

Darley F. Treatment of acquired aphasia. In: *Advances in Neurology* (volume 7) *Current Review of Higher Nervous System Dysfunction* (Friedlander W, ed.). New York: Raven Press, 1975.

David R, Enderby P, Bainton D. Treatment of acquired aphasia: speech therapists and volunteer compared. *J Neurol Neurosurg Psychiat* 1982; **45**: 957–61.

Hagen S. Communication abilities in hemiplegia: Effect of speech therapy. *Arch Phys Med Rehabil* 1973; **54**: 454–63.

Helm-Estabrooks N, Fitzpatrick PM, Baressi B. Visual action therapy for global aphasia. *J Speech Hear Dis* 1982; **47**: 385–9.

Holland AL. Treatment of aphasia after stroke. *Stroke* 1979; **10**: 475–7.

Howard D, Patterson K, Franklin S, Orchard-Lisle V, Morton J. Treatment of word retrieval deficits in aphasia: A comparison of two therapy methods. *Brain* 1985; **108**: 817–29.

Kertesz A, McCabe P. Recovery patterns and prognosis in aphasia. *Brain* 1977; **100**: 1–18.

Lincoln NB, Mulley GP, Jones AC, McGuirk E, Lendrem W, Mitchell JRA. Effectiveness of speech therapy for aphasic stroke patients: A randomized controlled trial. *Lancet* 1984; **i**: 1197–200.

Skelly R, Schinsky L, Smith R, Donaldson R, Griffin J. American Indian sign, a gestural communication system for the speechless. *Arch Phys Med Rehab* 1975; **56**: 156–60.

Sparks R, Helm N, Albert M. Aphasia rehabilitation resulting from melodic intonation therapy. *Cortex* 1974; **10**: 303–16.

Wertz RT, Weiss DG, Aten JL, Brookshire RH, Garcia-Bunuel L, Holland AL, Kurtzke JF, LaPointe LL, Milianti FJ, Brannegan R, Greenbaum H, Marshall RC, Vogel D, Carter J, Barnes NS, Goodman R. Comparison of clinic, home, and deferred language treatment for aphasia: A Veterans Administration cooperative study. *Arch Neurol* 1986; **43**; 653–8.

4
Amnesia

36. Bilateral lesions in the medial temporal–diencephalic circuit impair short-term memory

The limbic system is the anatomical core of memory. Like attention, however, memory is a distributed function not localized to a single center. Rather, memory is subserved by the integrated actions of a functional neuroanatomical network which includes both limbic and neocortical areas. In most cases of severe amnesia, bilateral lesions have damaged the medial temporal lobe, which includes the amygdala and hippocampus, or the diencephalon, which houses the dorsomedial nucleus and mamillary bodies (Zola-Morgan et al., 1982; Zola-Morgan and Squire, 1985; Victor et al., 1989).

The circuit of Papez (Maxim 61; Fig. 61.1) was originally described as a group of nuclei and their interconnections subserving emotion (Papez, 1937). However, these structures are also related to memory. In this circuit, neural communication travels from the hippocampus to the mamillary bodies via fornix, from the mamillary bodies to the anterior thalamic nuclei via the mamillothalamic tract, from the anterior thalamic nuclei to the cingulate gyrus via thalamocingulate fibers, and from the cingulate gyrus via cingulum back to the hippocampus. Although all structures in the Papez circuit play a role in memory, the hippocampus, fornix and mamillary bodies are most critical (Sweet et al., 1959; Milner, 1959; Brion et al., 1969; Gaffan, 1977; Moss et al., 1981; Holmes et al., 1983; Duyckaerts et al., 1985).

Diencephalic lesions are primarily responsible for the amnesia in the *Wernicke–Korsakoff syndrome*. This syndrome consists of two disorders: chronic severe impairment of anterograde memory, or Korsakoff's disease, and acute confusion, ataxia, nystagmus and ophthalmoplegia, or Wernicke's encephalopathy. The critical lesion site responsible for the memory disorder includes the dorsomedial (not the anterior) nuclei of the thalamus, with involvement of the mamillary bodies playing a controversial role (Mair et al., 1979; Victor et al., 1989).

The memory disorder in Korsakoff's disease may develop slowly or emerge *de novo* in the wake of Wernicke's encephalopathy. Thiamine deficiency is the cause of the Wernicke–Korsakoff syndrome; alcoholism is the most commonly associated condition, but other causes of nutritional compromise (e.g. advanced cancer) are not rare. Thiamine replacement is effective in reversing many of the features of Wernicke's encephalopathy, but has little or no effect on the memory disorder.

Patients with Korsakoff's disease have a severe problem with acquiring new information. Mild-to-moderate retrograde amnesia is a constant feature and confabulation is a common but not mandatory part of the syndrome. *Confabulation*, the creation of factitious responses by the patient to 'fill in' memory gaps, is by no means specific for Korsakoff's disease as it occurs in patients with frontal and, less often, left temporal lesions (Berlyne, 1972; Benson *et al.*, 1976; Mercer *et al.*, 1977; Kapur and Coughlan, 1980). Other behavioral problems in patients with Korsakoff's disease include euphoria, anosognosia (Maxim 63), disorientation, irritability and aggression.

Bilateral thalamic infarcts that involve the dorsomedial and paramedian nuclei produce both anterograde and retrograde memory disorders (McEntee *et al.*, 1976; Poirier *et al.*, 1981; Mehler, 1989). Most patients are acutely confused, and they may also display vertical gaze disorder, decreased spontaneity and aphasia. Unilateral infarction of the left anterolateral thalamus can cause amnesia with impaired verbal retrieval (Goldenberg *et al.*, 1983). For example, after a fencing foil passed through his right nostril into the left dorsal thalamic region, one patient developed anterograde amnesia that primarily affected verbal material (Squire and Moore, 1979). Disconnection, as well as destruction, of thalamic nuclei can produce amnesia in animals and humans (Mishkin, 1982; Warrington and Weiskrantz, 1982; von Cramon *et al.*, 1985).

Thalamic tumors may cause sudden or subacute onset of amnesia (Ziegler *et al.*, 1977). Hypothalamic tumors that invade the floor and adjacent walls of the third ventricle also cause amnesia (Williams and Pennybaker, 1954).

Medial temporal lesions are also associated with amnestic syndromes (Smith, 1989). Temporal lobectomy for medically intractable partial seizure disorders has provided a uniquely controlled setting to study human memory. Left anterior temporal lobectomy selectively impairs verbal memories, while right temporal lobectomy selectively impairs visuospatial and emotional memories (Corkin, 1965; Milner, 1968, 1973; Wechsler, 1973; Jones-Gotman, 1987; Smith, 1989). When bilateral medial temporal lobectomies were performed on one patient with epilepsy, he developed severe anterograde amnesia for both verbal and non-verbal materials (Scoville and Milner, 1957). Because of this dreaded complication, the bilateral procedure is no longer performed. Unilateral temporal lobe resection for seizure control can cause severe amnesia, presumably because of pre-existing damage in the unoperated hippocampus (Penfield and Milner, 1958; Milner, 1975). Use of the intracarotid sodium amytal (Wada) test prior to surgery tests memory function in each hemisphere, and has helped to prevent this devastating complication (Brown *et al.*, 1991).

Amnesia due to bilateral hippocampal damage may differ from the amnesia resulting from diencephalic lesions (Squire, 1982). With mesial temporal lesions, there is an accelerated rate of forgetting with impairment in both memory consolidation and retrieval. In contrast, there is a normal rate of forgetting in diencephalic amnesia, in which the deficit is principally in the encoding stage of memory.

Herpes simplex type I has a propensity for attacking the inferomedial portions of the temporal and frontal lobes, giving rise to prominent behavioral manifestations (e.g. confusion, temporal and frontal lobe seizures, and bizarre behavior) in the acute stage and a chronic amnesic syndrome (Maxim 61) (Rose and Symonds, 1960). The clinical characteristics of this memory disorder resemble that of bilateral anterior temporal lobectomies. When destruction of the anteromedial temporal lobes is severe, a full-blown Kluver–Bucy syndrome (Maxim 60) may develop.

Bilateral infarcts of the posterior cerebral arteries, which supply most of the hippocampus and parahippocampal areas, can produce a permanent amnesic disorder, as well as a transient or persistent confusional state (Symonds and MacKenzie, 1957; Victor *et al.*, 1961). Infarction of the left posterior cerebral artery can also cause confusion states and an amnesic syndrome, but the deficits are usually transient and any chronic memory dysfunction is mild (Benson *et al.*, 1974; Devinsky *et al.*, 1988).

Injury of the medial (limbic) temporal lobes by such mechanisms as anoxia, hypoglycemia, Alzheimer's and Pick's diseases, or focal neuronal loss in the amygdala and hippocampus can produce an amnesic syndrome (Duyckaerts *et al.*, 1985).

Damage to the basal forebrain regions, including the septal nuclei, nucleus accumbens, substantia innominata, caudal orbitofrontal areas and related pathways, can result in amnesia (Volpe and Hirst, 1983; Damasio *et al.*, 1985 a, b). The most common cause is rupture of anterior communicating artery aneurysms. Amnesia following basal forebrain damage can be both anterograde and retrograde. It is characterized by confabulation, improvement with cueing and inability to integrate learned items (e.g. associate a name and a face). Interruption of the robust interconnections between the basal forebrain and medial temporal lobe, as well as destruction of cholinergic and catecholaminergic neurons and pathways, probably causes the amnesic disorder. In addition, basal forebrain damage is associated with a behavioral syndrome that includes prominent personality changes affecting social judgment, affect, planning and executive functions.

Other lesions that cause memory impairment are less easily localized and result from a diverse group of disorders, procedures and substances. Causes of these structural or functional lesions include head trauma, epilepsy, depression, convulsive therapy, alcohol intoxication (as in blackouts), degenerative disorders (such as Alzheimer's disease and Huntington's chorea) and medications (including scopolamine and benzodiazepines).

The aging process is not a cause of amnesia *per se* but it reduces mnemonic powers, especially after the age of 60 years. Age-associated memory impairment (*Benign senescent forgetfulness*) is a slowly progressive, isolated memory disorder that is associated with aging but not with development of other cognitive impairments characteristic of dementia (Kral, 1962; Crook *et al.*, 1986). Individuals with benign senescent forgetfulness characteristically recall an experience, but have intermittent difficulty retrieving names, dates or places associated with the experience. This disorder of retrieval is an exaggeration of the normal forgetting of names and details that plagues all humans.

References

Benson DF, Gardner H, Meadows JC. Reduplicative paramnesia. *Neurology* 1976; **26**: 147–51.

Benson DF, Marsden CD, Meadows JC. The amnestic syndrome of posterior cerebral artery occlusion. *Acta Neurol Scand* 1974; **50**: 133–45.

Berlyne N. Confabulation. *Br J Psychiat* 1972; **120**: 31–9.

Brion S, Pragier C, Guerin R, Teitgen MMC. Korsakoff syndrome due to bilateral softening of fornix. *Rev Neurol (Paris)* 1969; **120**: 255–62.

Brown ER, Perrine K, Gershengorn J. Neuropsychological changes following temporal and frontal lobectomy. In: *Epilepsy and Behavior* (Devinsky O, Theodore WH, eds). New York: Alan R Liss, 1991, pp. 195–202.

Corkin S. Tactually-guided maze learning in man: Effects of unilateral cortical excisions and bilateral hippocampal lesions. *Neuropsychologia* 1965; **3**: 339–51.

Crook T, Bartus R, Ferris S *et al.* Age-associated memory impairment: Proposal diagnostic criteria and measures of clinical change – Report of a National Institute of Mental Health Work Group. *Dev Neuropsychol* 1986; **2**: 261–76.

Damasio AR, Eslinger PJ, Damasio H, Van Hoesen GW, Cornell S. Multimodal amnesic syndrome following bilateral temporal and basal forebrain damage. *Arch Neurol* 1985a; **42**: 252–9.

Damasio AR, Graff-Radford NR, Eslinger PJ, Damasio H, Kassell N. Amnesia following basal forebrain lesions. *Arch Neurol* 1985b; **42**: 263–71.

Devinsky O, Bear D, Volpe BT. Confusional states following posterior cerebral artery infarction. *Acta Neurol* 1988; **45**: 160–3.

Duyckaerts C, Derouesne C, Signoret JL, Gray F, Escourolle R, Castaigne P. Bilateral and limited amygdalohippocampal lesions causing a pure amnesic syndrome. *Ann Neurol* 1985; **18**: 314–19.

Gaffan D. Monkey's recognition memory for complex pictures and the effect of the fornix transection. *Q J Exp Psychol* 1977; **29**: 505–14.

Goldenberg G, Wimmer A, Maly J. Amnestic syndrome with a unilateral thalamic lesion: a case report. *J Neurol* 1983; **229**: 79–86.

Holmes EJ, Jacobson S, Stein BM, Butters N. Ablations of the mamillary nuclei in monkeys: effects on post-operative memory. *Exp Neurol* 1983; **81**: 97–113.

Jones-Gotman M. Psychological evaluation: testing hippocampal function. In: *Surgical Treatment of the Epilepsies* (Engel J, ed.). New York: Raven Press, 1987, pp. 203–11

Kapur N, Coughlan AK. Confabulation and frontal lobe dysfunction. *J Neurol Neurosurg Psychiat* 1980; **43**: 461–3.

Kral VA. Senescent forgetfulness: benign and malignant. *Can Med Assoc J* 1962; **86**: 257–60.

Mair WGP, Warrington EK, Weiskrantz L. Memory disorder in Korsakoff's psychosis. A neuropathological and neuropsychological investigation of two cases. *Brain* 1979; **102**: 749–83.

McEntee WJ, Biber MP, Perl DP, Benson DF. Diencephalic amnesia: A reappraisal. *J Neurol Neurosurg Psychiat* 1976; **39**: 436–41.

Mehler MF. The rostral basilar artery syndrome: Diagnosis, etiology, prognosis. *Neurology* 1989; **39**: 9–16.

Mercer B, Wapner W, Gardner H, Benson DF. A study of confabulation. *Arch Neurol* 1977; **34**: 429–33.

Milner B. Discussion of 'Loss of recent memory following section of the fornix'. *Trans Am Neurol Assoc* 1959; **84**: 78–9.

Milner B. Visual recognition and recall after right temporal-lobe excision in man. *Neuropsychologia* 1968; **6**: 191–209.

Milner B. Hemispheric specialization: Scope and limits. In: *The Neurosciences: Third Study Program* (Schnitt FO, Wordern FG, eds). Boston, MA: MIT Press, 1973, pp. 75–89.

Milner B. Psychological aspects of focal epilepsy and its neurosurgical management. In: *Advances in Neurology* (volume 8) (Purpura DP, Penry JK Walter R, eds), 1975, pp. 209–321.

Mishkin M. A memory system in the monkey. *Phil Trans Roy Soc B (London)* 1982; **298**: 83–95.

Moss M, Mahut H, Zola-Morgan SM. Concurrent discrimintation learning of monkeys after hippocampal, entorhinal or fornix lesions. *J Neurosci* 1981; **1**: 227–40.

Papez JW. A proposed mechanism of emotion. *Arch Neurol Psychiat* 1937; **38**: 725–43.

Penfield W, Milner B. Memory deficit produced by bilateral lesions in the hippocampal zones. *Arch Neurol Psychiat* 1958; **79**: 475–97.

Poirier J, Barbizet J, Gaston A, Meyrignac C. Demence thalamique. Lacunes expansives au territoire thalamo-mesencepahlique. paramedian. Hydrocephalie par stenose de l'aqueduc de Sylvius. *Rev Neurol* 1981; **139**: 349–58.

Rose FC, Symonds CP. Persistant memory defect following encephalitis. *Brain* 1960; **83**: 195–212.

Scoville WB, Milner B. Loss of recent memory after bilateral hippocampal lesions. *J Neurol Neurosurg Psychiat* 1957; **20**: 11–21.

Smith ML. Memory disorders associated with temporal-lobe lesions. In: *Handbook of Neuropsychology* (volume 3) (Boller F, Grafman J, eds). Amsterdam: Elsevier Science Publications 1989, pp. 91–106.

Squire LR. Comparisons between forms of amnesia: some deficits are unique to Korsakoff's syndrome. *J Exp Psychol Mem Learn Cog* 1982; **8**: 560–71.

Squire LR, Moore RY. Dorsal thalamic lesion in a noted case of chronic memory dysfunction. *Ann Neurol* 1979; **6**: 503–6.

Sweet WH, Tallande GA, Ervin FR. Loss of recent memory following section of the fornix. *Trans Am Neurol Assoc* 1959; **84**: 76–82.

Symonds C, MacKenzie I. Bilateral loss of vision from cerebral infarction. *Brain* 1957; **80**: 415–55.

Victor M, Adams RD, Collins GH. The Wernicke–Korsakoff syndrome and related neurologic disorders due to alcoholism and malnutrition. Philadelphia: FA Davis Company, 1989.

Victor M, Angevine JB, Mancall EL, Fisher CM. Memory loss with lesions of the hippocampal formation. *Arch Neurol* 1961; **5**: 244–63.

Volpe BT, Hirst W. Amnesia following rupture and repair of an anterior communicating artery aneurysm. *J Neurol Neurosurg Psychiat* 1983; **46**: 704–9.

von Cramon DY, Hebel N, Schuri U. A contribution to the anatomical basis of thalamic amnesia. *Brain* 1985; **108**: 993–1008.

Warrington EK, Weiskrantz L. Amnesia: a disconnection syndrome? *Neuropsychologia* 1982; **20**: 233–48.

Wechsler AF. The effect of organic brain disease on recall of remotionally charged vs. neutral narrative texts. *Neurology* 1973; **23**: 130–5.

Williams M, Pennybaker J. Memory disturbances in third ventricle tumors. *J Neurol Neurosurg Psychiat* 1954; **17**: 115–23.

Ziegler DW, Kaufman A, Marshall HE. Abrupt memory loss associated with thalamic tumor. *Arch Neurol* 1977; **34**: 545–8.

Zola-Morgan S, Squire LR. Amnesia in monkeys after lesions of the mediodorsal nucleus of the thalamus. *Ann Neurol* 1985; **17**: 558–64.

Zola-Morgan S, Squire LR, Mishkin M. The neuroanatomy of amnesia: Amygdala-hippocampal versus temporal stem. *Science* 1982; **218**: 1337–9.

37.   Memory is a complex process: there are different forms and multiple overlapping stages

Memory joins our past and present. Our memories allow us to interpret and react to new perceptions in the light of past experience. Disruption of mnemonic function is devastating when it prevents learning of any new information or recognizing one's home and family. Isolated disorders of memory may be generalized and encompass all classes of information or they may affect specific types of information, such as verbal or visual material.

The assessment of memory is difficult and requires an appreciation of the complexity of memory processing, as well as the differences between bedside and neuropsychological tests and real life. The inconsistent terminology of normal and abnormal memory functions has further clouded this area. Let us begin by exploring different classifications and divisions of memory processes.

Forms of memory

Memory has classically been divided into three forms, based on how long the information is stored: *immediate, short-term and long-term memory.*

Immediate memory is a misnomer; attention span more accurately describes this function. Patients with attentional disorders such as delirium have memory dysfunction, not because they are unable to recall information, but because of inability to focus or sustain their cognition. Indeed, if any patient is not listening or attending to your presentation of information, they will not recall it. The most common bedside test of attention measures the number of digits that a patient can repeat, or digit span (Maxim 6). Normal persons can repeat at least seven digits (Miller, 1956). When evaluating memory by other tests, such as asking a subject to recall several words or objects, it is important to have the patient repeat the words or cues immediately after presentation in order to ensure attentiveness. While delirious patients do poorly on digit span testing and immediate recall of word lists, patients with pure memory disorders typically have intact attention span (Sidman *et al.*, 1968; Baddeley and Warrington, 1970).

Short-term memory enables us to recall information over a period of minutes to days. The most vulnerable component of memory, it is tested at the bedside by asking the patient to repeat three or four words immediately and recall the same words five minutes later. After initial repetition of the words, other cognitive functions (e.g. calculations) should be tested to prevent the subject from silently repeating and memorizing the words. If the subject is unable to recall any of the words, the examiner should cue the subject to identify the word from a list. If a deficit is again registered, then visual memory is tested by pointing to three objects and asking the subject to point to the objects immediately and after five minutes. Visual memory testing is especially important if the patient is aphasic. While these tests, used in combination, constitute the most common bedside assessment of short-term memory, attention problems and anxiety due to the clinical setting occasionally produce false 'memory deficits'. Also, some patients will simply repeat the words over and over and perform poorly on intervening tests like simple subtraction, because they are focusing on the words to be recalled. They may then be incorrectly assessed as having intact short-term memory and impaired arithmetic skills. Thus, the 'three word – five minute' memory test is at best a crude indicator of short-term memory function.

Long-term memory refers to the recall of information and experiences from the remote past, such as childhood, historical dates and such general information as names of the months or the capital of France. Questions to test remote memories tend to be more general and encompass a broader time period than questions about recent memories. Documenting impairment is therefore easier in short-term rather than long-term memory (Squire, 1982).

The distinction between short- and long-term memory is controversial, and some consider it an artificial division of a continuous function (Craik and Lockart, 1972; Crowder, 1982). Also, one researcher's temporal criteria for short-term memory may fulfil another's definition for long-term memory (Klatzky, 1980; Delis, 1989). For clarity, it is best to describe how a patient performed on specific memory tests, rather than simply referring to a deficit in short-term or long-term memory. For example, describe the patient's impairment of immediate recall, of delayed recall after 3 or 20 minutes, or recall of information about historical events or persons.

A second theoretical system divides memory into two types, based on what kind of information is stored: *declarative and procedural memory*.

Declarative memory refers to the ability to remember names, faces, facts, events – all those items we were tested on in school (Squire and Cohen, 1984). Declarative memory is comprised of semantic and episodic components (Tulving, 1983). Semantic memory includes verbal information as well as pictorial images. Episodic memory includes personal and autobiographical memories, such as one's home address or activities yesterday. Semantic, visual and episodic memories are interrelated functionally and anatomically, but can demonstrate independence. In Huntington's disease, for example, patients may be significantly impaired in recalling personal, episodic memories but perform well on confrontational naming tests of semantic memory (Butters *et al.*, 1978; Albert *et al.*, 1981b).

Procedural memory refers to the ability to learn perceptual–motor tasks such as mirror reading (Cohen *et al.*, 1980; Squire and Cohen, 1982, 1984). The performance of these tasks is not mediated by conscious cognition. Patients with Korsakoff's psychosis, for example, suffer severe loss of declarative memory, but may have normal procedural memory and learning (Gardner *et al.*, 1973; Shimamura, 1986).

Stages of memory

The process of memory formation is divided into three sequential steps: *encoding, storage and retrieval.* Encoding is the formation of mental memory traces; storage refers to the laying down of more permanent memory traces; and retrieval refers to the process of remembering.

Encoding can be further divided into the processes of holding and acquisition (Signoret, 1985). Holding allows the temporary retention of information that exceeds the attention span. Interference (see below) disrupts the holding process of short-term memory in amnesics to a much greater extent than in normal persons (Huppert and Piercy, 1977). Acquisition is the process by which information is analyzed and organized. For example, telephone numbers are recalled by specific 'chunking' of digits or street names are recalled by linking them with associated stores. The encoding of memory often involves association with prior memories and cross-referencing among different sensory modalities and between language and emotional contexts. Thus, the childhood memories and emotions of a Thanksgiving meal may be evoked by a picture of grandma or the smell of sweet potatoes.

Storing is the process by which transient memory traces are consolidated and reconstructed into stable or long-term memories. Memory traces are dynamic phenomena. They do not simply sit in a storage bin, but are linked with other memories and integrated with new experiences.

Retrieving allows selective scanning and activation of memories from short- or long-term memory stores (Corballis, 1979). Failure to retrieve information leads to amnesia, in which the memories are intact but cannot be freely recalled. The simplest way to distinguish between amnesic disorders due to impaired retrieval and amnesic disorders due to impaired encoding and storage is to test both free recall and recognition. Recognition is tested by having patients choose the target stimulus from a group. Patients with defective encoding or storage will fail both to recall or to recognize stimuli, while those with defective retrieval will fail to recall freely but will succeed in recognizing stimuli. An impairment of retrieval may underlie the memory disorders associated with basal ganglia and frontal lesions (Butters *et al.*, 1985; Janowsky *et al.*, 1989).

Memory and learning are intimately related. 'Learning is the *process* of acquiring new information, while memory refers to the *persistence* of learning in a state that can be revealed at a later time' (Squire, 1987). In clinical practice, memory tests assess how much information can be recalled after a single presentation and a delay ranging from seconds (i.e. immediate recall) to days (i.e. long-term memory). In contrast, learning refers to the improvement of recall after successive presentations of the same information. Tests that assess learning include the Paired-Associate subtest of the Wechsler Memory Scale-Revised (Wechsler, 1987), the selective reminding procedure (Buschke, 1973), the Rey Auditory Verbal Learning Test (Lezak, 1983) and the California Verbal Learning Test (Delis *et al.*, 1987).

Dissociation can occur between memory and learning impairment. After unilateral temporal lobectomy patients may show selective deficits in learning tasks and verbal and non-verbal memory (Corkin, 1965; Corsi, 1972; Jones-Gotman, 1987; Smith, 1989). Patients with frontal lesions may demonstrate normal short-term memory by performing well with the first presentation and recall of material, but show impaired learning by failing to improve on subsequent presentations (Luria, 1981). Also, anxious subjects may perform poorly on the initial memory trial but then show significant improvement from learning on later trials (Lezak, 1983).

Interference occurs when a cognitive task has a negative effect on memory and learning. Proactive interference results when previously learned material intrudes on learning new items. For example, a medical student who has already memorized the nerve supply to the upper extremity may have difficulty learning the nerve supply to the lower extremity. As she studies, the already-learned names of muscles supplied by the radial and ulnar nerves become confused with those for muscles supplied by the peroneal and tibial nerves. In contrast, retroactive interference is the disruption of previously learned information by newly acquired material. In the above example, the student may have memorized all the upper extremity anatomy, but lost some of this hard-won data on learning the lower extremity.

The Rey Auditory Verbal Learning Test, in which the subject learns two word lists, is an effective means to assess retroactive and proactive interference (Lezak, 1983). If learning the first list impairs learning the second list, there is proactive interference. If learning the second list impairs later recall of the first, the interference is retroactive.

Memory disorders may be associated with both forms of interference, as in early Parkinson's disease or only one form, as in retroactive interference in Alzheimer's disease (Wilson *et al.*, 1983; Delis *et al.*, 1987).

Temporal components: anterograde and retrograde amnesias

Amnesic disorders may disrupt anterograde and retrograde knowledge. In *anterograde amnesia*, the holding and acquiring memory processes are impaired (Squire, 1982), and patients perform poorly on tests of short-term memory. In most patients with amnesia, the anterograde component is more severe and disabling (Hirst, 1982). The test battery most commonly used to assess anterograde memory is the Wechsler Memory Scale (WMS; Wechsler, 1945, 1987). The WMS provides a memory quotient that does not differentiate between specific memory tasks and is analogous to the intelligence quotient.

Anterograde amnesia may be restricted to new forms or patterns. Hanley *et al.* (1990) reported on a woman who sustained right hemisphere damage and was subsequently able to learn new visual information that related to a familiar visual form but was unable to learn unfamiliar faces or objects. In addition, she could identify faces of celebrities from before her injury, but was unable to identify the faces of individuals who became famous after her injury. She was also poor at remembering unfamiliar voices.

In *retrograde amnesia*, patients are unable to recall events occurring before the brain insult. Retrograde amnesia usually accompanies anterograde amnesia, but is often mild and affects memory for specific time periods of days, weeks, months or several years. Retrograde amnesia is usually assessed by asking the patient to recall major historical figures or events during their lifetime, as well as autobiographical information that can be confirmed by relatives or friends (Barbizet, 1970; Squire and Slater, 1975). The oldest memories are the most resistant to dissolution (Albert *et al.*, 1979). This temporal gradient, in which childhood memories are relatively preserved, is most often seen in cases with bilateral temporal lesions, Korsakoff syndrome and mild Alzheimer's disease (Albert *et al.*, 1979; Zola-Morgan *et al.*, 1982; Beatty *et al.*, 1987; Squire *et al.*, 1989; Victor *et al.*, 1989). In contrast, retrograde amnesia, in patients with Huntington's and moderate-to-severe Alzheimer's diseases does not show as much of a temporal gradient (Albert *et al.*, 1981a; Wilson *et al.*, 1981).

In conclusion, overlapping systems classify the mnemonic processes and amnesic disorders, further complicating our understanding of the intricate functions of memory. The limitations of bedside testing must be recognized. Indeed, the amnesias are one area in which the thorough and quantitative approach of neuropsychology may be most helpful in identifying the nature of the disorder and following its course over time.

References

Albert MS, Butters N, Brandt J. Patterns of remote memory in amnesic and demented patients. *Arch Neurol* 1981a; **38**: 495–500.

Albert MS, Butters N, Brandt J. Development of remote memory loss in patients with Huntington's disease. *J Clin Neuropsychol* 1981b; **3**: 1–12.

Albert MS, Butters N, Levin J. Temporal gradients in the retrograde amnesia with alcoholic Korsakoff's disease. *Arch Neurol* 1979; **36**: 211–16.

Baddeley AD, Warrington EK. Amnesia and the distinction between long- and short-term memory. *J Verbal Learn Verbal Behav* 1970; **9**: 176–89.

Barbizet J. *Human Memory and its Pathology*. San Francisco, CA: Freeman and Company, 1970.

Beatty WW, Salmon DP, Butters N, Heindel WC, Granholm EP. Retrograde amnesia in patients with Alzheimer's disease or Huntington's disease. *Neurobiol Aging* 1987; **9**: 181–6.

Buschke H. Selective reminding for analysis of memory and behavior. *J Verbal Learn Verbal Behav* 1973; **12**: 543–50.

Butters N, Sax D, Montgomery K, Tarlow S. Comparison of the neuropsychological deficits associated with early and advance Huntington's disease. *Arch Neurol* 1978; **35**: 585–9.

Butters N, Wolfe J, Martone M, Cranholm E, Cermak LS. Memory disorders associated with Huntington's disease: verbal recall, verbal recognition and procedural memory. *Neuropsychologia* 1985; **23**: 729–43.

Cohen NJ, Squire LR. Preserved learning and retention of pattern analyzing skill in amnesia: dissociation of knowing how and knowing what. *Science* 1980; **210**: 207–9.

Corballis MC. Memory retrieval and the problem of scanning. *Psychol Rev* 1979; **86**: 157–60.

Corkin S. Tactually-guided maze-learning in man: effects of unilateral cortical excisions and bilateral hippocampal lesions. *Neuropsychologia* 1965; **3**: 339–51.

Corsi P. *Human Memory and the Medial Temporal Region of the Brain* (unpublished PhD thesis). Montreal: McGill University, 1972.

Craik FIM, Lockhart RS. Levels of processing: a framework for memory research. *J Verbal Learn Verbal Behav* 1972; **11**: 671–84.

Crowder RG. The demise of short-term memory. *Acta Psychol* 1982; **50**: 291–323.

Delis DC. Neuropsychological assessment of learning and memory. In: *Handbook of Neuropsychology* (Volume 3) (Boller F, Grafman J, eds). Amsterdam, New York: Elsevier Science Publications, 1989, pp. 3–33.

Delis DC, Kramer JH, Kaplan E, Ober BA. *The California Verbal Learning Test*. New York: The Psychological Corporation, 1987.

Gardner H, Boller F, Moreines J, Butters N. Retrieving information from Korsakoff patients: effects of categorized cues and reference to the task. *Cortex* 1973; **9**: 165–75.

Hanley JR, Pearson NA, Young AW. Impaired memory for new visual forms. *Brain* 1990; **113**: 1131–48.

Hirst W. The amnestic syndrome: descriptions and explanations. *Psychol Bull* 1982; **91**: 435–60.

Huppert FA, Piercy M. Recognition memory in amnesic patients: A defect of acquisition? *Neuropsychologia* 1977; **15**: 643–52.

Janowsky JS, Shimamura AP, Squire LR. Source memory impairment in patients with frontal lobe lesions. *Neuropsychologia* 1989; **27**: 1043–56.

Jones-Gotman M. Psychologic evaluation: testing hippocampal function. In: *Surgical Treatment of the Epilepsies*, (Engel J Jr, ed.). New York: Raven Press, 1987, pp. 203–11.

Klatzky RL. *Human Memory: Structure and Processes*. San Francisco, CA: Freeman and Company, 1980.

Lezak MD. *Neuropsychological Assessment*. Oxford, New York: Oxford University Press, 1983.

Luria AR. *Higher Cortical Functions in Man*. New York: Basic Books, 1981.

Miller GA. The 'magical' number 7, plus or minus two: some limits on our capacity for processing information. *Psychol Rev* 1956; **63**: 81–97.

Shimamura AP. Priming effects in amnesia: evidence for a dissociable memory function. *Q J Exp Psychol* 1986; **38**: 619–44.

Sidman M, Stoddard LT, Mohr JP. Some additional quantitative observations of immediate memory in a patient with bilateral hippocampal lesions. *Neuropsychologia* 1968; **6**: 245–54.

Signoret JL. Memory and amnesias. In: *Principles of Behavioral Neurology* (Mesulam MM, eds). Philadelphia: FA Davis Company, 1985, pp. 169–92.

Smith ML. Memory disorders associated with temporal-lobe lesions. In: *Handbook of Neuropsychology* (volume 3) (Boller F, Grafman J, eds). Amsterdam, New York: Elsevier Publications, 1980, pp. 91–106.

Squire LR. The neuropsychology of human memory. *Ann Rev Neurosci* 1982; **5**: 241–73.

Squire LR. *Memory and Brain*. Oxford, New York: Oxford University Press, 1987, p. 3.

Squire LR, Cohen NJ. Remote memory, retrograde amnesia, and the neuropsychology of memory. In: *Human Memory and Amnesia* (Cermak LS, ed.). Hillsdale, NY: Erlbaum, 1982.

Squire LR, Cohen NJ. Human memory and amnesia. In: *Neurobiology of Learning and Memory* (Lynch G, McGaugh JL, Weinberger NM, eds). New York: Guilford Press, 1984.

Squire LR, Haist F, Shimamura AP. The neurology of memory: quantitative assessment of retrograde amnesia in two groups of amnestic patients. *J Neurosci* 1989; **9**: 828–39.

Squire LR, Slater PC. Forgetting in very long-term memory as assessed by an improved questionnaire technique. *J Exp Psychol Hum Learn Mem* 1975; **104**: 50–4.

Tulving E. *Elements of Episodic Memory*. Oxford: Clarendon Press, 1983.

Victor M, Adams RD, Collins GH. *The Wernicke–Korsakoff Syndrome*. Philadelphia: FA Davis Company, 1989.

Wechsler DA. A standardized memory scale for clinical use. *J Psychol* 1945; **19**: 87–95.

Wechsler DA. *Wechsler Memory Scale-Revised*. New York: The Psychological Corporation, 1987.

Wilson RS, Bacan LD, Fox JH, Kaszniak AW. Primary memory and secondary memory in dementia of the Alzheimer type. *J Clin Neuropsychol* 1983; **5**: 337–44.

Wilson RS, Kaszniak AW, Fox JH. Remote memory in senile dementia. *Cortex* 1981; **17**: 41–8.

Zola-Morgan S, Squire LR, Mishkin M. The neuroanatomy of amnesia: Amygdala-hippocampal versus temporal stem. *Science* 1982; **218**: 1337–9.

38.   *Transient global amnesia is a benign disorder, but it must be distinguished from other causes of temporary amnesia*

Originally reported by Bender in 1956, the clinical features associated with transient global amnesia (TGA) were expanded in 1958 by Fisher and Adams, who also coined the name. The syndrome has recently been reviewed (Caplan, 1985; Hodges and Warlow, 1990).

Transient global amnesia occurs in middle-aged and elderly adults, with such presenting symptoms as confusion, anxiety, mild-to-moderate agitation and amnesia. The patient typically repeats questions concerning location ('Where am I?', 'How did I get here?'), objects in the environment ('Whose car is that?'), and time. Episodes begin abruptly and usually last from two to four hours, although the duration can range from 30 minutes to 24 hours. During the attack, patients retain personal identity and can recall remote memories, but are unable to store or retrieve newly acquired information. Thus, when patients are told the location and date, they will often repeat the question a minute later having remembered neither the previous question nor the answer. During the attack, performance of complex motor tasks is preserved; the patient may skillfully drive a car, dress or throw a ball.

After the attack of TGA has resolved, patients often have retrograde amnesia spanning minutes to hours, during which they cannot recall events before the episode's onset. Patients also often experience anterograde amnesia lasting hours, in which they store and retrieve information in short-term memory, but are unable to recall it the following day (Meador et al., 1985; Kritchevsky et al., 1988).

The following case is typical:

> A 54-year-old man was returning home from a local supermarket with his son. As they approached the house, he continued to drive, and the son asked where they were going. The father replied, 'Where am I, what are we doing here?' When the patient was seen in the emergency room 30 minutes later, neurological examination was remarkable only for slight irritability, disorientation for time and place, and short-term memory loss. Symptoms resolved after three hours, although there was retrograde memory impairment for twenty minutes before and anterograde memory loss extending two hours after the attack.

In many cases, attacks follow specific precipitating factors. The most common precipitants (in order of decreasing frequency) are physical exertion, sexual intercourse, emotional stress, physical symptoms (e.g. pain, nausea, vomiting), exposure to cold temperatures and mild head trauma (Fisher, 1982a; Haas and Ross, 1986; Miller et al., 1987a,b).

The pathophysiology of TGA is uncertain. Multiple mechanisms have been implicated, including migraine, vasospasm and ischemia induced by thrombotic or embolic, structural lesions (Jensen and Olivarius, 1980; Caplan et al., 1981; Crowell et al., 1984); Leao's spreading depression (Olesen and Jorgensen, 1986); and partial epilepsy (Fisher and Adams, 1964; Greene and Bennett, 1974). In individual cases, evidence to support a specific mechanism is usually lacking. Migraine and vasospasm are the most likely causes when the disorder is associated with such precipitating factors as physical exertion and cold exposure. Curiously, however, TGA is not very common in younger persons with migraine or with partial epilepsy. In addition, the EEG is almost always normal both during and between attacks in TGA patients (Rowan and Protass, 1979; Miller *et al.*, 1987b).

Caplan (1986) proposed four criteria for the diagnosis of TGA: (1) onset of the attack should be witnessed; (2) dysfunction during the attack should be limited to repetitive queries and amnesia; (3) there should be no other major neurological signs and symptoms; and (4) the memory loss should be transient, usually lasting hours or up to one day. When these criteria are met, the diagnosis of TGA is certain and a good prognosis can almost always be assured.

Hodges and Warlow (1990) added a fifth criterion for benign outcome: attack duration of longer than one hour. In their study of 153 cases of transient amnesia, attacks that lasted less than one hour and rapidly recurred were often diagnosed as epilepsy.

Transient global amnesia episodes recur in only 10 to 20 percent of patients (Nausieda and Sherman, 1979; Shuping *et al.*, 1980). In addition, the incidence of subsequent transient ischemic attacks and strokes among TGA patients is not significantly different from that in the general population matched for age and sex (Nausdieda, 1979; Shuping *et al.*, 1980; Hinge *et al.*, 1986; Miller 1987a; Hodges and Warlow, 1990).

Although one neuropsychological follow-up study (Mazzucchi *et al.*, 1980) observed deficits in verbal long-term memory and in verbal IQ among TGA patients, others have found normal memory and IQ at follow-up (Matias-Guiu and Codina, 1985; Kritchevsky *et al.*, 1988).

When diagnosing TGA, it is important to keep in mind that fragmentary historical information concerning the episode or a neurological history and examination revealing additional signs or symptoms do not usually indicate classic TGA. Instead, the patient may have one of many alternative disorders that are associated with amnesia. Table 38.1 lists other conditions associated with transient amnesia that should be distinguised from TGA.

Among these other conditions that cause amnesia, head trauma is probably the most common culprit. When head trauma triggers disorientation and amnesia, the injury is often significant and associated with brief loss of consciousness, as well as with other neurological signs and symptoms. In some cases, however, relatively minor head injuries trigger prominent amnesia lasting up to 24 hours (Suping *et al.*, 1980). Amnesia can also occur with sudden head movements without trauma, i.e. whiplash amnesia. Whiplash amnesia is diagnosed only if (1) onset of amnesia was at the time of the whiplash injury; (2) cervical pain is present; (3) head trauma did not occur; and (4) attacks are otherwise typical of TGA (Fisher, 1982b; Matias-Guiu *et al.*, 1985).

Migraine may cause amnesia with or without other neurological abnormalities, and it is usually followed by headache (Croft *et al.*, 1973; Olivarius and Jensen, 1979; Caplan *et al.*, 1981).

Complex partial seizures always produce amnesia during the episode, and occasionally patients – usually those with right temporal foci – repetitively utter the same phrase or question (Serafetinides and Falconer, 1963).

Table 38.1   Disorders associated with transient amnesia.

Transient global amnesia
Head trauma
Whiplash
Migraine
Epilepsy
Convulsive therapy
Cerebral ischemia
Polycythemia vera
Coronary and cerebral angiography
Hypoglycemia
Drug intoxication
   Diazepam
   Digitalis
   Scopolamine
Alcoholic blackout
Brain tumor
Dissociative disorders

However, motor automatisms (e.g. lip smacking, swallowing, hand rubbing) and unresponsiveness (e.g. inability to follow a command such as 'Show me your hand') clearly distinguish most complex partial seizures from TGA (Theodore *et al.*, 1983). In addition, both spontaneous and electrically induced generalized tonic–clonic seizures are usually followed by transient amnesia (Fleminger *et al.*, 1970), and there may be an extremely small group of patients with partial epilepsy who have seizures that resemble TGA.

Patients with brain tumors may develop brief amnesic episodes that result from seizure activity or other mechanisms (Lisak and Zimmerman, 1977; Findler *et al.*, 1983).

Cerebral ischemia in the territory of the posterior cerebral artery, which affects the thalamus and mid-posterior hippocampus, produces transient or persistent amnesia (Benson *et al.*, 1974; Longridge *et al.*, 1979). Transient ischemic attacks, infarction and hemorrhagic strokes may produce transient amnesia (Shuttleworth and Wise, 1973; Jensen and Olivarius, 1980; Gorelick *et al.*, 1988; Moonis *et al.*, 1988).

Hypoglycemia often causes episodic confusion and amnesia (Service *et al.*, 1976). Drugs that can trigger transient amnesia include alcohol, which can cause 'blackouts', benzodiazepines and anticholinergics (Goodwin *et al.*, 1969). In fact, this property has led to the occasional criminal use of anticholinergic drugs for 'pharmacologic mugging' attacks, in which the mugger spikes a drink with scopolamine and wipes out the victim's memory of the drink, the hours before the drink and of the mugger.

Finally, dissociative disorders, including multiple personality disorder, psychogenic fugue and psychogenic amnesia, are characterized by disturbances of self and memory (American Psychiatric Association, 1987). Loss of personal identity in psychogenic fugue and amnesia distinguishes these disorders from TGA (Maxims 39 and 97).

References

American Psychiatric Association. *Diagnostic and Statistical Manual of Mental Disorders* (3rd edition, revised). Washington, DC: American Psychiatric Association Press, 1987.

Bender MB. Syndrome of isolated episode of confusion with amnesia. *J Hillside Hosp* 1956; **5**: 212–15.

Benson DF, Marsden CD, Meadows JC. The amnesic syndrome of posterior cerebral artery occlusion. *Acta Neurol Scand* 1974; **50**: 133–45.

Caplan LR. Transient global amnesia. In: *Handbook of Clinical Neurology* (volume 1 (45)) (Vinken P, Bruyn G, Klawans H, eds). Amsterdam: Elsevier Science Publishing, 1985, pp. 205–18.

Caplan LR. Transient global amnesia: criteria and classification. *Neurology* 1986; **36**: 441.

Caplan LR, Chedru F, Lhermitte F, Mayman C. Transient global amnesia and migraine. *Neurology* 1981; **31**: 1167–70.

Croft PB, Heathfield KWG, Swash M. Differential diagnosis of transient amnesia. *Br Med J* 1973; **4**: 593–6.

Crowell GF, Stump DA, Biller J, McHenry LC, Toole JF. The transient global amnesia–migraine connection. *Arch Neurol* 1984; **41**: 75–9.

Findler G, Feinsod M, Lijovetzky G, Hadani M. Transient global amnesia associated with a single metastasis in the non-dominant hemisphere. *J Neurosurg* 1983; **58**: 303–5.

Fisher CM. Transient global amnesia: Precipitating activities and other observations. *Arch Neurol* 1982a; **39**: 605–8.

Fisher CM. Whiplash amnesia. *Neurology* 1982b; **32**: 667–8.

Fisher CM, Adams R. Transient global amnesia. *Trans Am Neurol Assoc* 1958; **83**: 143–6.

Fisher CM, Adams RD. Transient global amnesia. *Acta Neurol Scand* 1964; **40**: 1–83 (Suppl 9).

Fleminger JJ, Horne JDL, Nott PN. Unilateral electroconvulsive therapy and cerebral dominance: effect of right- and left-sided electrode placement on verbal memory. *J Neurol Neurosurg Psychiat* 1970; **33**: 408–11.

Goodwin DW, Crane JB, Guze SB. Phenomenological aspects of the alcoholic 'blackout'. *Br J Psychiat* 1969; **115**: 1033–8.

Gorelick PB, Amico LL, Ganellen R, Benevento LA. Transient global amnesia and thalamic infarction. *Neurology* 1988; **38**: 496–9.

Greene HH, Bennett DR. Transient global amnesia with a previously unreported EEG abnormality. *EEG Clin Neurophys* 1974; **36**: 409–13.

Haas DC, Ross GS. Transient global amnesia triggered by mild head trauma. *Brain* 1986; **109**: 251–7.

Hinge H-H, Jensen TS, Kjaer M, Marquardsen J, Olivarius BDF. The prognosis of transient global amnesia: Results of a multicenter study. *Arch Neurol* 1986; **43**: 673–6.

Hodges JR, Warlow CP. Syndromes of transient amnesia: towards a classification. A study of 153 cases. *J Neurol Neurosurg Psychiat* 1990; **53**: 834–43.

Jensen TS, Olivarius BDF. Transient global amnesia as a manifestation of transient cerebral ischemia. *Acta Neurol Scand* 1980; **61**: 115–24.

Kritchevsky M, Squire LR, Zouzounis JA. Transient global amnesia: characterization of anterograde and retrograde amnesia. *Neurology* 1988; **38**: 213–19.

Lisak RP, Zimmerman RA. Transient global amnesia due to a dominant hemisphere tumor. *Arch Neurol* 1977; **34**: 317–18.

Longridge NS, Hackinski V, Barber HO. Brain stem dysfunction in transient global amnesia. *Stroke* 1979; **10**: 473–4.

Matias-Guiu J, Buenaventura I, Cervera C, Codina A. Whiplash amnesia. *Neurology* 1985; **35**: 1259.

Matias-Guiu J, Codina A. Neuropsychological functions in the follow-up of transient global amnesia (Letter). *J Neurol Neurosurg Psychiat* 1985; **48**: 713–25.

Mazzucchi A, Moretti G, Cafarra P, Parma M. Neuropsychological functions in the follow-up of transient global amnesia. *Brain* 1980; **103**: 161–78.

Meador KJ, Adams RJ, Flanigin HF. Transient global amnesia and meningioma. *Neurology* 1985; **35**: 769–71.

Miller JW, Petersen RC, Metter EJ, Millikan CH, Yanagihara T. Transient global amnesia: Clinical characteristics and prognosis. *Neurology* 1987a; **37**: 733–7.

Miller JW, Yanagihara T, Petersen RC, Klass DW. Transient global amnesia and epilepsy: Electroencephalographic distinction. *Arch Neurol* 1987b; **44**: 629–33.

Moonis M, Jain S, Prasad K, Mishra NK, Goulatia RD, Maheshwari MC. Left thalamic hypertensive haemorrhage presenting as transient global amnesia. *Acta Neurol Scand* 1988; **77**: 331–4.

Nausieda PA, Sherman IC. Long-term prognosis in transient global amnesia. *J Am Med Assoc* 1979; **241**: 392–3.

Olesen J, Jorgensen MB. Leao's spreading depression in the hippocampus explains transient global amnesia. *Acta Neurol Scand* 1986; **73**: 219–20.

Olivarius B, Jensen TS. Transient global amnesia with migraine. *Headache* 1979; **19**: 335–8.

Rowan AJ, Protass LM. Transient global amnesia: Clinical and electroencephalographic findings in 10 cases. *Neurology* 1979; **29**: 869–72.

Serafetinides E, Falconer M. Speech disturbances in temporal lobe seizures: A study of 100 epileptic patients submitted to anterior temporal lobectomy. *Brain* 1963; **86**: 333–46.

Service FJ, Dale AJD, Elveback LR, Jiang NS. Insulinoma: Clinical and diagnostic features of 60 consecutive cases. *Mayo Clin Proc* 1976; **51**: 417–29.

Shuttleworth EC, Wise GR. Transient global amnesia due to arterial embolism. *Arch Neurol* 1973; **29**: 340–3.

Shuping JR, Rollinson RD, Toole JF. Transient global amnesia. *Ann Neurol* 1980; **7**: 281–5.

Theodore WH, Porter RJ, Penry JK. Complex partial seizures: clinical characteristics and differential diagnosis. *Neurology* 1983; **33**: 1115–21.

39. *Amnesia for personal identity is virtually always psychogenic*

The chief disturbance in psychogenic amnesia is a sudden inability to recall important personal information that is too pervasive to be explained by ordinary forgetfulness. In psychogenic amnesia, this memory loss is not due to organic causes, as in alcoholic blackout and epilepsy, or to multiple personality disorder (American Psychiatric Association, 1987). Psychogenic memory loss is usually the result of an emotional trauma – as Freud put it, 'the forgetting of the disagreeable' (Freud, 1981). Common precipitating events include rape, criminal acts and such battle stresses as exhaustion, terror following the death of comrade or a bomb blast, and mild head trauma. In cases involving criminal and other wrongful acts linked to feelings of guilt, malingering must be considered as a possible cause (Pratt, 1977).

In organic amnesia, personal identity and memories (e.g. mother's name, home address) are usually preserved, and memory loss follows a temporal gradient, in which recently acquired memories are more severely affected than older memories (Russell and Nathan, 1932). Psychogenic amnesia, however, is organized primarily along affective, rather than temporal, dimensions (Schacter, 1982). Patients with psychogenic amnesia characteristically have normal acquisition of new information. They can remember physicians' names and faces and what they had for breakfast yesterday. Among retrograde memories, however, there are striking dissociations. For example, a patient may remember more about an American president's life than her own.

The most common form of psychogenic amnesia is circumscribed amnesia, in which the patient fails to recall all events during a brief time surrounding a traumatic event. In selective psychogenic amnesia, the patient recalls a limited number of events surrounding an emotional trauma. The least common but most dramatic forms of psychogenic amnesia are generalized amnesia, or failure to recall any personal events, and continuous amnesia, the failure to recall any events following a specific trauma (American Psychiatric Association, 1987).

With the exception of cases in military personnel, psychogenic amnesia is most common in young women. The memory loss typically begins and ends suddenly. Recovery is usually complete and recurrences are rare.

Psychogenic amnesia is one of the dissociative disorders (Maxim 97). These disorders are characterised by an alteration in the normal perception of self-identity and memory. When a patient with psychogenic loss of personal memories assumes a new identity and unexpectedly wanders away from home or work, the disorder is termed psychogenic fugue (American Psychiatric Association, 1987). In most cases of psychogenic fugue, mild disorientation is present, the new identity is partial and the episode is brief, lasting hours or days. Recovery is usually rapid and recurrences are rare. However, prolonged episodes with elaborate new identities (often with more extraverted personalities than the original personality) and the evolution of complex social situations also occur. Psychogenic fugue often follows severe psychic stress or heavy alcohol use, and it is more common in patients with a history of recurrent depression (Stengel, 1941).

Identifying the precipitating stress is often the key to treating patients with psychogenic amnesia and fugue. Interviewing the patient after administration of amobarbital (Amytal) is especially helpful. This test should only be done in patients who do not have increased intracranial pressure, porphyria or significant respiratory disease, such as emphysema. In the test, 100 to 400 mg amobarbital is infused slowly (< 50 mg/min) intra-venously to achieve a quiet and relaxed state. Patients with neurological causes of amnesia usually become disoriented and confused with low doses of amobarbital, while those with psychiatric disorders usually become more communicative and their symptoms may resolve. However, persistence of symptoms following amobarbital administration does not disprove a psychogenic etiology.

The amobarbitol interview may also be helpful in cases of malingering, although patients can continue to malinger after barbiturate adminis-tration.

The differential diagnosis of psychogenic amnesia and fugue from related conditions is shown in Table 39.1. Following head trauma, amnesia is common but usually follows a typical temporal gradient, with events occurring just before the trauma most often affected (Maxim 69). Also, in patients with head trauma, memory for personal identity is most resistant to loss, and short-term memory is most vulnerable.

Anticholinergic intoxication occurs accidently or intentionally, as in 'phar-macologic mugging'. It produces confusion and amnesia in association with pupillary dilatation, tachycardia and dry, warm skin.

The alcoholic blackout is a dense amnesia for events that occurred during a bout of heavy alcohol intake. The essential feature of such blackouts is that, while intoxicated, patients act relatively normally and lack a reduced level of consciousness. That is, they do not appear grossly intoxicated and are able to converse and perform complex acts (Jellinek, 1952). Alcoholic blackouts usually occur in poorly nourished, chronic alcoholics (Goodwin et al., 1969).

Epilepsy is often associated with memory disorders. Following complex partial and generalised convulsions, there is often brief retrograde and slightly longer anterograde memory loss. After repetitive seizures, the memory impairment and confusion are more prolonged. Non-convulsive status epilepticus, which is due to continuous or frequent recurrences of

Table 39.1 Differential diagnosis of psychogenic amnesia and fugue from related conditions.

Postconcussive amnesia
Anticholingeric intoxication
Benzodiazepine intoxication (especially triazolam)
Alcoholic blackout
Epilepsy
  Postictal state
  Non-convulsive status epilepticus
Confusional migraine
Catatonic stupor
Multiple personality
Malingering

absence or complex partial seizures, results in confusion or impaired con-sciousness and is often misdiagnosed as a psychiatric disorder. As a result, the electroencephalogram is critical for diagnosis. Rarely, 'poriomania' occurs with or, more likely, after complex partial seizures. Poriomania is characterized by episodes of wandering away from home or work with subsequent amnesia for the event (Mayeux, 1979). In epileptic poriomania, no psychosocial stressors or pre-existing psychiatric disorder is present.

Confusional migraine usually occurs in children or adolescents and consists of an altered sensorium, agitation and headache lasting less than 12 hours (Rothner, 1988).

Catatonic stupor is associated with mutism, which may suggest psycho-genic amnesia. In such cases, however, global impairment of motor and intellectual activity, rigidity, posturing and negativism are usually also present.

Malingering can present as a willful feigning of memory loss to avoid responsibility for wrongful deeds. It is not rare and may be difficult to distinguish from psychogenic cases. While the duration of feigned memory loss in malingering is often greater than that found in psychogenic amnesia, malingering is generally only substantiated once the wrongful deed is discovered.

References

American Psychiatric Association. *Diagnostic and Statistical Manual of Psychiatry* (3rd edition, revised). Washington, DC: American Psychiatric Association Press, 1987, pp. 269–77.

Freud S. On the theory of hysterical attacks. In: *The Standard Edition of the Complete Works of Sigmund Freud* (Volume 1) (Strachey J, transl.). London: Hogarth Press, 1981, pp. 151–4.

Goodwin DW, Crane JB, Guze SB. Alcoholic 'blackouts': A review and clinical study of 100 alcoholics. *Am J Psychiat* 1969; **126**: 191–8.

Jellinek EM. The phases of alcohol addition. *Q J Stud Alc* 1952; **13**: 673–84.

Mayeux R, Alexander MP, Benson DF, Brandt J, Rosen J. Poriomania. *Neurology* 1979; **29**: 1616–19.

Pratt TRC. Psychogenic loss of memory. In: *Amnesia*, (2nd edition) (Whitty CWM, Zangwill OL, eds). Boston: Butterworths, 1977, pp. 224–32.

Rothner AD. 'Not everything that shakes is epilepsy': The differential diagnosis of paroxysmal nonepileptiform disorders. *Cleve Clin Q* 1988; **56**: S206-S213 (Suppl part 2).

Russell WR, Nathan PW. Traumatic amnesia. *Brain* 1932; **69**: 280–300.

Schacter DL, Wang PL, Tulving E, Freedman M. Functional retrograde amnesia: A quantitative case study. *Neuropsychologia* 1982, **20**: 523–32.

Stengel E. The etiology of fugue states. *J Ment Sci* 1941; **87**: 572–99.

40.   *Behavioral training and pharmacotherapy have limited efficacy for memory disorders, but lists are quite helpful*

In the attempt to augment memory in amnesic patients, mnemonic training, rote drill, hypnosis and such conditioning paradigms as associating information with music have all played significant roles (Gianutsos and Gianutsos, 1979; Benson and Blumer, 1982; Dywan and Bowers, 1983; O'Connor and Cermak, 1987). Unfortunately, information acquired through conditioning or other behavioral techniques usually requires the appropriate cue for retrieval of the information. This constraint severely limits the practicality of these strategies, whether they are used in amnesic or normal subjects.

Visual imagery is an ancient mnemonic technique in which information is associated with specific images (Yates, 1966). Used in normal subjects, it can indeed augment memorization powers. In amnesic patients, however, it has little or no effect (Bower, 1970; Baddeley and Warrington, 1973; Glasgow *et al.*, 1977). Similarly, memory exercises and drills are often used to 'strengthen' memory (as if it were a muscle), but controlled studies have not shown any significant benefits to amnesic patients from the use of these techniques (Harris and Sunderland, 1981; Prigitano *et al.*, 1984; Godfrey and Knight, 1985). Finally, 'cognitive retraining' software packages sold for use on personal computers are aggressively marketed but they remain ineffective for treating amnesia.

Perhaps the most helpful suggestion for amnesic patients is to maintain lists. Patients should always carry a small notepad and pen, operating instructions should be placed on appliances and schedules of activities should be posted in frequently visited locations, such as the refrigerator door (Wilson and Moffat, 1984; Harris, 1984). Bell timers and watches with alarms may help remind the patient of the time, or that they should perform some function (Kurlychek, 1983). In addition, patients should always carry important telephone numbers and addresses around with them.

However, there are problems with all of these external aids. Patients often fail to consult the lists and notebooks. When notepads are used, patients often write cryptic, incomplete messages and fail to keep the lists current. A message from several weeks ago may be mistaken for one only several hours old (Glisky and Schacter, 1986). Bells go off and the patient knows he is supposed to do something, but can't remember what to do. Thus, to maximize benefit from these aids, someone must teach patients how to use them properly and should supervise their performance.

Hope for a pharmacological agent to augment memory has surged during the past decade as physicians, scientists and the public have witnessed an explosion of information regarding the biochemistry and neuropharmacology of memory. Investigations in animals and humans on acetylcholine, protein synthesis, adrenocorticotrophic hormone (ACTH), vasopressin, opioids and catecholamines have all shed light on the neurobiology of memory (Squire and Davis, 1981; Thal, 1989). Of the many potential memory pathways, the cholinergic memory system has been most extensively studied and will be the focus of this discussion.

A disorder of cortical cholinergic innervation has been proposed as a simplistic model of memory impairment in Alzheimer's disease (Coyle et al., 1983). Acetylcholine-synthesizing neurons in the basal nucleus of Meynert provide widespread innervation of the neocortical and limbic areas and selectively degenerate in Alzheimer's disease. Furthermore, pharmacological blockade of central cholinergic activity with scopolamine significantly impairs recall and recognition in memory tasks (Drachman and Leavitt, 1974; Nissen et al., 1987). These observations led to trials of cholinergic agonists including physostigmine and of the acetylcholine precursor, lecithin, for memory improvement. Although positive results have been reported with cholinergic pharmacotherapy (Drachman, 1977; Peters and Levin, 1977; Bartus, 1979; Thal et al., 1983), additional studies have demonstrated little or no benefit to normal or amnesic subjects (Davis et al., 1980; Jotkowitz, 1983).

In Korsakoff's disease, cerebrospinal fluid levels of the central noradrenergic metabolite, 3-methoxy 4-hydroxyphenyl glycol (MHPG), correlate inversely with memory function (McEntee and Mair, 1978). Preliminary studies have shown enhanced memory in patients with Korsakoff's disease who have been administered clonidine, a central alpha-noradrenergic agonist, although memory improvement was not shown when patients received D-amphetamine, which increases release and uptake of central norepinephrine, dopamine and serotonin (McEntee and Mair, 1980). Vasopressin administered by nasal spray has also been reported to enhance memory in Korsakoff's disease patients (LeBoeuf et al., 1978). Both findings demonstrating short-term improvement of memory are preliminary; they must be replicated and extended to long-term studies.

Despite the wealth of neurobiological and neuropharmacological data on memory and vigorous attempts by academic and pharmaceutical investigators to identify a drug for memory enhancement, no agent is clearly effective in the treatment of amnesia.

References

Baddeley AD, Warrington EK. Memory coding and amnesia. *Neuropsychologia* 1973; **11**: 159–65.

Bartus RT. Physostigmine and recent memory: Effects in young and aged non-human primates. *Science* 1979; **206**: 1087–9.

Benson DF, Blumer D. Amnesia: A clinical approach to memory. In: *Psychiatric Aspects of Neurologic Disease* (volume II) (Benson DF, Blumer D, eds). New York: Grune and Stratton, Inc., 1982, pp. 251–178.

Bower GH. Analysis of a mnemonic device. *Am Sci* 1970; **58**: 496–510.

Coyle JT, Price DL, DeLong MR. Alzheimer's disease: A disorder of cortical cholinergic innervation. *Science* 1983; **219**: 1184–90.

Davis KL, Mohs RC, Tinklenberg JR, Hollister LE, Pfefferbaum A, Kopell BS. Cholinominetics and memory: The effect of chlorine chloride. *Arch Neurol* 1980; **37**: 49–52.

Drachman DA. Memory and cognitive function in man: does the cholinergic system have a specific role? *Neurology* 1977; **27**: 783–90.

Drachman DA, Leavitt J. Human memory and the cholinergic system. *Arch Neurol* 1974; **30**: 113–21.

Dywan J, Bowers K. The use of hypnosis to enhance recall. *Science* 1983; **222**: 184–5.

Gianutsos R, Gianutsos J. Rehabilitating the verbal recall of brain-injured patients by mnemonic training: An experimental demonstration using single-case methodology. *J Clin Neuropsychol* 1979; **1**: 117–35.

Glasgow RE, Zeiss RA, Barrera M, Lewinsohn PM. Case studies on remediating memory deficits in brain-damaged individuals. *J Clin Psychol* 1977; **33**: 1049–54.

Glisky EL, Schacter DL. Remediation of organic memory disorders: Current status and future prospects. *J Head Trauma Rehabil* 1986; **1**: 54–63.

Godfrey HPD, Knight RG. Cognitive rehabilitation of memory functioning in amnesiac alcoholics. *J Consult Clin Psychol* 1985; **53**: 555–7.

Harris JE. Methods of improving memory. In: *Clinical Management of Memory Problems* (Wilson B, Moffat N, eds). London: Aspen, 1984, pp. 46–62.

Harris JE, Sunderland A. A brief survey of the management of memory disorders in rehabilitation units in Britain. *Int Rehabil Med* 1981; **3**: 206–9.

Jotkowitz S. Lack of efficacy of chronic oral physostigmine in Alzheimer's disease. *Ann Neurol* 1983; **14**: 690–1.

Kurlychek RT. Use of a digital alarm chronograph as a memory aid in early dementia. *Clin Gerontol* 1983; **1**: 93–4.

LeBoeuf A, Lodge J, Eames PG. Vasopressin and memory in Korsakoff syndrome. *Lancet* 1978; **ii**: 1370.

McEntee WJ, Mair RG. Memory impairment in Korsakoff's psychosis: A correlation with brain noradrenergic activity. *Science* 1978; **202**: 905–7.

McEntee WJ, Mair RG. Memory enhancement in Korsakoff's psychosis by clonidine: Further evidence for a noradrenergic deficit. *Ann Neurol* 1980; **7**: 466–70.

Nissen MJ, Knopmen DS, Schacter DL. Neurochemical dissociation of memory systems. *Neurology* 1987; **37**: 789–94.

O'Connor M, Cermak LS. Rehabilitation of organic memory disorders. In: *Neuropsychological Rehabilitation* (Meier MJ, Benton AL, Diller L, eds). New York: Guilford Press, 1987, pp. 260–79.

Peters BH, Levin HS. Memory enhancement after physostigmine treatment in the amnesia syndrome. *Arch Neurol* 1977; **34**: 215–19.

Prigitano GP, Fordyce DJ, Zeiner HK, Roueche JR, Pepping M, Wood BC. Neuropsychological rehabilitation after closed head injury in young adults. *J Neurol Neurosurg Psychiat* 1984; **47**: 505–13.

Squire LR, Davis HP. The pharmacology of memory: A neurobiological perspective. *Ann Rev Pharmacol Toxicol* 1981; **21**: 323–56.

Thal LJ. Pharmacological treatment of memory disorders. In: *Handbook of Neuropsychology* (volume 3) (Boller F, Grafman J, eds). Amsterdam: Elsevier Science Publishing, 1989, pp. 247–67.

Thal LJ, Fuld PA, Masur DM, Sharpless NS. Oral physostigmine and lecithin improve memory in Alzheimer's disease. *Ann Neurol* 1983; **13**: 491–6.

Wilson B, Moffat N. Rehabilitation of memory for everyday life. In: *Everyday Memory: Actions and Absentmindedness* (Harris JE, Morris PE, eds). London: Academic Press, 1984.

Yates F. *The Art of Memory*. Chicago: University of Chicago Press, 1966.

5
Alexia, Agraphia and Apraxia

---

41. *Agraphia is common and accompanies both aphasic and non-aphasic disorders*

Writing has been a very recent development for our species. Although writing was never necessary for survival in the savannas or woods, it has become indispensable in modern life. In agraphic patients, this crucial skill is lost or impaired by acquired brain disease.

Writing is the most painfully acquired language function for most people, and individual writing ability varies widely. Therefore, it is important to ask the patient with suspected agraphia about writing ability preceding the brain insult before estimating writing impairment.

To assess writing, use unlined paper and begin with the signature – the most elementary and overlearned written response. Then proceed with more complex writing skills by testing the patient's ability to copy and write numbers, letters, words and sentences on verbal command. Finally, ask the patient to write a paragraph on 'an average day in your life' or 'how to plan a vacation'. Observe the spontaneity, speed and ease of writing. When the patient has completed this task, check writing for quantity of output, form and size of letters, sentence length, accuracy of spelling, substantive words, grammar and paragraphias (the written equivalent of paraphasias). Assessment of writing is particularly important in aphasic patients because it can provide information on functional severity and lesion site, and it may reveal a relatively preserved avenue for communication.

Agraphia may be broadly separated into aphasic and non-aphasic forms, although components of both are present in many cases. Common non-aphasic causes of writing impairment include pyramidal and extrapyramidal motor disorders, sensory and sensorimotor integration disorders, visuospatial disorders and lower motor neuron lesions, as well as toxic and metabolic insults associated with confusional states (Chedru and Geschwind, 1972). Agraphia may also result from disorders of praxis (Maxim 43).

Aphasia is almost always accompanied by agraphia, as both result from impairment of language functions. Aphasic agraphia can be loosely divided functionally and anatomically into two forms analagous to those found in aphasia: (1) non-fluent anterior forms, which are associated with frontal lesions; and (2) fluent posterior forms, associated with parietotemporal lesions (Benson, 1967). Patients with non-fluent agraphia have difficulty when initiating writing and their output is effortful and slow with large, awkward and poorly formed letters. Their writing contains characteristic features: short phrase length, spelling errors and a lack of such grammatical words as 'if', 'and', 'or', 'but', and 'to' (Benson and Cummings, 1985). In contrast, patients with fluent agraphia write with ease; their calligraphy and sentence length are normal; their output contains abundant numbers of grammatical words. However, their writing lacks substantive words, such as basketball or computer, and is contaminated by paragraphias.

Aphasic agraphia is also divided into phonological and lexical forms (Shallice, 1981). In *phonological agraphia*, the patient is unable to write pro-nounceable non-words, due to disruption of the phoneme-to-grapheme conversion system, which correlates sounds with letters. For example, when the patient with phonological agraphia hears the sound 'ba' (a pho-neme), he is unable to write the letters 'ba' (a grapheme). In *lexical agraphia*, however, the patient is unable to retrieve and motorically conceptualize whole words and demonstrates impaired writing of familiar, but atypical, words (Friederici *et al.*, 1981). The impairment lies within the lexical system, which is important for writing words with irregular or ambiguous spell-ings. For example, such patients may have difficulty with the irregular words 'kerchief' and 'circuit', because they contain unusual spellings that prevent simple phoneme-to-grapheme conversion. Additionally, they may stumble over such ambiguous words as 'cotton' and 'city', which require lexical interpretation because they contain sounds that correspond to mul-tiple graphemes. The differing functional impairment between these two agraphias may correspond to varying lesion sites: Roeltgen and Heilman (1984) reported that patients with lexical agraphia have lesions in the angular gyrus, while those with phonological agraphia have lesions in the supramarginal gyrus or subjacent insula.

Another form of aphasic agraphia is *agraphia with alexia*, or *acquired illiter-acy*. This results from lesions in the dominant inferior parietal lobe (angular gyrus) and is often accompanied by anomic aphasia and components of the Gertsmann syndrome (Maxim 64), which includes agraphia, acalculia, right–left disorientation and finger agnosia (Benson and Geschwind, 1969). Agraphia associated with alexia is characteristically fluent.

Aphasic agraphia restricted to the left hand occurs in patients who have language dominance in the left hemisphere and lesions in the anterior corpus callosum (Geschwind and Kaplan, 1962). On verbal command, such patients cannot write with the left hand, because of an inability to transfer language information from the dominant to the non-dominant hemisphere (Geschwind, 1965). However, they can copy well with the left hand. Agra-phia of the left hand commonly occurs in patients with Broca's aphasia (sympathetic apraxia), whose inability to perform left-handed movements on verbal command extends beyond agraphia to encompass all learned

motor actions, because language areas are disconnected from motor association areas in the right hemisphere. In addition, Broca's aphasia patients
often have an aphasic component that contributes to their agraphia.

Aphasic professional musicians may also have musical agraphia and
alexia, affecting both pitch and rhythm (Brust, 1980).

Pure or isolated agraphia is defined as impaired writing without apraxia or
other language disorders. This rare condition is usually associated with
dominant hemisphere lesions in the superior parietal region (Kinsbourne
and Rosenfield, 1974; Auerbach and Alexander, 1981; De Bastiani *et al.*,
1983). However, left posterior frontal and temporal lesions have also been
reported in pure agraphia (Dubois *et al.*, 1969; Rosati and De Bastiani, 1979;
Rapcsak *et al.*, 1988).

Non-aphasic agraphia results from weakness and from disorders of
movement, visuospatial function and conversion. It is not associated with
spelling or language errors nor with the absence of substantive or grammatical words.

In *paretic agraphia*, the lesion may be located in the muscle, neuromuscular junction, peripheral nerve, plexus, root, anterior horn cell or upper
motor neuron. *Micrographia*, or 'small writing', occurs in two forms, as
distinguished by Wilson (1925). The first form is characterized by consistently small writing and follows *corticospinal lesions*, while the second form
is associated with progressively smaller writing and *parkinsonism*. Parkinsonism is also associated with decreased initiative to write, slow writing,
crowding of letters and difficulty maintaining a straight line; dopaminergic
therapy improves micrographia and other writing problems in these
patients. In *hyperkinetic movement disorders* such as tremor, chorea, tics and
dystonia, intrusion of pathological movements disrupts writing (Benson
and Cummings, 1985). *Writer's cramp*, a focal dystonia, usually appears
between 20 and 50 years of age and is often associated with abnormal
posture and tone in the affected arm (Sheehy and Marsden, 1982). *Visuospatial dysfunction* can also impair writing. Patients with lesions in the right
parietal lobe frequently have left-sided neglect (Maxim 63). As a result,
their writing is displaced toward the right side of the page, and the normal
spacing and arrangement of letters and sentences is disrupted. Among
patients with *conversion disorders*, isolated agraphia is rare, but paralysis of
the dominant hand to give agraphia is more common.

Hypergraphia is a tendency toward extensive and, in some cases, compulsive writing. It can occur in patients with schizophrenia, mania and, interictally, complex partial seizures (Waxman and Geschwind, 1974; Hermann
et al., 1988).

References

Auerbach SH, Alexander MP. Pure agraphia and unilateral optic ataxia associated
   with a left superior parietal lobule lesion. *J Neurol Neurosurg Psychiat* 1981; **44**:
   430–2.

Benson DF. Fluency in aphasia: correlation with radioactive scan localization. *Cortex* 1967; **3**: 373–94.

Benson DF, Cummings JL. Agraphia. In: *Handbook of Clinical Neurology* (volume 1 (45)) *Clinical Neuropsychology* (Frederiks JAM, ed.). New York: Elsevier Science Publishing Company, 1985, pp. 457–72.

Benson DF, Geschwind N. The alexias. In: *Handbook of Clinical Neurology* (volume 4) (Vinken PJ, Bruyn, eds). Amsterdam: North-Holland Publishing Company, 1969, pp. 112–140.

Brust JCM. Music and language: Musical alexia and agraphia. *Brain* 1980; **103**: 367–92.

Chedru F, Geschwind N. Writing disturbances in acute confusional states. *Neuropsychologia* 1972; **10**: 343–53.

De Bastiani PE, Monetti VC, Boldrini P, Rosati G. Pure 'aphasic' agraphia due to damage of the left superior parietal lobule. *Ictal J Neurol Sci* 1983; **2**: 233–7.

Dubois J, Hecaen H, Marcie P. L'agraphie pure. *Neuropsychologia* 1969; **7**: 271–86.

Friederici AD, Schoenle PW, Goodglass H. Mechanisms underlying writing and speech in aphasia. *Brain Lang* 1981; **13**: 212–22.

Geschwind N. Disconnexion syndromes in animals and man. *Brain* 1965; **88**: 237–94; 585–644.

Geschwind N, Kaplan EF. A human cerebral deconnection syndrome. *Neurology* 1962; **12**: 675–85.

Hermann BP, Whitman S, Wyler AR, Richey ET, Dell J. The neurological, psychosocial and demographic correlates of hypergraphia in patients with epilepsy. *J Neurol Neurosurg Psychiat* 1988; **51**: 203–8.

Kinsbourne M. Rosenfield RB. Agraphia selective for written spelling. *Brain Lang* 1974; **1**: 215–26.

Rapcsak SZ, Arthur SA, Rubens AB. Lexical agraphia from focal lesions of the left precentral gyrus. *Neurology* 1988; **38**: 1119–23.

Roeltgen DP, Heilman KM. Lexical agraphia: Further support for the two-system hypothesis of linguistic agraphia. *Brain* 1984; **107**: 811–27.

Rosati G, De Bastiani P. Pure agraphia: a discrete form of aphasia. *J Neurol Neurosurg Psychiat* 1979; **42**: 266–9.

Shallice T. Phonological agraphia and the lexical route in writing. *Brain* 1981; **104**: 413–29.

Sheehy MP, Marsden CD. Writer's cramp – a focal dystonia. *Brain* 1982; **105**: 461–80.

Waxman SG, Geschwind N. Hypergraphia in temporal lobe epilepsy. *Neurology* 1974; **24**: 629–36.

Wilson SAK. Disorders of motility and muscle tone with special reference to the corpus striatum. *Lancet* 1925; **ii**: 1–10.

42.   *Alexia usually results from disconnection of visual input from language areas (alexia without agraphia) or from lesions of the angular gyrus (aphasic alexia or alexia with agraphia)*

Alexia is acquired reading impairment due to brain damage, and dyslexia is a congenital or developmental reading disorder. Dyslexia should not be used to describe partial reading impairment which is acquired.

Assessment of reading begins with an inquiry about premorbid skills. After determining how well the patient read before the onset of neurological dysfunction, silent reading for comprehension, and reading aloud should be tested. One should listen for paralexias (reading errors), including verbal (semantic) paralexias in which a related word is substituted for the target word (e.g. 'town' for 'village'), phonemic paralexias (mispronunciations similar to the phonemic paraphasias in Broca's aphasia) and visual paralexias (misreading a portion of the word, usually the left half due to visual neglect). Language function, color naming, visual field responses to unilateral and double simultaneous stimuli, and dominant parietal lobe functions (writing, right–left orientation, finger gnosis, calculations and constructional praxis) must be carefully tested.

Alexia without agraphia (pure alexia) results from a lesion in the left occipital lobe and adjacent splenium (posterior corpus callosum) that disconnects visual input from language areas (Fig. 42.1). These patients have a right hemianopsia; the visual information from the intact left field is received and processed by the right visual areas, but cannot be transferred to the contralateral language areas. The most common pathological process is infarction in the territory of the left posterior cerebral artery (PCA), usually occlusion by thrombi and emboli, although PCA compression during tentorial herniation may also cause the syndrome (Caplan and Hedley-White, 1974; Cohen *et al.*, 1976; Kirshner *et al.*, 1982). Occipitotemporal white matter lesions deep to the angular gyrus disconnect this language area from visual association cortices and thereby cause alexia without agraphia (Greenblatt, 1976; Damasio and Damasio, 1983). A single lesion in the left occipital paraventricular white matter can result in pure alexia. It has been theorized that pure alexia results when left occipital lesions interrupt interhemispheric, and destroy or interrupt intrahemispheric, visual pathways (Damasio and Damasio, 1983). However, the disconnection hypothesis has been criticized because many patients with pure alexia can read and name single letters. To account for this preserved function, others have postulated that pure alexia is a visual disorder in which only limited data can be simultaneously processed, i.e. 'simultagnosia' (Kinsbourne and Warrington, 1962a; Petterson and Kay, 1982). Both mechanisms may be relevant in pure alexia.

Patients with pure alexia usually have right hemianopsia or superior quadrantanopsia, but visual fields may be complete (Greenblatt, 1973). In some cases, only color vision in the right hemifield is defective (hemiachromatopsia). Motor and somatosensory deficits are usually lacking, but can occur when the lesion extends into the cerebral peduncle, internal capsule or thalamus (Benson and Tomlinson, 1971). Such patients often have anomia for colors (lesions in the medial occipitotemporal junction of the left hemisphere), optic ataxia, or impaired visually guided reaching in the intact left field with the right hand (interruption of left occipital–parietofrontal connections), short-term memory loss (lesions in the dominant hippocampus) and, less often, visual agnosia (lesions in the bilateral

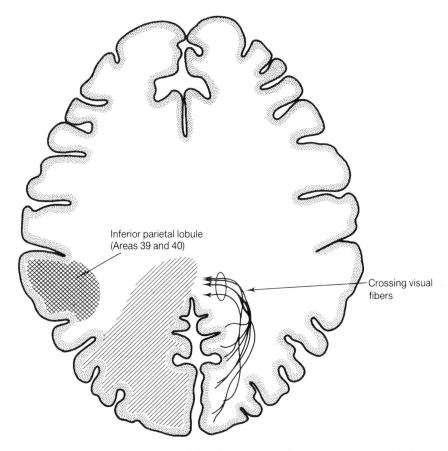

Fig. 42.1 Alexia without agraphia. The cross-hatched area represents infarction of the left visual cortex and the posterior portion of the corpus callosum. The visual information from the right visual cortex (arrow) is unable to reach the left inferior parietal lobule (39 and 40) because of the callosal lesion.

visual association cortices) (Geschwind and Fusillo, 1966; Lhermitte and Beauvois, 1973; Benson *et al.*, 1974; Damasio and Damasio, 1983).

Alexia with agraphia (aphasic or deep alexia) is acquired illiteracy (i.e. inability to read or write) and usually results from lesions in the angular gyrus. These patients often make abundant semantic paralexias (e.g. reading 'dog' for 'mutt'), a finding referred to as deep dyslexia (Marshall and Newcombe, 1973). A mild fluent aphasia with anomia and paraphasias is also often present (Benson, 1982). The defect in deep dyslexia appears to lie in the conversion of graphemes (written syllables) to phonemes (syllable sounds). Patients extract word meaning without translating written words into sounds. This syndrome is distinguished from Wernicke's aphasia by preserved auditory comprehension and repetition. Lesions of the angular gyrus also cause constructional apraxia and the Gertsmann syndrome (agraphia, acalculia, right–left orientation and finger agnosia) (Maxims 43 and 64). Associated elementary neurological findings include right-sided hemianopsia or inferior quadrantanopsia and less often, right-sided hemisensory loss or hemiparesis. The most often common etiology is infarction in the posterior division of the left middle cerebral artery, although tumors, arteriovenous malformations and other lesions also produce alexia with agraphia.

Frontal alexia occurs in patients with dominant frontal lesions that also produce Broca's (anterior) aphasia (Benson, 1977; Boccardi *et al.*, 1984). These patients comprehend meaningful content words but have difficulty with syntactic or relational words that are critical for comprehension of written passages. For example, patients have difficulty following a sentence such as 'The loss of Jeff's uncle's cat caused concern about the rat problem in the house and Jeff's aunt was petrified'. Patients with frontal alexia may conclude that it was Jeff's cat that was lost and have no idea why the aunt was upset. Lack of syntactic comprehension probably underlies frontal alexia, although gaze paresis, failure to maintain verbal sequences and literal paralexias may also contribute. Because both alexia with agraphia and frontal alexia have been called 'aphasic alexia', use of the latter, confusing term is discouraged.

Spatial alexia results from visual neglect, usually of the left visual field (Kinsbourne and Warrington, 1962). This is not aphasia, it is a disorder of attention. Patients usually have right parietal lesions, and there is also neglect of left visual stimuli on presentation of a double, simultaneous stimulus. These patients may read the word 'cocktail' as 'tail'. Efforts to retrain patients to scan the left visual field more effectively may be beneficial (Weinberg *et al.*, 1977).

References

Benson DF. The third alexia. *Arch Neurol* 1977; **34**: 327–31.

Benson DF. The alexias: a guide to the neurologic basis of reading. In: *The Neurology of Aphasia* (Kirshner HS, Freemon FR, eds). Amsterdam: Swets, 1982, pp. 139–61.

Benson DF, Marsden CD, Meadows JC. The amnestic syndrome of posterior cerebral artery occlusion. *Acta Neurol Scand* 1974; **50**: 133–45.

Benson DF, Tomlinson E. Hemiplegic syndrome of the posterior cerebral artery. *Stroke* 1971; **2**: 559–64.

Boccardi DF, Bruzzone MG, Vignolo LA. Alexia in recent and late Broca's aphasia. *Neuropsychologia* 1984; **22**: 745–74.

Caplan LR, Hedley-White T. Cueing and memory dysfunction in alexia without agraphia. *Brain* 1974; **97**: 251–62.

Cohen D, Salanga V, Hully W, Steinberg M, Hardy R. Alexia without agraphia. *Neurology* 1976; **26**: 455–9.

Damasio AR, Damasio H. The anatomical basis of pure alexia. *Neurology* 1983; **33**: 1573–83.

Geschwind N, Fusillo M. Color-naming deficits in association with alexia. *Arch Neurol* 1966; **15**: 137–46.

Greenblatt SH. Alexia without agraphia or hemianopsia. *Brain* 1973; **96**: 307–16.

Greenblatt SH. Subangular alexia without agraphia. *Brain Lang* 1976; **3**: 229–45.

Kinsbourne M, Warrington EK. A disorder of simultaneous form perception. *Brain* 1962a; **85**: 461–86.

Kinsbourne M, Warrington EK. A variety of reading disability associated with right hemisphere lesions. *J Neurol Neurosurg Psychiat* 1962b; **25**: 339–44.

Kirshner HS, Staller J, Webb W, Sachs P. Transtentorial herniation with posterior cerebral artery territory infarction: a new mechanism of the syndrome of alexia without agraphia. *Stroke* 1982; **13**: 243–6.

Lhermitte F, Beauvois MF. A visual–speech disconnexion syndrome–report of a case with optic aphasia, agnosia, alexia and color agnosia. *Brain* 1973; **96**: 695–714.

Marshall JG, Newcombe F. Patterns of paralexia: a psycholinguistic approach. *J Psycholinguist Res* 1973; **2**: 175–200.

Petterson K, Kay J. Letter-by-letter reading: psychological descriptions of a neurological syndrome. *Q J Exp Psychol* 1982; **34A**: 411–41.

Weinberg J, Diller L, Gordon WA *et al.* Visual scanning training effect on reading-related tasks in acquired right brain damage. *Arch Phys Med Rehab* 1977; **58**: 479–86.

43. *Apraxia is the inability to perform movements in response to commands and results from disconnection or destruction of dominant hemisphere association areas*

Apraxia, by definition, cannot be explained by weakness, sensory loss, incoordination, poor comprehension or inattention. This common disorder often coexists with Broca's and conduction aphasias, but is often overlooked unless specifically sought. Apraxia is usually considered only when the deficit involves learned or skilled movements. However, apraxia includes such deficits as failure to protrude the tongue on command, despite ability to perform this motor act by imitation or spontaneous action (e.g. licking an ice cream cone).

Apraxia is divided into various types: ideomotor, ideational, limb-kinetic, constructional, ocular, gait and dressing. Ideomotor (motor) apraxia is the principal form and is often referred to simply as apraxia; it will be the focus of this discussion. Other forms are controversial, and calling them apraxia may imprecisely characterize the disorder, as they are often accompanied by other neurological deficits. For example, so-called 'apraxia of eyelid opening', (Goldstein and Cogan, 1965) is actually an extrapyramidal motor disorder with involuntary inhibition of the levator palpebrae, not an apraxia (Lepore and Duvoisin, 1985).

Ideomotor apraxia may involve buccofacial, limb or truncal (axial) musculature.

Buccofacial apraxia is tested by asking the patient to imitate various motor acts, including 'Blow out a match', 'Drink with a straw', or 'Stick out your tongue'. Patients should be discouraged from pretending to hold the match or straw in the above examples, as it makes the task easier. One should look for incomplete, unrelated or opposite motor acts. For example, the patient may inhale while blowing out the imaginary match.

Limb apraxia can involve the upper or lower limbs and may be unilateral. Therefore, all four extremities should be tested. Test by asking the patient to 'Salute with your left hand', 'Put out a cigarette with your left foot', 'Kick a ball with your right foot', and 'Brush your teeth holding the imaginary toothbrush with your right hand'. Observe for such errors as the use of a finger for the toothbrush or failure to open the mouth. Vary the commands on subsequent sides, since visual cues can artificially enhance performance. However, if the patient fails to perform one of the above tasks, then repeat the task with the contralateral extremity after an interval of at least several minutes.

Truncal apraxia is tested with commands such as 'bow' or 'stand like a boxer'. Axial movements are typically preserved in apraxic patients, probably because these movements can be mediated through non-pyramidal pathways.

The severity of ideomotor apraxia can be graded from mildest (failure to perform behavior to verbal command) to moderate (failure to imitate the behavior) to most severe (failure to imitate or perform behavior with an actual object, for example, a lit match).

Liepmann, who introduced the term apraxia in 1900, correctly posited that the left hemisphere in right-handed individuals contains a special repository for movement patterns or engrams (Liepmann, 1900a).

Support for Liepmann's hypothesis comes from observation of motor impairment in various disorders. For example, some patients with Broca's aphasia or callosal lesions fail to imitate movements of the left arm or leg. Since such mimetic movements do not rely on transmission of verbal input from the left hemisphere to motor areas in the right hemisphere, this phenomenon demonstrates that disconnection of language and motor areas cannot account for all apraxic deficits (Geschwind, 1975). Furthermore, these patients probably would not display mimetic deficits if engrammatic storage took place in the right hemisphere. A left hemisphere storehouse of acquired movements, however, would explain their deficits. Further support for this notion is found among patients with right-sided hemiplegia due to cortical lesions. When using left-sided limbs, these patients are often clumsy and very poor at acquiring new motor skills. In contrast, normal individuals who have their right arm immobilized in a cast after injury may become dextrous with their left arm. In this setting, the repository of motor skills in the left hemisphere assists right hemisphere motor control. Indeed Liepmann (1900b) theorized that the normal left hand may be even less dextrous than we think, 'because much of its skill may be borrowed from the left hemisphere across the corpus callosum'.

The left hemisphere may contain two repositories of motor engrams, one in the frontal lobe largely containing information needed for motor execution, and a second in the parietal lobe storing visuokinesthetic movements (Liepmann, 1900b; Heilman *et al.*, 1982). The extent of left hemisphere dominance for motor tasks is variable in individuals, but is more prominent for verbal than visuomotor tests of praxis (Graff-Radford *et al.*, 1987).

Ideomotor apraxia can result from disconnection of pathways that subserve Wernicke's area, engram storage areas in the left hemisphere, motor areas of the left hemisphere and motor areas in the right hemisphere (Geschwind, 1965). Alternatively, destruction of the left hemisphere's frontal or parietal motor engram repositories, described above, can produce apraxic deficits (Liepmann, 1977; Heilman *et al.*, 1982). Figure 43.1 shows the anatomical lesions associated with apraxia.

Ideomotor apraxia is often present in patients with Broca's aphasia. In this disorder, called *sympathetic apraxia* (Geschwind, 1963), a left hemisphere lesion in the motor association areas or white matter disconnects motor regions of the two hemispheres. As a result, fibers from the motor areas of the dominant hemisphere do not reach the non-dominant motor cortex. Patients are unable to carry out commanded movements with their non-hemiplegic left arm.

Callosal apraxia is related to sympathetic apraxia and usually results from a lesion in the anterior corpus callosum disconnecting the motor areas of the two hemispheres (Maxim 52). In callosal apraxia, patients are unable to perform movements on command with their left arm or leg, although they execute commands easily with right-sided limbs (Graff-Radford,

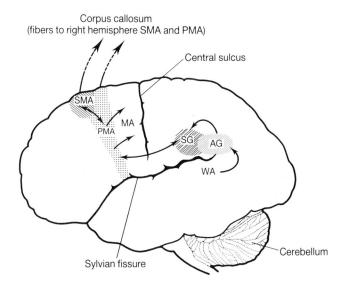

Fig. 43.1 Pathways for praxis in the left hemisphere. WA, Wernicke's area. AG, angular gyrus. SG, supramarginal gyrus. PMA, premotor area. SMA, supplementary motor area. MA, motor area.

1987). In these cases, visual cueing may occur if the patient first performs the task with the right-sided limb and is subsequently asked to perform the same task with the left-sided limb. In addition, lesions in the posterior corpus callosum can impair coordination and execution of hand movements ipsilateral to the hemisphere receiving the visual, non-verbal stimulation (Volpe *et al.*, 1982).

Ideomotor, *parietal apraxia* results from lesions in the supramarginal and angular gyri and underlying white matter. Among patients with parietal apraxias, those with lesions of the supramarginal and angular gyri cannot distinguish between well-performed and poorly performed movements in others, while those with lesions in the deep parietal white matter can make the correct discrimination (Heilman *et al.*, 1982; Graff-Radford *et al.*, 1987).

Finally, ideomotor apraxia also occurs with lesions in the *supplementary motor area of the dominant hemisphere* (Watson *et al.*, 1986). These patients are apraxic for limb movements bilaterally, but have no buccofacial apraxia. Imitation and use of the actual object usually improve the movement.

Non-ideomotor, *ideational apraxia*, refers to 'a disruption in the logical and harmonious succession of separate elements' in a movement (Hecaen and Albert, 1978). Patients with ideational apraxia may successfully perform individual components of a complex sequence, but fail to execute the correct series of actions. Ideational apraxia usually results from parietal lesions in the dominant, left hemisphere and is often associated with fluent aphasia and components of Gerstmann's syndrome (DeRenzi *et al.*, 1982; Lehmkuhl and Poeck, 1981).

The diagnosis of ideational apraxia must be made with great caution in the presence of prominent comprehension deficits. Such patients must demonstrate impairment of non-verbal motor sequences that are not initiated after verbal command, such as spontaneous lighting of a cigarette. Secondly, this apraxia is difficult to distinguish from the impairment of planning and sequential behaviors seen in the frontal lobe syndrome. In general, frontal patients have greater difficulty with more complex multi-step tasks, such as making dinner or planning a vacation, while those with ideational apraxia fail at simpler sequential behaviors, such as boiling water.

Limb-kinetic apraxia refers to the loss of fine, skilled movements following premotor lesions. Patients are clumsy, slow and awkward in executing motor tasks that were performed more rapidly and precisely prior to cerebral insult. Differentiation of true apraxia and a primary motor deficit is often difficult. Not surprisingly, limb-kinetic apraxia is a controversial entity, as many believe the deficit merely reflects destruction of corticospinal fibers or their cells of origin in premotor cortex.

Constructional apraxia (Maxim 50), another controversial entity, refers to impaired spatial manipulation of objects. Visual–spatial agnosia may be a more appropriate description (McFie *et al.*, 1950; Oxbury *et al.*, 1974; Yim *et al.*, 1984), especially for those deficits that follow right hemisphere injury

(Warrington *et al.*, 1966; Ratcliff, 1979). The lesions that cause constructional apraxia are usually posterior (mostly parietal) and are right-sided in two-thirds of patients (Arrigoni and DeRenzi, 1964; Black and Strub, 1976).

Constructional apraxia is tested by having the patient copy or spontaneously draw figures, arrange blocks in patterns, and construct or mentally manipulate three-dimensional structures. Patients with right-sided lesions often demonstrate left-sided neglect and, when copying and constructing, they produce replicas that lack the original's general outline, or gestalt. In contrast, patients with left-sided lesions often make impoverished copies that lack detail but preserve the outline and general structure. Also, visual cues are of greater benefit to patients with left-sided lesions. Indeed, the constructional deficits found patients with left-sided lesions may be more aptly described as an executive motor disorder than as constructional apraxia.

Reference

Arrigoni G, DeRenzi E. Constructional apraxia and hemispheric locus of lesion. *Cortex* 1964; **1**: 170–94.

Black FW, Strub RL. Constructional apraxia in patients with discrete missile wounds of the brain. *Cortex* 1976; **12**: 212–20.

DeRenzi E, Faglioni F, Sargata P. Modality specific and supramodal mechanisms of apraxia. *Brain* 1982; **105**: 301–12.

Geschwind N. Sympathetic dyspraxia. *Trans Am Neurol Assoc* 1963; **88**: 219–20.

Geschwind N. Disconnection syndromes in animals and man. *Brain* 1965; **88**: 237–94.

Geschwind N. The apraxias: Neural mechanisms of disorders of learned movements. *Am Sci* 1975; **63**: 188–95.

Goldstein JE, Cogan DG. Apraxia of lid-opening. *Arch Ophthalmol* 1965; **73**: 155–9.

Graff-Radford NR, Welsh K, Godersky J. Callosal apraxia. *Neurology* 1987; **37**: 100–5.

Hecaen H, Albert M. *Human Neuropsychology*. New York: John Wiley and Sons, 1978.

Heilman KM, Rothi LJ, Valenstein E. Two forms of ideomotor apraxia. *Neurology* 1982; **32**: 342–6.

Lehmkuhl G, Poeck K. A disturbance in the conceptual organization of actions in patients with ideational apraxia. *Cortex* 1981; **17**: 153–8.

Lepore FE, Duvoisin RC. 'Apraxia' of eyelid opening: An involuntary levator inhibition. *Neurology* 1985; **35**: 423–7.

Liepmann H. *Das Krankheitsbild der Apraxie ('motorischen Asymbolie')*. Berlin: Karger, 1900a.

Liepmann H. *Monatschrift Psychiatrie Neurologie* 1900b; **8**: 15–44.

Liepmann H. The syndrome of apraxia (motor asymboly) based on a case of unilateral apraxia. In: *Neurologic Classics in Modern Translation* (Rottenberg RA, Hochberg FH, eds; Bohne WHO, Liepmann K, Rottenberg DA, transl.). New York: Hafner Press, 1977, pp. 155–84.

McFie J, Piercy MF, Zangwill OL. Visual spatial agnosia associated with lesions of the right hemisphere. *Brain* 1950; **73**: 167–90.

Oxbury JM, Campbell DC, Oxbury SM. Unilateral spatial neglect and impairments of spatial analysis and visual perception. *Brain* 1974; **97**: 551–65.

Ratcliff G. Spatial thought, mental rotation and the right cerebral hemisphere. *Neuropsychologia* 1979; **17**: 49–54.

Volpe BT, Sidtis JJ, Hotzman JD, Wilson DH, Gazzaniga MS. Cortical mechanisms involved in praxis: Observations following partial and complete section of the corpus callosum in man. *Neurology* 1982; **32**: 645–50.

Warrington EK, James M, Kinsbourne M. Drawing disability in relation to laterality of cerebral lesion. *Brain* 1966; **89**: 53–82.

Watson RT, Fleet WS, Rothi LG, Heilman KM. Apraxia and the supplementary motor area. *Arch Neurol* 1986; **43**: 787–92.

Yim Y, Morrow L, Passafiume D, Boller F. Visuoperceptual and visuomotor abilities and locus of lesion. *Neuropsychologia* 1984; **22**: 177–85.

6
Disorders of Visual Processing

---

44. *Cortical blindness is caused by bilateral lesions of the primary visual cortex or optic radiations*

Blindness results from bilateral lesions in the visual system at any site from the eyes to the primary visual cortex (striate cortex, area 17), including the lenses, retinas, optic nerves and tracts, lateral geniculate bodies, optic radiations and striate cortices.

Cortical blindness is distinguished from other forms of blindness because the pupillary light reflexes are preserved. This is because the lesions underlying cortical blindness spare those fibers exiting the optic tracts to reach the midbrain and subserving the pupillary light reflex.

Among patients with cortical blindness, extraocular movements are full, unless there is damage to the brainstem, and optokinetic nystagmus is absent.[1] The latter finding is helpful in distinguishing blindness with conversion disorder from that following cortical lesions. Pupillary light reflexes are preserved in both conditions, but optokinetic nystagmus is present only with conversion disorder. However, the absence of optokinetic nystagmus does not exclude conversion blindness, since patients may not foveate on the stimulus.

Visual imagination while awake and while dreaming is usually normal in patients with cortical blindness. Visual hallucinations may occur as ictal phenomena or release hallucinations (Maxim 45; Russell and Whitty, 1955; Cogan, 1973; Lance, 1976). When onset of cortical blindness is acute, patients are often confused and agitated (Symonds and Mackenzie, 1957; Horenstein *et al.*, 1967). Impairment of memory may occur when the lesion extends to medial temporal areas in the dominant hemisphere or bilaterally (Benson *et al.*, 1974).

Patients with cortical blindness are occasionally unaware of their visual loss, a phenomenon known as Anton's syndrome or visual anosognosia. These patients act as if their vision is intact: they walk into walls, bump

---

[1] Cogan observed that with unilateral occipital lobe lesions, optokinetic nystagmus is often lost (towards the side of the hemianopia) if the cause is a mass lesion, but preserved if the cause is vascular (Smith, 1963).

into furniture and attempt to walk outside without the usual precautions a blind person would take. When confronted with their actions and apparent visual impairment, they may confabulate about what they are 'seeing' or offer excuses such as 'The lighting is poor in this room', or 'These are my bad glasses'. In Anton's syndrome, the lesion often extends beyond the striate cortex to involve medial temporal or visual association areas. Many of these patients also have impairment of memory, which may contribute to the anosognosia.

Despite the absence of conscious visual perception, patients with cortical blindness may possess 'blind sight'. Eye movements may be directed toward objects that the patient cannot see (Poppel et al., 1973). Patients may also detect brightness, movement and gross size of objects, but they do not perceive finer visual features such as color, shape or depth (Brindley et al., 1969; Perenin et al., 1980). Blind sight is most likely subserved by fibers from the optic tracts that pass to the midbrain, and possibly by other subcortical structures, such as the lateral geniculate bodies. However, the possibility of a small island of preserved cortical function is difficult to exclude. Merrill and Kewman (1986) reported a successful training of color and form recognition in a young girl with cortical blindness and global cognitive impairment after a cardiopulmonary arrest. This suggests that specific procedures can enhance the function of preserved visual input in these patients.

Bergman (1957) reported loss of alpha activity in the electroencephalogram (EEG) of patients with cortical blindness and reappearance of the activity with improvement in vision. Absence of alpha activity is a consistent finding in cortical blindness. Visual evoked potentials (VEP) recorded in patients with cortical blindness are abnormal in approximately 75 percent of cases, but the findings do not correlate with the severity of visual loss or outcome (Aldrich et al., 1987). The EEG, therefore, is a more sensitive test of cortical blindness than evoked potentials. Unfortunately, neither VEP nor EEG are useful predictors of recovery after cortical blindness (Duchowny et al., 1974; Robertson et al., 1976; Frank and Torres, 1979).

Cortical blindness usually occurs suddenly from a single vascular insult, but may occur gradually or with successive lesions affecting each hemifield (Symonds and Mackenzie, 1957). Bogousslavsky et al. (1983) prospectively studied 58 patients with unilateral occipital infarction and found that 13 developed cortical blindness. In addition to arterial and venous occlusive vascular disorders, permanent cortical blindness also results from cerebral hemorrhage, tumors, cardiopulmonary arrest (especially in children), cardiac bypass surgery, air and fat embolism, uncal herniation, demyelination and the Heidenhain variant of Creutzfeldt–Jakob disease (Gilman, 1965; Nepple et al., 1978; Aldrich et al., 1987). Prognosis is poor in patients with stroke, greater than 40 years of age, a history of diabetes mellitus or hypertension, or cognitive deficits (Aldrich et al., 1987). In contrast, young patients with hypoxic cortical blindness have a better prognosis, especially those in whom neuroimaging studies reveal normal visual radiations (Lambert *et al.*, 1987). Transient causes of cortical blindness include cerebral arteriography, migraine, head trauma, seizures and myelography (Barnet *et al.*, 1970; Greenblatt, 1973; Hachinski *et al.*, 1973; Stoddard *et al.*, 1981; Smirniotopoulos *et al.*, 1984).

References

Aldrich MS, Alessi AG, Beck RW, Gilman S. Cortical blindness: etiology, diagnosis, and prognosis. *Ann Neurol* 1987; **21**: 149–58.

Barnet AB, Manson JI, Liner E. Acute cerebral blindness in childhood: six cases studied clinically and electrophysiologically. *Neurology* 1970; **20**: 1147–56.

Benson DF, Marsden CD, Meadows JC. The amnestic syndrome of posterior cerebral artery occlusion. *Acta Neurol Scand* 1974; **50**: 133–45.

Bergman PS. Cerebral blindness: an analysis of twelve cases, with special reference to the electroencephalogram and patterns of recovery. *Arch Neurol Psychiat* 1957; **78**: 568–84.

Bogousslavsky J, Regli F, Van Melle G. Unilateral occipital infarction: evaluation of the risks of developing bilateral loss of vision. *J Neurol Neurosurg Psychiat* 1983; **46**: 78–80.

Brindley GS, Gautier-Smith PC, Lewin W. Cortical blindness and the function of the non-geniculate fibers of the optic tracts. *J Neurol Neurosurg Psychiat* 1969; **32**: 259–64.

Cogan DG. Visual hallucinations as release phenomena. *Albrecht Graefes Arch Klin Exp Ophthal* 1973; **188**: 139–50.

Duchowny MS, Weiss IP, Majlessi H *et al.* Visual evoked responses in childhood cortical blindness after head trauma and meningitis. *Neurology* 1974; **24**: 933–40.

Frank Y, Torres F. Visual evoked potentials in the evaluation of 'cortical blindness' in children. *Ann Neurol* 1979; **6**: 126–9.

Gilman S. Cerebral disorders after open-heart operations. *N Engl J Med* 1965; **272**: 489–98.

Greenblatt SH. Post traumatic transient cerebral blindness: association with migraine and seizure diathesis. *JAMA* 1973; **225**: 1073–6.

Hachinski VC, Porchawka J, Steele JC. Visual symptoms in the migraine syndrome. *Neurology* 1973; **23**: 570–9.

Horenstein S, Chamberlain W, Conomy J. Infarctions of the fusiform and calcarine regions: Agitated delirium and hemianopia. *Trans Am Neurol Assoc* 1967; **92**: 85–9.

Lambert SR, Hoyt CS, Jan JE, Barkovich J, Flodmark O. Visual recovery from hypoxic cortical blindness during childhood: Computed tomography and magnetic resonance imaging predictors. *Arch Ophthalmol* 1987; **105**: 1371–7.

Lance JW. Simple formed hallucinations confined to the area of a specific visual field defect. *Brain* 1976; **99**: 719–34.

Merrill MK, Kewman DG. Training of color and form identification in cortical blindness: A case study. *Arch Phys Med Rehabil* 1986; **67**: 479–83.

Nepple EW, Appen RE, Sackett JF. Bilateral homonymous hemianopsia. *Am J Ophthalmol* 1978; **86**: 536–43.

Perenin MT, Ruel J, Hecaen H. Residual visual capacities in a case of cortical blindness. *Cortex* 1980; **16**: 605–12.

Poppel E, Held R, Frost D. Residual visual functions after brain wounds involving the central visual pathways in man. *Nature* 1973; **243**: 295–6.

Robertson R, Jan JE, Wong PKH. Electroencephalograms of children with permanent cortical visual impairment. *Can J Neurol Sci* 1976; **13**: 256–1.

Russel WR, Whitty CWM. Studies in traumatic epilepsy 3. Visual fits. *J Neurol Neurosurg Psychiat* 1955; **18**: 79–96.

Smirniotopoulos JG, Murphy FM, Schellinger D, Kurtzke JF, Borts FT. Cortical blindness after metrizamide myelography. *Arch Neurol* 1984; **41**: 224–6.

Smith JL. *Optokinetic Nystagmus*. Springfield, IL: Charles C Thomas Publishers, 1963, pp. 69–92.

Stoddard WE, David DD, Young SW. Cortical blindness after cerebral angiography: case report. *J Neurosurg* 1981; **54**: 240–4.

Symonds C, Mackenzie I. Bilateral loss of vision from cerebral infarction. *Brain* 1957; **80**: 415–55.

45.   *Visual hallucinations and illusions are caused by destructive and irritative lesions in any portion of the visual system*

Visual hallucinations are visual sensations independent of concurrent external light stimulation; the patient sees something the examiner cannot (Lessell, 1975). The hallucinations may be simple (e.g. spots of light, diffuse color, geometric forms) or complex (e.g. a face), localized (e.g. right superior quadrant) or throughout the visual field, and can occur with a clear or clouded sensorium (Bender *et al.*, 1988). Table 45.1 shows the various forms and causes of visual hallucinations. Visual illusions, in contrast, are distortions of external stimuli, such as a book appearing as a telephone.

Simple (elementary) visual hallucinations

Photopsias – sparks or flashes – are the most common type of simple visual hallucinations. Elementary visual hallucinations arise from dysfunction in the visual pathways running between the eye and the primary visual cortex or, less often, from irritative lesions in the visual association cortex and medial temporal lobe. Electrical stimulation of the visual radiations and cortex (Brodman areas 17 and 18) produces simple visual hallucinations, usually flashes of lights or colors (Foerster, 1931; Adams and Rutkin, 1970).

Elementary hallucinations have little localizing value, but lateralization is usually ipsilateral with lesions anterior to the chiasm and contralateral with optic pathway more posteriorly situated lesions. Patients with homonymous hemianopsia and simple visual hallucinations often incorrectly describe the image as occurring solely in the contralateral eye. It is important to ask the patient if they tested vision in each eye with the other eye closed and to instruct them to do so with future episodes if there is doubt.

In patients with calcarine cortex lesions, visual hallucinations usually occur in areas of visual loss and tend to be continuous and unformed. These hallucinations are often associated with an element of movement,

Table 45.1   Visual hallucinations.

	Type	
	Simple (elementary)	Complex (formed)
	Photopsia (light flashes) Phosphenes (blue lights) Scintillations (zigzags) Geometric forms Checkerboard patterns Positive scotomas*	People Objects Scenes and landscapes Animals (zoopsia)

Etiology	Sleep/sensory deprivation
	Febrile states
	Nutritional deficiencies
	Drugs (e.g. LSD)
	Alcohol withdrawal
	Pressure on globe
	Glaucoma
	Macular degeneration†
	Retinal ischemia†.
	Incipient retinal detachment
	Migraine
	Release
	Irritative visual cortex lesions†
		Sleep/sensory deprivation
		Febrile states
		Nutritional deficiencies
		Drugs (e.g. LSD)
		Alcohol withdrawal
		Temporal or parietal-occipital
		  visual association area
		  lesions† (Release)
		Irritative temporal lesions†
		Irritative occipitoparietal
		  lesions

*Seen with eyes closed and in the dark.
†Most common lesion sites are listed, but they may occur with lesions in any part of the visual pathways.

such as in weaving patterns, zigzag lights and a shower of sparks or colored clouds (Russel and Whitty, 1955). However, interrupted flashes of light are not typical of hallucinations arising in primary visual cortex. Unformed visual hallucinations also occur with cerebral lesions outside the calcarine cortex. Stimulation of the hippocampus evokes colored balls or flashing lights (Adams and Rutkin, 1970; Halgren *et al.*, 1978), and patients with temporal lobe epilepsy may 'see' flashing lights (Russel and Whitty, 1955).

Scintillating scotomas and zigzag lines are most often found in classic migraine, but also occur with posterior cerebral structural lesions, such as tumors or arteriovenous malformations (Bender and Furlow, 1945). Basilar artery migraine is usually a benign disorder in young women (Bickerstaff, 1961; Swanson and Vick, 1978). However, it occurs in both sexes, a wide age range and is associated with posterior circulation strokes in some patients (Caplan, 1991). Scotomas are usually negative phenomena resulting from loss of normal sensory input, although they may be associated with such positive symptoms as halos of color, opacity or 'heat waves' surrounding the black hole. In some patients, however, scotomas are positive phenomena that persist even in the dark or when the eyes are closed

(Bender and Furlow, 1945). Scotomata and these surrounding phenomena usually result from optic nerve or striate cortex lesions.

Complex (formed) visual hallucinations

Formed visual hallucinations usually occur with lesions in the temporal or parieto-occipital association areas, but have been reported with lesions throughout the visual system (Weinberger and Grant, 1940). The images may appear to be moving, multiple or abnormal in size (most often, the images are perceived as smaller than their real counterparts, a phenomenon known as 'lilliputian hallucinations'). Hallucinations caused by seizure discharges are typically brief, lasting less than three minutes and often less than 30 seconds, and are often associated with illusions or hallucinations in other sensory modalities. However, this association also occurs among patients with systemic illness or under the influence of hallucinogenic drugs. Ictal simple visual hallucinations may transform into complex forms, as Dewhurst and Pearson (1955) reported in a man with seizures from a shrapnel wound in the right temporal lobe. Initially, he saw multicolored lights, but he later reported approaching and receding 'crowds of tiny figures all the colors of the rainbow – all myself.'

Autoscopy is the hallucination or psychic experience of seeing oneself. There are two principal forms of autoscopic phenomena. The first is a 'complex psychosensorial hallucinatory perception of one's own body image projected into external visual space', or seeing one's double (Lukianowicz, 1958). The second, an out-of-body experience, is the feeling of leaving one's body and viewing it from another vantage point, usually from above. Autoscopic phenomena occur in healthy persons, especially with anxiety and fatigue, and in those patients experiencing near-death phenomena, systemic illnesses, migraine and ictal discharges from temporal or parietal lobes without lateralized preference (Devinsky *et al.*, 1989).

Peduncular hallucinosis is a rare disorder in which vivid, well-formed visual hallucinations, such as a brightly colored parrot, follow infarction in the distal basilar territory (Lhermitte, 1922; van Bogaert, 1924). Among these patients, infarction is usually embolic and variably affects the midbrain, diencephalon and occipitotemporal cortex (posterior cerebral artery distribution). Although complex visual hallucinations predominate among such patients, unformed visual hallucinations are also reported. The pathological anatomy and physiology of these hallucinations is not clear, but they are probably related to a sleep abnormality, which is present in most cases (Caplan, 1980). Evening hallucinations in elderly subjects with cognitive deficits, sometimes called 'sun-downing', may be a related disorder.

Pathophysiology of visual hallucinations

Visual hallucinations result from a variety of pathophysiological mechanisms (West, 1962). When cortical in origin, simple visual hallucinations usually result from irritation of the striate cortex, while complex visual hallucinations usually result from stimulation of temporal or occipitoparietal association cortices (Baldwin, 1970).

Epileptic phenomena, discussed above, are characteristically paroxysmal in onset and brief in duration.

Sensory deprivation or prolonged darkness can cause simple and complex hallucinatory experiences (Bliss and Clark, 1962).

Release hallucinations occur after lesions of the visual pathway impair normal inhibitory visual mechanisms and are typically continuous, non-stereotyped and influenced by such purposeful acts as changing the direction of gaze (Cogan, 1973). They are more common in the acute stage and among those patients who have visual acuity of 20/50 or less in both eyes (Cogan, 1973; Lepore, 1990). Release hallucinations have less localizing value than those due to cortical irritation (Cogan, 1973; Lepore, 1990). Among patients with visual release hallucinations, simple forms are more than twice as common as complex hallucinations (Lepore, 1990).

However, simple sensory deprivation cannot explain all release hallucinations. Following enucleation, simple visual hallucinations may occur despite normal vision in the remaining eye (Gillmore, 1980). Also, simple and complex visual hallucinations occur in patients with pseudotumor cerebri with only slightly enlarged blind spots (Lepore, 1990).

It is uncertain if the confabulatory visual reports of patients with Anton's syndrome (denial of cortical blindness; Maxim 63) represent release hallucinations or fabrications.

Delirium, drug intoxication and withdrawal states are commonly associated with hallucinations, in addition to an altered sensorium. These hallucinations often occur in several sensory modalities and tend to be continuous. Disruption of the normal mechanisms of selective attention may permit subliminal visual experiences to rise into consciousness (Bender *et al.*, 1988).

Visual illusions

In visual illusions, the image may be altered in size (micropsia or macropsia), shape (dysmorphopsia or metamorphopsia), position (telopsia), number (polyopia), color or movement (Bender and Savitsky, 1943; Teuber and Bender, 1949; Bender *et al.*, 1957). Visual illusions may be restricted to areas with partial visual loss or affect the entire visual field.

In confused patients, images of real objects may be perceived as more complex and familiar. For example, a patient in alcohol withdrawal may 'see' a spot on the wall as a spider, or a sock as a rat. Vestibular or oculomotor disorders may cause illusions with altered depth perception, tilting and changes in shape (e.g. straight edges become curved). Brainstem lesions involving vestibulo-ocular integrative functions can cause a 180 degree reversal of the visual world, effectively turning it upside down (Steiner *et al.*, 1987; Hornsten, 1974).

Palinopsia is the persistence or recurrence of visual images after the excitatory stimulus has been removed (Bender *et al.*, 1968). Critchley (1951) reported a patient with palinopsia who had difficulty shaving: 'I have shaved one side so that it is beautifully clean to my fingers. I looked back to find that the beard seemed to be still there. Because of that I sometimes shave myself twice, for no earthly reason'. Whether one considers palinopsia as a hallucination is a question of nomenclature, since one can define hallucinations according to whether there is no real stimulus or, alternatively, based on the absence of a stimulus at the time the image is perceived.

Palinopsia occurs with structural lesions in the parietal and occipital lobes of either hemisphere, but most often the right hemisphere (Meadows and Munro, 1977; Michel and Troost, 1980; Cummings *et al.*, 1982). It is usually a transient phenomenon occurring during the progressive evolution or resolution of a homonymous visual field defect, and it appears in the area of visual loss. Rarely, however, palinopsia may persist for years. Palinopsia is probably related to the phenomenon of illusory visual spread, in which the visual perception extends over a greater area than that which the stimulus would be expected to excite. For example, the subject looks at a clock and sees the area between 7 and 12 o'clock as being twice as large as the area between 1 and 6 o'clock (Critchley, 1951).

Possible mechanisms for palinopsia include sensory seizures, psychogenic elaborations and release hallucinations (Bender *et al.*, 1968). Palinopsia can result from epileptic discharges. This mechanism is supported by the recording of epileptiform discharges during palinopsia, occurrence of palinopsia with other epileptic symptoms and resolution of palinopsia with antiepileptic medications (Swash, 1979; Jacobs, 1980). Psychogenic mechanisms may contribute to palinopsia, as patients report that 'things they think about a lot do not go out of vision as quickly, as if they were slow in being switched off' (Critchley, 1951). Most cases of palinopsia are probably release hallucinations.

Visual dysesthesiae are unpleasant visual sensations precipitated by looking at an object in a defective homonymous visual hemifield. These rare phenomena usually occur following lesions in the visual radiations (Bender *et al.*, 1949a).

Visual synesthesiae are optic percepts induced by stimuli in other sensory modalities, e.g. auditory or tactile (Jacobs *et al.*, 1981). Patients may see shapes or colors in response to hearing specific sounds. Visual synesthesia occurs with lesions throughout the visual pathways.

The *Tullio phenomenon* is a rare condition in which loud sounds cause a rapid shift of gaze. The postulated mechanism is abnormal mechanical connection between the auditory and vestibular end-organs (Bender *et al.*, 1988).

Visual allesthesia is transposition of visual images from one homonymous half-field to another. This rare phenomenon usually occurs in patients with bilateral cerebral lesions, but may occur with focal seizures (Bender *et al.*, 1948, 1949b; Jacobs, 1980; Heilman and Howell, 1980). Allesthesia often occurs with auditory and somatic sensations as well as visual images.

References

Adams JE, Rutkin BB. Visual responses to subcortical stimulation in the visual and limbic systems. *Confin Neurol* 1970; **32**: 158–64.

Baldwin F. Neurologic syndromes and hallucinations. In: *Origin and Mechanisms of Hallucinations* (Keup W, ed.). New York: Plenum Press, 1970, pp. 3–12.

Bender MB, Feldman M, Sobin AJ. Palinopsia. *Brain* 1968; **91**: 321–38.

Bender MB, Furlow LT. Visual disturbances produced by bilateral lesions of the occipital lobes with central scotomas. *Arch Neurol Psychiat* 1945; **53**: 165–70.

Bender MB, Furlow LT, Teuber HL. Alterations in behavior after massive cerebral trauma (intraventricular foreign body). *Confin Neurol* 1949a; **9**: 140–57.

Bender MB, Postel DM, Krieger HP. Disorders in oculomotor function in lesions of the occipital lobe. *J Neurol Neurosurg Psychiat* 1957; **20**: 139–43.

Bender MB, Rudolph SH, Stacy CB. The neurology of the visual and oculomotor systems. In: *Clinical Neurology* (volume 1, Chapter 12) (Joynt RJ, ed.). Philadelphia: JB Lippincott Company, 1988, pp. 1–132.

Bender MB, Savitsky N. Micropsia and telopsia limited to the temporal fields of vision. *Arch Ophthalmol* 1943; **29**: 904–8.

Bender MB, Shapiro MF, Teuber HL. Allesthesia and disturbance of the body schema. *Arch Neurol Psychiat* 1949b; **62**: 222–35.

Bender MB, Wortis SB, Cramer J. Organic mental syndrome with phenomena of extinction and allesthesia. *Arch Neurol Psychiat* 1948; **59**: 273–91.

Bickerstaff ER. Basilar artery migraine. *Lancet* 1961; **i**: 15–17.

Bliss EL, Clark LD. Visual hallucinations. In: *Hallucinations* (West LJ, ed.). New York: Grune and Stratton, 1962.

Caplan LR. 'Top of the basilar' syndrome. *Neurology* 1980; **30**: 72–9.

Caplan LR. Migraine and vertebrobasilar ischemia. *Neurology* 1991; **41**: 55–61.

Cogan DG. Visual hallucinations as release phenomena. *Albrecht von Graefes Arch Klin Exp Ophthalmol* 1973; **188**: 139–50.

Critchley M. Types of visual perseveration: 'Paliopsia' and 'illusory visual spread'. *Brain* 1951; **74**: 267–99.

Cummings JL, Syndulko K, Goldberg Z, Treiman DM. Palinopsia reconsidered. *Neurology* 1982; **32**: 444–7.

Devinsky O, Feldmann E, Burrowes K, Bromfield E. Autoscopic phenomena with seizures. *Arch Neurol* 1989; **46**: 1080–8.

Dewhurst K, Pearson J. Visual hallucinations of the self in organic disease. *J Neurol Neurosurg Psychiat* 1955; **18**: 53–7.

Foerster O. The cerebral cortex in man. *Lancet* 1931; **ii**: 309–12.

Gillmore CS. Visual images observed following an ennucleation. *Perception* 1980; **9**: 493–502.

Halgren E, Walter RD, Cherlow DG, Crandall PH. Mental phenomena evoked by electrical stimulation of the human hippocampal formation and amygdala. *Brain* 1978; **101**: 83–117.

Heilman KM, Howell GJ. Seizure-induced neglect. *J Neurol Neurosurg Psychiat* 1980; **43**: 1035–40.

Hornsten G. Wallenberg's syndrome. I. General symptomatology with special reference to visual disturbances and imbalance. *Acta Neurol Scand* 1974; **50**: 434–46.

Jacobs L. Visual allesthesia. *Neurology* 1980; **30**: 1059–63.

Jacobs L, Karpik A, Bozian D, Gothgen S. Auditory–visual synesthesia. *Arch Neurol* 1981; **38**: 211.

Lepore FE. Spontaneous visual phenomena with visual loss: 104 patients with lesions of retinal and neural afferent pathways. *Neurology* 1990; **40**: 444–7.

Lessell S. Higher disorders of visual function: positive phenomena. In: *Neuro-ophthalmology* (volume 8) (Glaser JS, Smith JL, eds). St Louis: CV Mosby Company, 1975, pp. 27–44.

Lhermitte J. Syndrome de la calotte du pedoncle cerebral: Les troubles psycho-sensoriels dans les lesions du mesocephale. *Rev Neurol (Paris)* 1922; **38**: 1359–65.

Lukianowicz N. Autoscopic phenomena. *Arch Neurol Psychiat* 1958: **80**: 199–220.

Meadows JC, Munro SSF. Palinopsia. *J Neurol Neurosurg Psychiat* 1977; **40**: 5–8.

Michel EM, Troost BT. Palinopsia: cerebral localization with computed tomography. *Neurology* 1980; **30**: 887–9.

Russel WR, Whitty CWM. Studies in traumatic epilepsy. 3. Visual fits. *J Neurol Neurosurg Psychiat* 1955; **18**: 79–96.

Steiner I, Shahin R, Melamed E. Acute 'upside down' reversal of vision in transient vertebrobasilar ischemia. *Neurology* 1987; **37**: 1685–6.

Swanson JW, Vick NA. Basilar artery migraine. *Neurology* 1978; **28**: 782–6.

Swash M. Visual perseveration in temporal lobe epilepsy. *J Neurol Neurosurg Psychiat* 1979; **42**: 569–71.

Teuber HL, Bender MB. Alterations in pattern vision following trauma of occipital lobes in man. *J Gen Psychol* 1949; **40**: 37–57.

van Bogaert L. L'hallucinose pedonculaire. *Rev Neurol (Paris)* 1924; **40**: 416–23.

Weinberger L, Grant FC. Visual hallucinations and their neuro-optic correlates. *Arch Ophthalmol* 1940; **23**: 166–99.

West LJ. *Hallucinations*. New York: Grune and Stratton, 1962.

46.   *Normal visual perception must be established before the diagnosis of visual agnosia is made*

Visual agnosia is the failure to recognize visual stimuli despite normal attention, intelligence, language and visual perception (Ettlinger and Wyke, 1961; Albert *et al.*, 1975). As in all agnosias, the patient is unable to derive meaning from the preserved primary sensory input. Visual agnosia is commonly divided into two principal forms: apperceptive, resulting from impairment in higher order visual perception, and associative, which is the true form (Alexander and Albert, 1983). In visual apperceptive agnosia, patients often complain of blurred or unclear vision and are unable accurately to copy a drawing or match related visual stimuli. Therefore, this disorder is not truly an agnosia and will not be discussed further.

Associative visual agnosia consists of two subsyndromes: object agnosia, or the inability to recognize objects, and prosopagnosia, the inability to recognize faces (Maxim 47) (Rubens and Benson, 1971). Patients with visual object agnosia also have prosopagnosia, but those with prosopagnosia do not necessarily have visual object agnosia.

The diagnosis of visual agnosia can only be made after normal visual perception is established. In visual agnosia, visual acuity is normal or near normal, visual fields are normal or mildly abnormal, and complaints of hazy or otherwise altered vision should not be present. There are several means by which to judge normal visual perception.

The first and most important criterion is the patient's description of the visual world. The patient should be able to give a detailed description of visual stimuli, since aphasia is mild or absent. Ask about shape, size, edges and contour, position and number of stimuli. Most patients with visual agnosia are unable to describe colors, because usually they have achromatopsia, an abnormality of color recognition and discrimination among hues that is not a primary naming defect (Maxim 49). Normal visual perception can also be demonstrated by copying a complex figure, matching similar figures or matching an object with a drawing of the object. Despite success with verbal descriptions, drawing and matching of visual stimuli, it is possible that subtle defects in primary visual perception exist and contribute to the impaired recognition found in visual agnosia.

Once normal visual perception is established, one must then rule out anomia. Because agnosic patients are often misdiagnosed with anomic aphasia (the inability to name) and vise versa, it is essential to use both verbal and non-verbal tests of object recognition. First, ask the patient to describe what she sees. Agnosic patients can describe the features and shape of an object, but fail to recognize it. When shown a picture of a car, for example, the patient is unable to state what the object is, what you do with it or what you put in it to make it go. In contrast, an anomic patient shown the same picture might respond 'It's that thing you get in and drive'. Secondly, test such non-verbal tasks as matching of pictures with functionally related objects. In non-verbal tasks, anomic patients do well – they easily match pictures of a hammer and of a nail – but agnosic patients fare poorly.

In addition, the recognition defect in visual agnosia is often incomplete. Patients with visual agnosia recognize real objects better than line drawings of objects. They also recognize common objects like a fork or pen more easily than such objects as a stethoscope or city skyline, which are uncommon or complex.

Visual agnosia is caused by bilateral damage to the inferior temporo-occipital junction and subjacent white matter (Figure 47.1) (Benson et al., 1974; Mack and Boller, 1977; Albert et al., 1979). The functional basis of visual agnosia can be destruction of higher order visual associative cortices in the occipital lobe or disconnection of visual association and temporo-limbic memory areas. The inferior longitudinal fasciculus, which connects the occipital association cortex and medial temporal lobe, is usually destroyed bilaterally in visual associative agnosia. The pathogenesis is most often bilateral posterior cerebral artery infarction. In many cases, infarction on one side is followed months or years later by a stroke on the other side, giving rise to the agnosic defect. Other causes include tumor, hemorrhage and demyelination.

References

Albert ML, Reches A, Silbergerg R. Associative visual agnosia without alexia. *Neurology* 1975; **25**: 322–6.

Albert ML, Soffer D, Silverberg R, Reches A. The anatomical basis of visual agnosia. *Neurology* 1979; **29**: 876–9.

Alexander MP, Albert ML. The anatomical basis of visual agnosia. In: *Localization in Neuropsychology* (Kertesz A, ed.). Orlando, FL: Academic Press, Inc., 1983, pp. 393–415.

Benson DF, Segarra J, Albert ML. Visual agnosia-prosopagnosia. *Neurology* 1974; **30**: 307–10.

Ettlinger G, Wyke M. Defects in identifying objects visually in a patient with cerebrovascular disease. *J Neurol Neurosurg Psychiat* 1961; **24**: 254–9.

Mack JL, Boller F. Associative visual agnosia and its related deficits: The role of the minor hemisphere in assigning meaning to visual perceptions. *Neuropsychology* 1977: **15**: 345–9.

Rubens AB, Benson DF. Associative visual agnosia. *Arch Neurol* 1971; **24**: 305–16.

47. *Prosopagnosia, or defective facial recognition, is caused by bilateral occipital or occipitotemporal lesions*

Prosopagnosia, a distinct form of visual agnosia, is characterized by the inability to recognize previously known faces and an impairment in learning and recognizing new faces (Bodamer, 1947). Because prosopagnosia is a form of visual agnosia, the criteria of normal attention, intelligence, language and visual perception must be met (Maxim 46).

These patients look in the mirror and don't recognize their own image. When patients with prosopagnosia look at a face, they can identify the nose, eyes, cheek and mouth, and can describe the whole as a face, but they cannot tell you whose face it is.

Although prosopagnosia is defined by this impairment in recognizing human faces, the defect affects visually triggered memory more generally (Damasio, 1985), extending to other classes of visually related stimuli. Thus, there is not only a defect in visual identification of relatives and friends, but also in recognition of specific types of cars (e.g. Cadillac versus Volkswagen), birds (e.g. eagle versus owl), trees (e.g. pine versus oak) and so on.

In contrast to visual object agnosia, recognition of classes of objects in prosopagnosia is preserved. Despite inability to recognize specific members within a class of objects, patients with prosopagnosia correctly identify the class itself, e.g. 'car' versus 'tree'.

Prosopagnosia usually develops suddenly, and patients realize that a relative's or their own face appears unfamiliar. Patients can identify their spouses by voice, perfume, body shape or clothes, but they perceive spouses' faces as foreign. The recognition of familiar individuals by voice and other clues indicates that intelligence and memory are intact.

Other deficits associated with prosopagnosia include constructional apraxia, dressing apraxia, left hemianopia and left-sided neglect (Hecaen and Angelergues, 1962). In addition, Pallis (1955) reported the association of prosopagnosia and geographical disorientation. Patients with geographic disorientation are unable to identify correct spatial relations (e.g. New York City is northeast of Los Angeles), recall directions or learn new routes.

The mechanism underlying prosopagnosia may vary with the location of the lesion. Hecaen and Angelergues (1962) and Warrington and James (1967) suggested that mnenomic processes specific for certain visual information are disrupted in prosopagnosia. Levine et al. (1985) described a patient with prosopagnosia who could not visually describe objects from memory, especially faces and animals. Damasio et al. (1982) proposed a model in which three possible abnormalities in complex visual processing could produce prosopagnosia: (1) interference with arrival of visual input at the 'facial template system'; (2) destruction of the facial template system, located in the mesial occipitotemporal visual association cortex (lingual and fusiform gyri); or (3) destruction of the white matter pathways that connect the facial template system with multimodal memory banks.

Controversy persists over the site of the lesions that produce prosopagnosia. Some propose that bilateral mesial occipitotemporal lesions are always present, while others argue that right-sided mesial occipitotemporal lesions are sufficient to produce permanent prosopagnosia (Meadows, 1974). DeRenzi (1986) reported two cases of persistent prosopagnosia in which computed tomography (CT) demonstrated only a right medial occipitotemporal lesion, and Sergent and Villemure (1989) reported a woman with right-sided hemispherectomy and persistent prosopagnosia who was unaware of her deficit. In general, however, most patients with unilateral, right-sided lesions and prosopagnosia have transient, mild-to-moderate deficits. Damasio et al. (1982) found that the vast majority of cases with persistent prosopagnosia have bilateral lesions in the inferomesial visual association cortices (lingual and fusiform gyri) and subjacent white matter (Fig. 47.1). To support further this bilateral lesion localization, Damasio et al. (1975) point out that some patients with right-sided hemispherectomy recognize faces normally. Also, following corpus callosotomy, patients are able to recognize faces in each hemifield (Levy et al., 1972).

Lesions that cause prosopagnosia occupy similar territory to those found in visual object agnosia, but they are usually less extensive. The most common pathogenesis is embolic infarction in the posterior cerebral artery (PCA) distribution. When the infarct is restricted to the right hemisphere, the deficit often resolves within several months. In some cases, a unilateral PCA stroke is followed months or years later by a contralateral infarct that

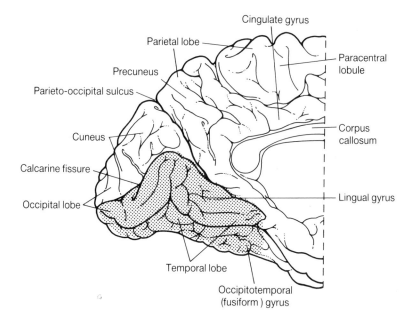

Fig. 47.1   Medial view of the brain: areas involved (bilaterally) in patients with visual agnosia and prosopagnosia.

causes prosopagnosia, visual object agnosia or cortical blindness (Maxims 44 and 46). In addition, butterfly gliomas that traverse the splenium of the corpus callosum to involve the white matter of both hemispheres posteriorly can cause prosopagnosia. Prosopagnosia has been reported as an ictal phenomenon in one patient with left posterior temporal–occipital focus; the deficit most likely resulted from bilateral spread of the seizure activity (Agnetti *et al.*, 1978).

References

Agnetti V, Carreras M, Pinna L, Rosati G. Ictal prosopagnosia and epileptogenic damage of the dominant hemisphere: A case history. *Neuropsychologia* 1978; **14**: 50–7.

Bodamer J. Die prosopagnosie. *Arch Psychiatr Nervenkr* 1947; **179**: 6–54.

Damasio AR. Disorders of complex visual processing. In: *Principles of Behavioral Neurology* (Mesulam M-M, ed.). Phildelphia: FA Davis Company, 1985, pp. 259–88.

Damasio AR, Damasio H, Van Hoesen GW. Prosopagnosia: Anatomic basis and behaviorial mechanisms. *Neurology* 1982; **32**: 331–41.

Damasio AR, Lima PA, Damasio H. Nervous function after right hemispherectomy. *Neurology* 1975; **25**: 89–93.

DeRenzi E. Prosopagnosia in two patients with CT evidence of damage confined to the right hemisphere. *Neuropsychologia* 1986; **24**: 385–9.

Hecaen H, Angelergues R. Agnosia for faces. *Arch Neurol* 1962; **7**: 92–100.

Levine DN, Warach J, Farah M. Two visual systems in mental imagery. *Neurology* 1985; **35**: 1010–18.

Levy J, Trevarthen C, Sperry RW. Perception of bilateral chimeric figures following hemispheric disconnection. *Brain* 1972; **95**: 61–78.

Meadows JC. The anatomical basis of prosopagnosia. *J Neurol Neurosurg Psychiat* 1974; **37**: 489–501.

Pallis CA. Impaired identification for faces and places with agnosia for colors. *J Neurol Neurosurg Psychiat* 1955; **18**: 218.

Sergent J, Villemure JG. Prosopagnosia in a right hemispherectomized patient. *Brain* 1989; **112**: 979–95.

Warrington EK, James M. An experimental investigation of facial recognition in patients with unilateral cerebral lesions. *Cortex* 1967; **3**: 317–26.

48.   *Balint's syndrome – the triad of simultanagnosia, oculomotor apraxia and optic ataxia – results from bilateral occipitoparietal lesions*

Balint's syndrome is rare and presents as one of the most dramatic behavioral disorders. Patients appear blind at first glance; they are unable visually to detect new stimuli approaching them, fail to see a car pass in front of them, bump into walls and furniture, and make wild, inaccurate movements when reaching for things. However, they can often describe minute visual details that require normal visual acuity. Formal visual field testing reveals full fields or inconsistent partial defects (Hecaen and Ajuriaguerra, 1954).

The paradox of what can and cannot be seen in Balint's syndrome is explained by the central feature of the syndrome: *simultanagnosia*. Simultagnosia is the inability to perceive the visual field as whole, sometimes called 'piecemeal vision' (Rizzo and Robin, 1990). For example, a patient with simultanagnosia may look out the window on a scene of snow, sidewalk, street, trees, bushes and children but see only a small piece of the picture, such as a part of a tree. Suddenly, the patient's gaze is uncontrollably shifted to another fragment of the scene (e.g. a child's lower body) and shifted again (e.g. a patch of snow). Thus, patients with simultanagnosia are unable to see more than one or two objects at one time (Kinsbourne and Warrington, 1962); they usually see only with macular vision, which provides good acuity but only captures a tiny fraction of the visual field; and experience unpredictable jumping of focus from sector to sector, which does not allow detailed or systematic analysis of a particular region or object. Patients complain that just when they find the target stimulus, it disappears. A defect in sustained visual attention may underly simultanagnosia (Rizzo and Robin, 1990).

The Cookie Theft Picture (Fig. 48.1), from the Boston Diagnostic Aphasia

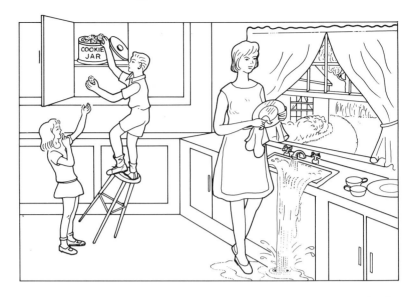

Fig. 48.1 The cookie thief. (From the Boston Naming Text; Lea and Febiger, with permission.)

Examination, is an excellent stimulus to test simultanagnosia (Rizzo and Hurtig, 1987). Patients often report seeing only the mother, the stool or a hand and the cookie jar.

Oculomotor apraxia or psychic paralysis of gaze, is the inability voluntarily to direct gaze toward a specific part of the visual field (Cogan and Adams, 1953). Thus, even if the patient is told where to look to see an object, he has difficulty directing foveal vision to that spot. This disorder is more accurately described as an impairment of visuomotor integration and generation of saccades, rather than apraxia. Normally, when a novel stimulus enters our peripheral vision, we make a saccadic eye movement to bring foveal vision in line with that stimulus. In oculomotor apraxia, however, absent or inaccurate saccades render the subject functionally blind. Tyler (1968) demonstrated that the visual perceptual deficit in Balint's syndrome is largely due to deficient eye movements when scanning a complex scene. Thus, the simultanagnosia and oculomotor apraxia are related deficits.

Optic, or visuomotor, ataxia is the inability to direct movement of an extremity using visual guidance. The patient sees the pen she wants to pick up, and the right hand moves to grasp it, but the pen eludes her. In contrast, hand and arm movements under proprioceptive guidance (e.g. 'close your eyes and touch the tip of your left index finger to the tip of your nose') are performed accurately.

There is often diagnostic confusion between Balint's syndrome and visual agnosia or alexia. This occurs because patients with Balint's syndrome complain that, although they can see, they cannot recognize what

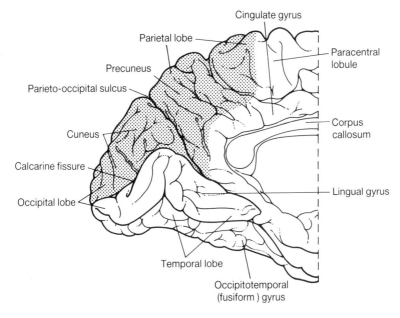

Fig. 48.2 Medial view of the brain: areas involved (bilaterally) in patients with Balint's syndrome.

they are seeing and cannot read (Damasio, 1985). It is therefore important to test patients with small visual stimuli, making sure to test foveal vision. Under these conditions, recognition will occur. Patience is required, since it may take time for the fovea to locate the test stimulus. Balint's syndrome may also be mistaken for a visual conversion reaction since a patient may report seeing 'features of the nurse's face across the room but . . . not . . . the examiner's hand when it was held one foot in front of him' (Juergens *et al.*, 1986).

Balint's syndrome results from bilateral occipitoparietal lesions, specifically within the dorsal, superior, visual system (Hecaen and Ajuriaguerra, 1954; Hausser *et al.*, 1980; Damasio, 1985). In contrast, the lesions in visual agnosia are found in the ventral, inferior occipitotemporal, visual system. The cause is most often stroke resulting from hypotension (e.g. myocardial infarction with diffuse cerebral atherosclerosis or cardiac bypass surgery) with infarction encompassing the watershed between the territories of the anterior, posterior and middle cerebral arteries. Multiple emboli, venous infarction (e.g. postpartum), multiple metastases and butterfly gliomas extending bilaterally across the splenium and posterior body of the corpus callosum also cause Balint's syndrome.

Partial forms of Balint's syndrome, with isolated simultanagnosia, optic ataxia, or oculomotor apraxia have been reported. In patients with isolated simultanagnosia, stationary objects in direct view disappear, despite normal visual acuity and ocular motility and scanning (Rizzo and Hurtig, 1987). The disappearance of stationary objects most probably results from the defect in sustained visual attention that accompanies and contributes to simultanagnosia (Rizzo and Robin, 1990). In such patients, the lesion involves superior visual association cortices in the occipital lobes but spares the parietal visual centers needed for visuomotor control. Patients with left-sided occipital lesions and alexia without agraphia may also develop simultanagnosia (Levine and Calvanio, 1978), having an inability to read entire words despite normal reading of individual letters (Kinsbourne and Warrington, 1962; Levine and Calvanio, 1978).

Isolated optic ataxia causes a severe impairment in visually guided movements and results from destruction of visual association areas, parietal visuomotor centers, or disconnection of the projections from visual and visuomotor areas to the frontal lobe (Rondot and de Recondo, 1974; Boller *et al.*, 1975; Damasio and Benton, 1979). In a patient with a right-sided parietal tumor, optic ataxia was reported for all movements of the left hand and for movements of the right hand within the left hemifield (Levine *et al.*, 1978).

Isolated oculomotor apraxia is rare (Cogan and Adams, 1953; Waltz, 1961). These patients can move their eyes on command but the ocular movements are random and aimless. They are unable to follow a moving stimulus. This deficit has been reported with unilateral lesions in the frontal or frontoparietal lobes (Cogan and Adams, 1953; Waltz, 1961).

References

Boller F, Cole M, Kim Y, Mack JL, Patawaren C. Optic ataxia: Clinical–radiological correlations with the EMI scan. *J Neurol Neurosurg Psychiat* 1975; **38**: 954–8.

Cogan DG, Adams RD. A type of paralysis of conjugate gaze (ocular motor apraxia). *Arch Ophthalmol* 1953; **50**: 434–42.

Damasio AR. Disorders of complex visual processing. In: *Principles of Behavioral Neurology* (Mesulam M-M, ed.). Philadelphia: FA Davis Company, 1985, pp. 259–88.

Damasio AR, Benton AL. Impairment of hand movements under visual guidance. *Neurology* 1979; **29**: 170–8.

Hecaen H, Ajuriaguerra J. Balint's syndrome (psychic paralysis of gaze) and its minor forms. *Brain* 1954; **77**: 373–400.

Hausser CO, Robert F, Giard N. Balint's syndrome. *Can J Neurol Sci* 1980; **7**: 157–61.

Juergens SM, Fredrickson PA, Pfeiffer FE. Balint's syndrome mistaken for visual conversion reaction. *Psychosomatics* 1986; **27**: 597–9.

Kinsbourne M, Warrington EK. A disorder of simultaneous form perception. *Brain* 1962; **85**: 461–86.

Levine DN, Calvanio R. A study of the visual defect in verbal alexia-simultanagnosia. *Brain* 1978; **101**: 65–81.

Levine DN, Kaufman KJ, Mohr JP. Inaccurate reaching associated with a superior parietal tumor. *Neurology* 1978; **28**: 556–61.

Rizzo M, Hurtig R. Looking but not seeing: Attention, perception, and eye movements in simultanagnosia. *Neurology* 1987; **37**: 1642–8.

Rizzo M, Robin DA. Simultanagnosia: A defect of sustained attention yields insights on visual information processing. *Neurology* 1990; **40**: 447–55.

Rondot P, de Recondo J. Ataxie optique: Trouble de la coordination visuo-motrice. *Brain Res* 1974; **71**: 367–75.

Tyler HR. Abnormality of perception with defective eye movements (Balint's syndrome). *Cortex* 1968; **4**: 154–71.

Waltz AG. Dyspraxias of gaze. *Arch Neurol* 1961; **5**: 74–83.

49.   *Distinguish achromatopsia from color anomia*

Achromatopsia is an acquired disorder characterized by loss of color perception in part or all of the visual field, and it results from lesions that affect visual association cortex in the occipitotemporal area or damage to subjacent white matter. In contrast, patients with color anomia have normal color perception and can discriminate hues non-verbally, although they are unable to name colors or to point to a color when given its name (Damasio, 1985).

Although they are designed for testing color blindness, pseudoisochromatic plates (Ishihara or American Optical) are helpful in diagnosing patients with achromotopsia. These plates contain numbers or geometric designs formed by dots of related hues and varying sizes juxtaposed against a random background composed of dots with a different hue. These plates are also useful in the assessment of optic nerve disease (e.g. retrobulbar neuritis) with impaired color vision.

Achromatopsia usually develops suddenly, and patients are often aware that their world has faded from color to black and white (Meadows, 1974). Color loss varies in degree. For some patients, the world may appear washed-out or bleached and color identification may still be possible. Others may only see shades of gray that even render green and red tomatoes indistinguishable. Visual acuity and ability to distinguish subtle differences in form and depth are well preserved (Pearlman *et al.*, 1979), and patients have no difficulty reciting the names of colors. Loss of color perception from cerebral lesions can be transient or permanent.

Hemiachromatopsia, or loss of color perception in half the visual field, may occur without other visual defects (Albert *et al.*, 1975). Right hemiachromatopsia results from left occipitotemporal lesions that involve the lingual and fusiform gyri (Damasio *et al.*, 1980). It is often accompanied by alexia (Maxim 42) and right superior quadrantanopsia when lesions involve the inferior optic radiations or, less often, inferior calcarine cortex. Left hemiachromatopsia usually occurs as an isolated deficit.

Full-field achromatopsia is often associated with prosopagnosia and field defects involving one or both upper quadrants. Less commonly, it is accompanied by visual object agnosia. As with prosopagnosia, the lesion in full-field achromatopsia (i.e. loss of color vision in those areas in which vision is preserved) are bilateral and involve the occipitotemporal areas. The etiology is usually embolic stroke in the territory of the posterior cerebral arteries. In some cases of cortical blindness, achromatopsia develops as vision improves. However, return of color vision often occurs early during the recovery from cortical blindness, especially in infants and children following hypoxia (Lambert *et al.*, 1987).

Color anomia is almost always associated with right homonymous hemianopsia and alexia (Geschwind and Fusillo, 1966). It is tested simply by asking the patient to name the color of an object to which the examiner points or to point to a color when the examiner names the color. There may be a dissociation between these two tasks; often patients have greater difficulty in supplying the color name. Color perception, as demonstrated by color matching tasks, is intact in the preserved left visual field. In contrast to patients with achromatopsia, those with color anomia are able to discriminate hues on testing with pseudoisochromatic plates. The lesion in patients with color anomia is located in the left mesial occipitotemporal region, inferior to the splenium. The associated right field cut results from involvement of the optic radiations, striate cortex or lateral geniculate body.

References

Albert ML, Reches A, Silverberg R. Hemianopic color blindness. *J Neurol Neurosurg Psychiat* 1975; **38**: 546–9.

Damasio AR. Disorders of complex visual processing. In: *Principles of Behavioral Neurology* (Mesulam M-M, ed.). Philadelphia: FA Davis Company, 1985.

Damasio AR, Yamada T, Damasio H, Corbett J, McKee J. Central achromatopsia: Behavioral, anatomic, and physiologic aspects. *Neurology* 1980; **30**: 1064–71.

Geschwind N, Fusillo M. Color-naming defects in association with alexia. *Arch Neurol* 1966; **15**: 137–46.

Lambert SR, Hoyt CS, Jan JE, Barkovich J, Flodmark O. Visual recovery from hypoxic cortical blindness during childhood: Computed tomography and magnetic resonance imaging predictors. *Arch Ophthalmol* 1987; **105**: 1371–7.

Meadows JC. Disturbed perception of colors associated with localized cerebral lesions. *Brain* 1974; **97**: 615–32.

Pearlman AL, Birch J, Meadows JC. Cerebral color blindness: An acquired defect in hue discrimination. *Ann Neurol* 1979; **5**: 253–61.

7
Right Hemisphere Disorders

50. *The right hemisphere is dominant for tasks requiring spatial and constructional skills, as well as for directed attention and body image*

Lesions of the right hemisphere do not affect linguistic functions (in right-handed subjects), but they do cause deficits not observed after injury to homologous areas of the left hemisphere. In over 90% of the population, the left hemisphere is dominant for language and motor functions, as well as linguistic thought and reasoning, analytical and mathematical skills, and temporal sequencing of stimuli (Efron, 1963; Albert *et al.*, 1972; Luria, 1980; Sperry, 1982; Vignolo, 1983; Heilman *et al.*, 1983). Left hemisphere language and motoric dominance led to the unfair designation of the right hemisphere as the non-dominant, minor or 'dumb' hemisphere. However, the 'non-dominant' hemisphere is vital for human cognitive and emotional functions and is 'dominant' for a variety of cortical functions.

Right hemisphere injury results in a wide range of behavioral disorders: visuospatial and constructional disorders include constructional apraxia, dressing apraxia, topographical disorientation and loss of topographic memory; amusia (Maxim 59); prosopagnosia (Maxim 47); anosognosia; impersistence; unilateral spatial neglect (Maxim 63); attentional deficits and delirium (Maxims 12 and 62); and emotional indifference (Maxim 53).

The right parietal lobe is dominant for *non-linguistic visuospatial functions*. Patients with right parietal lesions have impairment of simple and complex visuospatial perceptual and motor tasks (McFie *et al.*, 1950; Warrington *et al.*, 1966; DeRenzi *et al.*, 1977; Kase *et al.*, 1977; Benton, 1978b; Fisher, 1982; Meerwaldt and Van Harskamp, 1982; Kertesz, 1983). Impaired visuospatial abilities affect a wide range of tasks, including: visual orientation of lines or patterns, orientation of clothing and body (e.g. top versus bottom, front versus back), geometric block design and assembly, visual maze performance, learning and recall of geographical relations, and drawing of complex figures.

The two hemispheres make different contributions to drawing and copying (Warrington *et al.*, 1966; Benson and Barton, 1970). The right hemisphere is critical for the visuospatial perception and overall gestalt of figures, whereas the left hemisphere is more concerned with detail and executive motor functions, i.e. praxis. Copies of the Rey–Ostereich complex Fig. 50.1 show characteristic patterns after unilateral parietotemporal injury 50.2 (a–b). Patients with left hemisphere lesions tend to produce simplified copies that lack detail but preserve the overall shape and spatial relations. Patients with right hemisphere lesions make copies that are spatially disorganized but preserve details. For example, patients with right-sided lesions asked to draw a rectangle may start in one corner and draw four, poorly formed squares to duplicate the original rectangle, rather than tracing an outline. Copying and immediate recall of a given figure is disrupted most by right parietal lesions, whereas failure on immediate, and especially, delayed recall is most often associated with right temporal lesions. Thus, constructional deficits with right parietal lesions impair the ability to copy the complex figure. In contrast, mnemonic deficits in patients with right temporal lesions do not disrupt copying, but ability to recall the figure and make another copy is impaired. Gainotti *et al.* (1972) found that providing a model improved the figures of patients with left-sided lesions who were asked to draw a figure, but it did not improve the performance of those with right-sided lesions. Table 50.1 summarizes the principal differences between left and right hemisphere lesions and is derived from the work of Warrington *et al.* (1966) and Benson and Barton (1970).

The right hemisphere is also dominant for certain *non-visuospatial perceptual domains*, including somesthetic (tactile rod orientation), auditory (melody and tone discrimination) and emotional functions (comprehension of emotional tone in voice and body gestures) (Benton *et al.*, 1978a; Heller and Levy, 1981; McFarland and Fartrin, 1982; Mazziotta *et al.*, 1982; Zoccolotti *et al.*, 1982; Benowitz *et al.*, 1983).

The right hemisphere's dominant role in *attention* is reviewed in Maxim

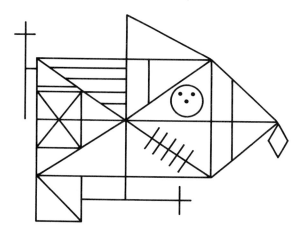

Fig. 50.1   Rey complex figure.

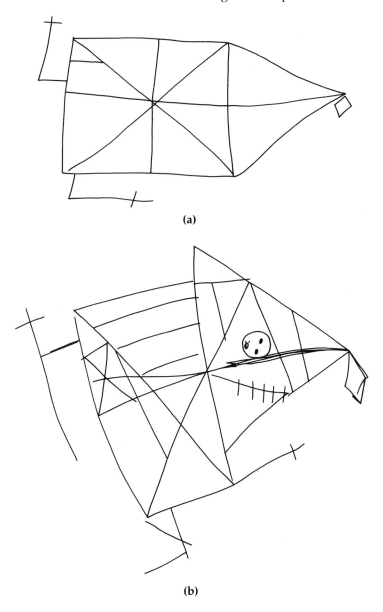

(a)

(b)

Fig. 50.2(a) Copy of the Rey Complex figure by a patient with a left temporoparietal stroke – note the paucity of detail. (Courtesy of Bonnie Levin, PhD.); **(b)** Copy of the Rey Complex figure by a patient with a right parietal stroke – note the lack of organisation and poor representation of the overall configuration. (Courtesy of Kenneth Perrine, PhD.)

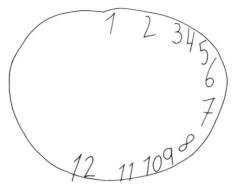

Fig. 50.3   Drawing of a clock made by a patient with a right parietal stroke.

62. The attentional network includes the parietal lobe, as well as the right cingulate, prefrontal, striatal and thalamic areas. Although the left hemisphere contributes to attentional processes, the right brain is dominant. Neglect and inattention to the left are common after right hemisphere lesions and include both sensory and motor components. Because humans are visual animals, visuospatial neglect is often the most prominent manifestation. When asked to draw a clock or copy a figure patients often neglect the left half (Fig. 50.3). The clock's numbers are only drawn on, or are skewed towards the right half.

The attentional deficit in right hemisphere lesions also has a motor

Table 50.1   Drawing and copying: effects of lateralized cerebral lesions.

Feature	Left-sided lesions	Right-sided lesions
Overall shape	Preserved	Fragmented, disrupted
Orientation	Preserved	Impaired
Spatial relations	Preserved	Disrupted
Detail	Lacking	Preserved
Motor performance	Slow, effortful	Fluent
Effect of model on copying	Improvement	No improvement

component: *impersistence* and *motor neglect* (Maxim 63). Fisher (1956) introduced the term impersistence to describe the failure of patients with left hemiplegia to persist in a motor act, and a higher prevalence of impersistence with right hemisphere lesions has since been confirmed (Joynt *et al.*, 1964; Hier *et al.*, 1983b). These patients can perform a requested motor act for brief periods but then spontaneously cease. In many cases, despite repeated requests by the examiner, they cannot persist in keeping their eyes closed, protruding their tongue, holding up their arms, etc. Hier *et al.* (1983b) found impersistence was associated with large right middle cerebral artery strokes and that its presence correlated with other deficits, including severe hemiparesis, prosopagnosia, left-sided neglect, constructional apraxia and anosognosia. Resolution of impersistence is often slow and incomplete (Hier *et al.*, 1983a). The mechanism underlying impersistence is probably a defect in sustained attention, and this deficit is consistent with the presumed right hemisphere dominance for directed attention (Heilman and Van Den Abell, 1980).

Anosognosia refers to the patient's lack of awareness of his own deficit. Anosognosia is most common in patients with left hemiplegia, and the term was first used by Babinski (1914) in reference to this group. However, patients may also be unaware of other deficits, including cortical blindness (Anton's syndrome), unilateral spatial neglect, memory disorder, Wernicke's aphasia and dementia. Anosognosia is more fully described in Maxim 62.

Confabulation – elaboration of imaginary facts and experiences to fill in gaps of knowledge or memory – occurs in Korsakoff's disease and right hemisphere lesions. The most common hemispheric lesion site associated with confabulation is the right frontal lobe (Stuss *et al.*, 1978; Shapiro *et al.*, 1981; Joseph, 1986). Patients with right frontal lesions are disinhibited with excessive, circumstantial and occasionally bizarre language output. When asked simple questions, these patients may respond with an emotional and hypomanic style. When unsure of an answer to the examiner's question they cannot answer, they pause to reflect on the question and then blurt out a confabulatory response. Confabulation also occurs with posterior right hemisphere and callosal lesions that interrupt transfer of sensory input to the dominant hemisphere. The language hemisphere either denies having perceived the stimulus or confabulates (Geschwind, 1965; Joseph, 1988). For example, a man with a posterior callosal lesion may be shown a naked woman's body in the left visual field, smile, and when asked what he saw may reply 'nothing' or 'a tree'.

Disorders of body image are more common with right than left hemisphere lesions. The right hemisphere is dominant for somesthetic, proprioceptive sensibility and perceptual integration of visuospatial and body position input. The right parietal lobe is superior to the left in perceiving tactile stimuli such as geometric and complex shapes, and in making directional, pressure and two-point discriminations based on tactile input (Semmes *et al.*, 1960; Weinstein and Sersen, 1961; Carmon and Benton, 1969; Corkin *et al.*, 1970; Franco and Sperry, 1977; Bradshaw *et al.*, 1982). Body image disturbances following right hemisphere lesions result from a combination of attentional, emotional, visuospatial and somatosensory body perceptual disorders. Patients may put their shirts on backwards or place pants' legs over their arms, groom only the right half of their body, fail to perceive or incorrectly lateralize left-sided sensory stimuli, and even deny that their left arm is indeed theirs! These disturbances often occur together in the same patient and are based on complex and interrelated functions for which the right hemisphere is dominant.

References

Albert ML, Sparks R, Strockert T, Sax D. A case of auditory agnosia: linguistic and nonlinguistic processing. *Cortex* 1972; **8**: 427–43.

Babinski J. Contribution a l'etude des troubles mentaux dans l'hemiplegie organique cerebrale (anosognosie). *Rev Neurol* 1914; **27**: 845–8.

Benowitz LI, Bear DM, Rosenthal R, Mesulam MM, Zaidel E, Sperry RW. Hemispheric specialization in nonverbal communication. *Cortex* 1983; **19**: 5–11.

Benson DF, Barton M. Constructional disability. *Cortex* 1970; **6**: 19–46.

Benton AL, Varney NR, Hamsher K de S. Lateral differences in tactile directional perception. *Neuropsychologia* 1978a; **16**: 109–14.

Benton AL, Varney NR, Hamsher K de S. Visuospatial judgment. *Arch Neurol* 1978b; **35**: 364–7.

Bradshaw JL, Nettleton NC, Spher K. Braille reading and left and right hemispace. *Neuropsychologia* 1982; **20**: 493–500.

Carmon A, Benton AL. Tactile perception of direction and number in patients with unilateral cerebral disease. *Neurology* 1969; **19**: 525–32.

Corkin S, Milner B, Rasmussen T. Somatosensory thresholds: Contrasting effects of post-central gyrus and posterior parietal-lobe excisions. *Arch Neurol* 1970; **23**: 41–58.

DeRenzi E, Faglioni P, Villa P. Topographical amnesia. *J Neurol Neurosurg Psychiat* 1977; **40**: 498–505.

Efron R. The effect of handedness on the perception of simultaneity and temporal order. *Brain* 1963; **86**: 261–84.

Fisher CM. Left hemiplegia and motor impersistence. *J Nerv Ment Dis* 1956; **123**: 201–18.

Fisher CM. Topographic disorientation. *Arch Neurol* 1982 **39**: 33–6.

Franco L, Sperry RW. Hemispheric lateralization for cognitive processing of geometry. *Neuropsychologia* 1977; **15**: 107–11.

Gainotti G. Emotional behavior and hemispheric side of lesion. *Cortex* 1972; **8**: 41.

Geschwind N. Disconnection syndromes in animals and man. *Brain* 1965; **88**: 585–644.

Heilman KM, Van Den Abell. Right hemisphere dominance for attention: the mechanism underlying hemispheric asymmetries of inattention (neglect). *Neurology* 1980; **30**: 327–30.

Heilman KM, Rothi L, Kertesz A. Localization of apraxia-producing lesions. In: *Clinical Neuropsychology* (Kertesz A, ed.). Oxford, New York: Oxford University Press, 1983, pp. 300–20.

Heller W, Levy J. Perception and expression of emotion in right-handers and left-handers. *Neuropsychologia* 1981; **19**: 263–72.

Hier DB, Mondlock J, Caplan LR. Recovery of behavioral abnormalities after right hemisphere stroke. *Neurology* 1983a; **33**: 345–50.

Hier DB, Mondlock J, Caplan LR. Behavioral abnormalities after right hemisphere stroke. *Neurology* 1983b; **33**: 337–44.

Joseph R. Confabulation and delusional denial: Frontal and lateralized influences. *J Clin Psychol* 1986; **42**: 507–18.

Joseph R. The right cerebral hemisphere. *J Clin Psychol* 1988; **44**: 630–73.

Joynt RL, Benton AL, Fogel ML. Behavioral and pathologic correlates of motor impersistence. *Neurology* 1964; **12**: 876–81.

Kase CS, Troncoso JF, Court JE, Tapia JF, Mohr JP. Global spatial disorientation. *J Neurol Sci* 1977; **34**: 267–78.

Kertesz A. Right hemisphere lesions in construction apraxia and visuospatial deficit. In: *Localization in Neuropsychology* (Kertesz A, ed.) Orlando, FL: Academic Press, 1983, pp. 455–70.

Luria A. *Higher Cortical Functions in Man*. New York: Basic Books, 1980.

Mazziotta JC, Phelps ME, Carson RE, Kuhl DE. Tomographic mapping of human cerebral metabolism: Auditory stimulation. *Neurology* 1982; **32**: 921–37.

McFarland HR, Fartrin D. Amusia due to right temporoparietal infarct. *Arch Neurol* 1982; **32**: 725–7.

McFie J, Piercy MF, Zangwill OL. Visual spatial agnosia associated with lesions of the right cerebral hemisphere. *Brain* 1950; **73**: 167–90.

Meerwaldt JD, Van Harskamp F. Spatial disorientation in right-hemisphere infarction. *J Neurol Neurosurg Psychiat* 1982; **45**: 586–90.

Semmes J, Weinstein S, Ghent L, Teuber HL. *Somatosensory Changes After Penetrating Head Wounds in Man*. Cambridge, MA: Harvard University Press, 1960.

Shapiro BE, Alexander MP, Gardner H, Mercer B. Mechanisms of confabulation. *Neurology* 1981; **31**: 1070–6.

Sperry R. Some effects of disconnecting the cerebral hemispheres. *Science* 1982; **217**: 1223–6.

Stuss DT, Alexander MP, Lieberman A, Levine H. An extraordinary form of confabulation. *Neurology* 1978; **28**: 1166–72.

Vignolo LA. Modality-specific disorders of written language. In: *Localization in Neuropsychology* (Kertesz A, ed.). Orlando, FL: Academic Press, 1983, pp. 357–70.

Warrington EK, James M, Kinsbourne M. Drawing disability in relation to laterality of cerebral lesion. *Brain* 1966; **89**: 53–82.

Weinstein EA, Sersen EA. Tactual sensitivity as a function of handedness and laterality. *J Compar Physiol Psychol* 1961; **54**: 665–9.

Zoccolotti P, Scabini D, Violani C. Electrodermal responses in patients with unilateral brain damage. *J Clin Neuropsychol* 1982; **4**: 143–50.

51.   *The right hemisphere modulates non-verbal communication and prosody*

Human communication is often mistakenly equated with verbal language. Words can convey remarkably complex concepts, but a glance into someone's eyes often reveals more about their intentions than their words. The information transmitted through eye contact is difficult to quantify and study, as are many other forms of non-verbal behavior, such as gestures, facial expression, and the intonation, melody and accent of speech prosody. Other behaviors, such as changes in heart and respiratory rates and perspiration, are more easily measured and form the basis of the polygraph, or lie detector test. We tend to study what we can measure and ignore what is non-metrical.

Hughlings Jackson (1878–79) recognized that, following left hemisphere lesions and aphasia, patients can communicate emotions through right hemisphere 'nervous arrangements'. 'He smiles, laughs, frowns and varies his voice properly. His recurring utterance comes out now in one tone and now in another, according as he is vexed, glad, etc. . . . he may swear when excited, or get out more innocent interjections, simple or compound (acquired parts of emotional language).' (Jackson, 1878–79.)

The non-dominant, right hemisphere plays a major role in the emotional modulation of verbal and non-verbal communication (Blonder *et al.*, 1991). Speech is rich in emotion. The words 'I'm going to kill you' may be said with a soft rising tone and a playful smile or with violent anger. Survival demands that one comprehend and express both the linguistic and emotional meanings of speech.

Prosody is the variation in speech rhythm, pitch, melody and distribution of stress. In addition to semantic and grammatical elements of speech, prosody plays an important role in conveying the message. Monrad-Krohn (1945, 1947) first systematically studied prosody, focusing on patients with left hemisphere lesions. He defined prosody (1947) as the aspect of speech that conveys shades of meaning through variations in stress and pitch, independent of words (semantics) and organization (grammar). Monrad-Krohn described four components of prosody relating to (1) dialectic and inflectional changes, which are intrinsic (e.g. a rising voice at the end of a sentence implies a question); (2) attitudinal changes that impart meaning and are intellectual (as in the above, 'I'm going to kill you', scenario); (3) affective tone, which is emotional; and (4) non-linguistic components, such as grunts and moans, which are inarticulate.

The right hemisphere plays an important role in prosody, especially in regulating and understanding emotional components. Dichotic auditory tests[1] in normal subjects reveal that the right hemisphere (left ear) is superior in comprehending intonational aspects of speech (Zuriff, 1974). Furthermore, patients with right hemisphere injury have greater difficulty understanding emotional intonation in semantically neutral sentences than patients with left-sided lesions (Heilman *et al.*, 1975; Tucker *et al.*, 1977; Ross, 1981). Although the right hemisphere is dominant for affective prosody, both hemispheres make important contributions to non-affective, propositional prosody, such as the rising pitch at the end of a sentence that indicates a question (Weintraub *et al.*, 1981; Heilman *et al.*, 1984).

Ross and Mesulam (1979) reported two patients with right frontoparietal strokes who were unable to express emotional color in their speech and gestures. Ross (1981) subsequently proposed a functional–anatomical organization of affective components of language in the right hemisphere that mirrored the organization of language in the left hemisphere. He classified disturbances of prosody into motor, sensory, transcortical and global categories, which parallel those for aphasia. He based this categorization on patients' ability to (1) use affective prosody and gesturing spontaneously; (2) imitate linguistically neutral sentences with affective tone; (3) comprehend spoken affective prosody; and (4) comprehend affective gestures (Ross, 1985). This classification (Table 51.1) of the aprosodias remains preliminary and is probably an oversimplification.

Eye contact is another important route of emotional communication that

---

[1] Although both cerebral hemispheres receive auditory input from both ears, the predominant input to the hemispheres is from the contralateral ear.

Table 51.1 The aprosodias.

	Spontaneous affective prosody and gesturing	Affective prosodic repetition	Affective prosodic comprehension	Comprehension of emotional gesturing
Motor	Poor	Poor	Good	Good
Sensory	Good	Poor	Poor	Poor
Global	Poor	Poor	Poor	Poor
Transcortical sensory	Good	Good	Poor	Poor
Mixed transcortical	Poor	Good	Poor	Poor

Modified from Ross (1985) with permission.

may be disrupted by brain injury. Lesions of the right hemisphere disrupt both the understanding and transmission of affective messages delivered through the eyes, although complete dissociation of emotions expressed in the eyes from other facial expressions is unusual.

Gestural behaviors may be divided into those that communicate linguistic (semiotic or pantomime) and emotional components. Patients with left hemisphere lesions have difficulty comprehending symbolic, non-emotional gestures such as pantomime (Gainotti and Lemmo, 1976; De Renzi *et al.*, 1980). Jackson (1878–79) recognized that emotional gesturing was often increased in patients with aphasia. On the other hand, patients with right-sided lesions have significant deficits in comprehension of emotional gestures, especially facial expression (DeKosky *et al.*, 1980; Benowitz *et al.*, 1983). Ross and Mesulam (1979) observed an almost complete loss of spontaneous gestural behavior in patients with right frontal opercular lesions. Therefore, both the comprehension and expression of emotional gestures appear to be dominant functions of the right hemisphere.

References

Benowitz LI, Bear DM, Rosenthal R, Mesualm MM, Zaidel E, Sperry RW. Hemispheric specialization in nonverbal communication. *Cortex* 1983; **19**: 5–11.

Blonder LX, Bowers D, Heilman KM. The role of the right hemisphere in emotional communication. *Brain* 1991; **114**: 115–27.

DeKosky ST, Heilman KM, Bowers D, Valenstein E. Recognition and discrimination of emotional faces and pictures. *Brain Lang* 1980: **9**: 206–14.

De Renzi E, Motti F, Nichelli P. Imitating gestures: A quantitative approach to ideomotor apraxia. *Arch Neurol* 1980; **37**: 6–10.

Gainotti G, Lemmo M. Comprehension of symbolic gestures in aphasia. *Brain Lang* 1976; **3**: 451–60.

Heilman KM, Bowers D, Speedie L, Coslett HB. Comprehension of affective and nonaffective prosody. *Neurology* 1984; **34**: 917–21.

Heilman KM, Scholes R, Watson RT. Auditory affective agnosia: disturbed comprehension of affective speech. *J Neurol Neurosurg Psychiat* 1975; **38**: 69–72.

Jackson JH. On affections of speech from disease of the brain. *Brain* 1878–79; **1**: 716.

Monrad-Krohn GH. Dysprosody or altered 'melody of language'. *Brain* 1945; **70**: 405.

Monrad-Krohn GH. The prosodic quality of speech and its disorders. *Acta Psychiat Neurol* 1947; **22**: 255–69.

Ross ED. The aprosodias: functional–anatomic organization of the affective components of language in the right hemisphere. *Arch Neurol* 1981; **38**: 561–9.

Ross ED. Modulation of affect and nonverbal communication by the right hemisphere. In: *Principles of Behavioral Neurology* (Mesulam M-M, ed.). Philadelphia: FA Davis Company, 1985, pp. 239–57.

Ross ED, Mesulam M-M. Dominant language functions of the right hemisphere? Prosody and emotional gesturing. *Arch Neurol* 1979; **36**: 144–8.

Tucker DM, Watson RT, Heilman KM. Affective discrimination and evocation in patients with right parietal disease. *Neurology* 1977; **27**: 947–50.

Weintraub S, Mesulam M-M, Kramer L. Disturbances in prosody: A right hemisphere contribution to language. *Arch Neurol* 1981; **38**: 742–4.

Zuriff EB. Auditory lateralization: Prosodic and syntactical factors. *Brain Lang* 1974; **1**: 391–404

52.   *The corpus callosum interconnects the associative areas of the two hemispheres*

I believe it then to be entirely unphilosophical, and tending to important errors, to speak of the cerebrum as one organ . . . The two hemispheres of the brain are really . . . two distinct and entire organs . . . as fully perfect in all its parts . . . as the two eyes. The corpus callosum, and the other commissures between them, can with no more justice be said to constitute the two hemispheres into one organ than the optic commissure can be called an union of the *two eyes* into one organ.

(Wigan, 1844)

Phylogenetically, the corpus callosum increases with development of the associative neocortical areas. It is the principal interhemispheric commissure in placental, but not marsupial animals (Heath and Jones, 1971). Callosal fibers interconnect homologous association areas of the two hemispheres, but make no significant connections between primary motor and sensory areas (Welker and Seidenstein, 1959). Other interhemispheric connections in humans include: (1) the hippocampal commissure or psalterium, which interconnects homologous and non-homologous hippocampal and entorhinal areas (Blackstad, 1956); (2) the anterior commissure, which interconnects the olfactory bulbs, amygdalae, entorhinal and other temporal areas (Brodal, 1981); (3) the posterior commissure; and (4) the habenular commissure. The massa intermedia (thalamic adhesion) is a nucleus that may be absent in humans and does not contain commissural fibers in humans (Toncray and Krieg, 1946; Rosales *et al.*, 1968). In the brainstem,

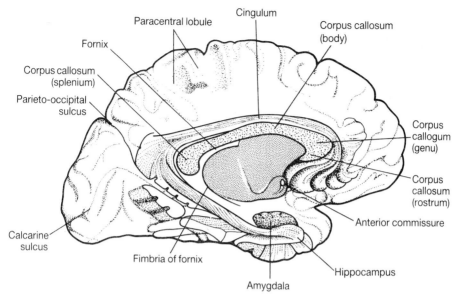

Fig. 52.1   Medial surface of the left cerebral hemisphere exposing the cingulum. The diencephalon has been removed.

the left and right sides of the reticular formation have extensive connections.

The corpus callosum is divided into four parts (from anterior to posterior): the rostrum, genu, body and splenium (Fig. 52.1). The rostrum is the thin anterior portion, the genu is the curve that joins the rostrum with the large body, and the splenium is the enlarged posterior end of the callosum. The blood supply to the corpus callosum is primarily from the anterior (rostrum, genu and body) and posterior (splenium) cerebral arteries. Surprisingly, nearly 40 percent of callosal fibers are unmyelinated, suggesting that the corpus callosum does not exclusively function to inform one hemisphere rapidly of what is happening on the other side (Selnes, 1974). Rather, these slowly conducting fibers may serve to both inhibit and modulate activity on the other side.

The massive size of the human corpus callosum is paradoxical in the light of the difficulties defining its functions. Individuals who are born without this commissure (agenesis of the corpus callosum) and those in whom the interhemispheric pathway is severed to control seizures may have normal intellect, behavior and emotions (Akelitis, 1944; Sperry, 1966; Ettlinger *et al.*, 1972; Ledoux *et al.*, 1977; Sergent, 1987). However, destruction of corpus callosum can produce very severe behavioral disorders.

Agenesis of the corpus callosum has not provided a good model of callosal function. These patients often have a variety of cerebral malformations, epilepsy and hydrocephalus; thus, intellectual and behavioral disorders cannot be attributed to the absence of a corpus callosum. The intelligence quotient in patients with agenesis of the callosum is often low and appears to result from the associated neurological disorders, not callosal agenesis (Parrish *et al.*, 1979; Milner, 1983; Lacey, 1985). However, these patients develop independent language function in both hemispheres (Gott and Saul, 1978), which suggests that hemispheric specialization is at least partly dependent on callosal functions.

Our knowledge of how the corpus callosum functions and of the deficits that follow its destruction is based on studies of patients with strokes and, most importantly, with elective division of the corpus callosum to treat medically refractory seizures. What follows is a summary of this literature.

In patients with callosal lesions, the *alien hand sign* is a dramatic neuro-behavioral phenomenon in which each hand interferes with the actions of the other hand. The patient is often astonished and embarrassed by the discordant actions that are most often expressed by the left hand (right hemisphere). The alien hand sign is most common after anterior callosal (and often medial frontal) lesions, but may occur with posterior callosal lesions as well (Van Wagenen and Herren, 1940; Akelitis, 1945; Goldberg *et al.*, 1981; Degos *et al.*, 1987; Maganini *et al.*, 1987; McNabb *et al.*, 1988; Leiguarda *et al.*, 1989). The hemispheric form of the alien hand sign always appears in the hand contralateral to the lesion, regardless of the pattern of cerebral dominance. In contrast, the callosal form of the alien hand sign develops in the hand ipsilateral to the language-dominant hemisphere (Leiguarda *et al.*, 1989).

Akelitis (1945) described his experience with a female patient who had undergone callosotomy: 'In tasks requiring bimanual activity, the left hand would frequently perform oppositely to what she desired to do with the right hand. For example, she would be putting on clothes with her right hand and pulling them off with her left, opening a door or drawer with her right hand and simultaneously pushing it shut with the left. These uncontrollable acts made her increasingly irritated and depressed'. Another typical case was described by McNabb *et al.* (1988) in a woman following left anterior cerebral artery infarction with medial frontal and anterior callosal injury: when she attempted 'to write with her left hand, the right hand would reach over and attempt to take the pencil. The left hand would respond by grasping the right and trying to restrain it'. Joseph (1988a, b) observed similiar behavior following callosotomy for intractable seizures: one patient's 'left hand would not allow him to smoke and would pluck lit cigarettes from his mouth, whereas another patient's left hand (right brain) preferred different foods and even television shows and would interfere with the choices made by the right hand (left hemisphere)'.

Callosal apraxia (unilateral ideomotor apraxia) occurs with lesions in the genu and body of the corpus callosum (Geschwind and Kaplan, 1962; Volpe *et al.*, 1982; Watson and Heilman, 1983; Watson *et al.*, 1985; Graff-Radford *et al.*, 1987). Callosal apraxia is most severe when the patient is asked to perform skilled movements of the left hand and leg to verbal command (e.g salute, kick a ball). In many cases, there is an initial impairment in imitating left-hand postures and demonstrating use of objects with the left hand. However, these non-verbal tasks often improve over several months. As Liepmann (1977) suggested, there appears to be a left hemisphere repository for skilled motor actions (Maxim 43).

Unilateral agraphia, loss of left-handed writing ability, results from both anterior and posterior callosal lesions (Degos *et al.*, 1987; Leiguarda *et al.*, 1989). Unilateral agraphia can occur with or without callosal apraxia (Sugishita *et al.*, 1980; Gersh and Damasio, 1981). Anterior callosal lesions are associated with both left-handed agraphia and apraxia while posterior lesions are associated only with left-handed agraphia.

Hemialexia occurs with splenial lesions that disconnect the right visual cortex (left hemifield) from left hemisphere language areas. The patient can only read in the right visual field. Posterior callosal lesions also cause visual anomia for objects seen only in the left visual field.

Callosal lesions prevent interhemispheric transfer of tactile information between the somatosensory association areas, resulting in impaired ability to (1) copy hand postures using only position sensation, to identify correctly homologous contralateral (non-facial) body parts that are touched, (2) name objects that are palpated in the left hand, and (3) identify left-sided body parts (other than the face) that are touched by the examiner (*left tactile anomia*) (Bogen, 1979; Degos *et al.*, 1987; Leiguarda *et al.*, 1989). Left tactile anomia and other somatosensory transfer disorders occur primarily with mid callosal lesions, since somesthetic fibers traverse the body of the corpus callosum (Jeeves *et al.*, 1979). However, the caudal third of the callosal body may be the critical site for transfer of tactile information required for naming (Degos *et al.*, 1987; Leiguarda *et al.*, 1989).

In patients with posterior callosal body lesions, there is impairment of right-handed copying and visuospatial constructions (*unilateral constructional apraxia*) (Bogen, 1969; LeDoux *et al.*, 1978; Degos *et al.*, 1987; Graff-Radford *et al.*, 1987). This deficit results from disconnection of the left hemisphere (right hand) from intact visuospatial perceptual functions of the right parietal lobe.

Sustained directed attention (*vigilance*) may be impaired after callosal lesions (Dimond, 1979).

Wigan's (1844) view of two brains in one cranial vault cannot be upheld. The most remarkable aspect of patients with callosal lesions is the apparent unity of consciousness and the capacity to perform complex cognitive functions requiring input from both hemispheres (Gazzaniga *et al.*, 1975; LeDoux *et al.*, 1977; Sergent, 1987). In some patients, however, the alien hand sign demonstrates that each hemisphere is capable of independent perception as well as consciousness. Furthermore, the non-dominant right hemisphere may have its own behavioral agenda – an agenda that is normally brought 'in line' with the goals and actions of the left hemisphere when the callosum is intact.

Language and motor dominance within a single hemisphere is probably no coincidence. Dissociation of language and motor dominance could produce a self-conscious language hemisphere and a relatively independent emotional consciousness that directs actions. Indeed, evidence from corpus callosotomy suggests that patients who are most likely to suffer the most severe language and behavioral disorders are those in whom the hemisphere dominant for language is opposite the hemisphere dominant for motor control (Sass *et al.*, 1990; Westerveld *et al.*, 1991).

The growth of the corpus callosum in concert with the development of hemispheric specialization suggests that the callosum may serve both to integrate the two halves of the brain and to preserve their functional independence. However, there may be aspects of intellectual and emotional life that one hemisphere may be unable or 'unwilling' to tell the other side. The experience of emotions (e.g. sad, irritable, happy) for no apparent reason or performance of impulsive and embarrassing acts may result from actions of the right hemisphere for which the left hemisphere has no awareness (Joseph, 1980, 1982, 1986).

The mystery of the corpus callosum persists. I suggest that what initially developed as a telephone line between two relatively equipotential hemispheres in early placental mammals became a vital component in the evolution of human language by allowing a dissociation of hemispheric function, as well the capacity of one hemisphere to inhibit the other.

References

Akelitis AJ. A study of gnosis, praxis and language following section of the corpus callosum and anterior commissure. *J Neurosurg* 1944; **1**: 94–102.

Akelitis AJ. Studies on the corpus callosum. IV. Diagnostic dyspraxia in epileptics following partial and complete section of the corpus callosum. *Am J Psychiat* 1945; **101**: 594–9.

Blackstad TW. Commissural connections of the hippocampal region in the rat, with special reference to their mode of termination. *J Comp Neurol* 1956; **105**: 417–537.

Bogen JE. The other side of the brain. I. Dysgraphia and dyscopia following cerebral commissurotomy. *Bull LA Neurol Soc* 1969; **34**: 73–105.

Bogen JE. The callosal syndrome. In: *Clinical Neuropsychology* (Heilman KM, Valenstein E, eds). Oxford, New York: Oxford University Press, 1979, pp. 308–59.

Brodal A. *Neurological Anatomy*. Oxford, New York: Oxford University Press, 1981, p. 658.

Degos JD, Gray F, Louarn F, Ansquer JC, Poirier J, Barbizet J. Posterior callosal infarction: clinicopathologic correlation. *Brain* 1987; **110**: 1155–71.

Dimond SJ. Performance of split-brain humans on lateralized vigilance tasks. *Cortex* 1979; **15**: 43–50.

Ettlinger G, Blakemore CB, Milner AD, Wilson J. Agenesis of the corpus callosum: a further behavioral study. *Brain* 1972; **97**: 225–34.

Gazzaniga MS, Risse GL, Springer SP, Clark E, Wilson DH. Psychologic and neurologic consequences of partial and complete cerebral commissurotomy. *Neurology* 1975; **25**: 10–15.

Gersch R, Damasio AR. Praxis and writing of the left hand may be served by different callosal pathways. *Arch Neurol* 1981; **38**: 634–6.

Geschwind N, Kaplan E. A human cerebral deconnection syndrome: a preliminary report. *Neurology* 1962; **12**: 675–85.

Gott PS, Saul RE. Agenesis of the corpus callosum: limits of functional compensation. *Neurology* 1978; **28**: 1272–9.

Graff-Radford NR, Welsh K, Godersky J. Callosal apraxia. *Neurology* 1987; **37**: 100–5.

Goldberg G, Meyer NH, Toglia JU. Medial frontal cortex infarction and the alien hand sign. *Arch Neurol* 1981; **38**: 683–6.

Heath CJ, Jones EG. Interhemispheric pathways in the absence of a corpus callosum. An experimental study of commissural connections in the marsupial phalanger. *J Anat* 1971; **109**: 253–70.

Jeeves MA, Simpson DA, Geffen G. Functional consequences of the transcallosal removal of intraventricular tumours. *J Neurol Neurosurg Psychiat* 1979; **42**: 134–42.

Joseph R. Awareness, the origin of thought and the role of conscious self-deception in resistance and repression. *Psychol Rep* 1980; **46**: 767–81.

Joseph R. The neuropsychology of development: Hemispheric laterality, limbic language and the origin of thought. *J Clin Psychol* 1982; **38**: 4–33.

Joseph R. Confabulation and delusional denial. Frontal lobe and lateralized influences. *J Clin Psychol* 1986; **42**: 507–18.

Joseph R. The right cerebral hemisphere: Emotion, music, visual–spatial skills, body-image, dreams and awareness. *J Clin Psychol* 1988a; **44**: 630–73.

Joseph R. Dual mental functioning in a 'split-brain' patient. *J Clin Psychol* 1988b; **44**: 770–9.

Lacey DJ. Agenesis of the corpus callosum: clinical features in 40 children. *Am J Dis Child* 1985; **139**: 953–5.

LeDoux JE, Risse GL, Springer SP, Wilson DH, Gazzaniga MS. Cognition and commissurotomy. *Brain* 1977; **100**: 87–104.

LeDoux JE, Wilson DH, Gazzaniga MS. Block design performance following callosal sectioning. *Arch Neurol* 1978; **35**: 506–8.

Liepmann H. The syndrome of apraxia (motor asymboly) based on a case of unilateral apraxia. In: *Neurologic Classics in Modern Translation* (Rottenberg RA, Hochberg FH, eds); (Bohne WHO, Liepmann K, Rottenberg DA, transl.). New York: Hafner Press, 1977, pp. 155–84.

Leiguarda R, Starkstein S, Berthier M. Anterior callosal hemorrhage: partial interhemispheric disconnection syndrome. *Brain* 1989; **112**: 1019–37.

Maganini G, Mazzucchi A, Poletti A, Souccuti U, Parma M. Involuntary grasping and grouping responses to space-related visual stimuli. *Movement Dis* 1987; **2**: 9–23.

Milner D. Neuropsychological studies of callosal agenesis. *Psychol Med* 1983; **13**: 721–5.

McNabb AW, Carroll WM, Mastaglia FL. 'Alien hand' and loss of bimanual coordination after dominant anterior cerebral artery territory infarction. *J Neurol Neurosurg Psychiat* 1988; **51**: 218–22.

Parrish ML, Roessmann U, Levinsohn MW. Agenesis of the corpus callosum: a study of the frequency of associated malformations. *Ann Neurol* 1979; **6**: 349–54.

Rosales RK, Lemay MJ, Yakovlev PI. The development and involution of the massa intermedia with regard to age and sex. *J Neuropath Exp Neurol* 1968; **27**: 166.

Sass KJ, Novelly RA, Spencer DD, Spencer SS. Postcallosotomy language impairments in patients with crossed cerebral dominance. *J Neurosurg* 1990; **72**: 85–90.

Selnes OA. The corpus callosum: Some anatomical and functional considerations with special reference to language. *Brain Lang* 1974; **1**: 111–39.

Sergent J. A new look at the human split brain. *Brain* 1987; **110**: 1375–92.

Sperry RW. Brain bisection and mechanisms of consciousness. In: *Brain and Conscious Experience* (Eccles JC, ed.). Berlin: Springer-Verlag, 1966, pp. 298–308.

Sugishita M, Toyokura Y, Yoshioka M, Yamada R. Unilateral agraphia after section of the posterior half of the trauncus of the corpus callosum. *Brain Lang* 1980; **9**: 215–25.

Toncray JE, Krieg WJS. The nuclei of the human thalamus: a comparative approach. *J Comp Neurol* 1946; **85**: 421–59.

Van Wagenen WP, Herren RY. Surgical division of commissural pathways in the corpus callosum: relation to spread of an epileptic attack. *Arch Neurol Psychiat* 1940; **44**: 740–59.

Volpe BT, Sidtis JJ, Holtzman JD, Wilson DH, Gazzaniga MS. Cortical mechanisms involved in praxis: observations following partial and complete section of the corpus callosum in man. *Neurology* 1982; **32**: 645–50.

Watson RT, Heilman KM. Callosal aprasia. *Brain* 1983; **106**: 391–403.

Watson RT, Heilman KM, Bowers D. Magnetic resonance imaging (MRI, NMR) scan in a case of callosal apraxia and pseudoneglect. *Brain* 1985; **108**: 535–6.

Welker WI, Seidenstein S. Somatic sensory representation in the cerebral cortex of the raccoon (*Procyon lotor*). *J Comp Neurol* 1959; **111**: 469–501.

Westerveld M, Sass KJ, Spencer SS, Spencer DD. Neuropsychological function following corpus callosotomy for epilepsy. In: *Epilepsy and Behavior* (Devinsky O, Theodore WH, eds). New York: Alan R Liss, 1991, pp. 203–12.

Wigan AL. *Duality of the Mind*. London: Longman, Brown, Green and Longmans, 1844, pp. 24–5.

53. *Emotional changes follow right hemisphere lesions*

The right cerebrum dominates the regulation of emotional perception and expression in right-handed people (Gianotti, 1972; Bear, 1983). Table 53.1 summarizes some of the contrasting emotional and cognitive functions within the hemispheres.

Normal subjects consistently identify facial emotions presented tachisto-scopically into the left visual field (right hemisphere) more accurately than those presented to the right field (Rizzolatti *et al.*, 1971; Ley and Bryden, 1979). Frightening films are judged more horrible and cause greater heart rate changes when projected to the right hemisphere of normal subjects

Table 53.1   Behavioral features of the right and left hemispheres.*

Behavior	Right hemisphere	Left hemisphere
Language	Primitive or absent	Dominant
Consciousness	'Unconscious'	Self-conscious
Attention	Attentive, vigilant towards both sides and periphery	Inattentive, directed only to center and right side
Emotion	Affective, biased for negative emotions	Unemotional, biased for positive emotions
Cognitive style	Spatial, holistic	Temporal, logical
Information processing	Simultaneous	Sequential
Response style	Impulsive	Reflective

*Modified from Bear (1983) with permission.

(Dimond *et al.*, 1976; Dimond and Farrington, 1977). The right hemisphere is also superior in the discrimination of non-verbal auditory stimuli in dichotic listening studies (Carmon and Nachson,1973). Facial emotions are expressed with greater motor activity in the left lower face compared to the right lower face, consistent with a dominant role of the right hemisphere in the expression of emotion (Sackeim *et al.*, 1978).

This right hemisphere dominance in emotional regulation is further supported by observations in patients with unilateral brain lesions. Intracarotid sodium amobarbital injection on the right side produces unconcern and euphoria, but left-sided injections cause feelings of sadness, presumably mediated by the awake, right hemisphere (Terzian, 1964; Serafetinides *et al.*, 1965; Rossi and Rosadini, 1967). Patients with right hemisphere lesions show deficits in the appreciation of emotional stimuli in visual and auditory modalities (Heilman *et al.*, 1974; Benowitz *et al.*, 1980) and in the expression of emotional prosody (Maxim 51) (Tucker *et al.*, 1977; Ross and Mesulam, 1979).

Anosognosia or denial of illness was the first reported lateralized emotional deficit (Babinski, 1914). This striking behavioral phenomenon includes both cognitive and emotional components. The cognitive disorder is primarily attentional (Maxim 50). If a person has no conscious awareness that their left arm belongs to them, then it follows that they may be quite perplexed when the doctor asks them about left arm weakness. Patients do not recognize their condition or fail to display the usual emotional reactions to such devastating deficits as left hemiplegia or hemianopia. Failure to recognize the deficit may be primary, and lack of emotional response secondary, but many patients acknowledge the deficit and display none of the expected emotional responses. When asked if they are worried about loss of strength in their left arm and leg, a patient may jokingly respond, 'It doesn't bother me, never liked that arm anyway' or simply acknowledge their deficit in a matter-of-fact manner, without any evidence of distress.

Emotional indifference is most common after right frontal lesions (Robinson, 1984). Destruction of limbic areas in the non-dominant temporal lobe also contributes to blunted affect. During the weeks after right temporal lobectomy, patients may report that they lack their usual interests and feelings, e.g. 'It's like I'm a bump on a log'.[1] After a stroke in the right frontotemporal region, patients may learn that a close family member has died and show little sadness; their first question after learning of such a tragedy may be 'What's for lunch?' This unconcern stands in sharp contrast

---

[1] However, other patients are euphoric shortly after right temporal lobectomy, reporting that they have never been in such a 'good mood'. This paradoxical contrast of emotional states after the same area is resected may result from individual differences in the hemispheric specialization of emotional function. Epilepsy is often used as a model to study neurobehavioral deficits since elective surgery allows investigators to study carefully specific behavioral changes resulting from a well-demarcated excision. However, many patients with medically refractory epilepsy have the onset of seizures in childhood, and their brains may have anomalous localizations and distributions of behavioral functions, including language dominance.

to the exaggerated emotional responses seen following left hemisphere lesions.

Goldstein described the '*catastrophic reaction*' to *left frontal injuries* in which non-fluent aphasia is associated with profound depression, anxiety and withdrawal (Goldstein, 1948). Right-sided lesions are characterized by an opposite emotional reaction, including anosognosia, minimization, indifference and a tendency to joke (Gainotti, 1972; Gasparrini *et al.* 1978). Patients with right hemisphere lesions and indifference have normal dexamethasone suppression tests, suggesting that both biochemical and clinical markers of depression are absent in these patients (Finklestein *et al.*, 1982).

Depression occurs with right hemisphere lesions, but is more common after left cerebral insults. Patients with major depression after right hemisphere strokes are more likely to have family members with psychiatric illness and *parietal lesions*, compared to those with right hemisphere strokes without depression (Starkstein *et al.*, 1989).

Sackeim *et al.* (1982) reviewed the literature on *pathological laughing and crying* with destructive and irritative cerebral lesions and on mood changes following hemispherectomy. Pathological laughing was associated with predominantly right-sided destructive lesions and left-sided seizure foci. Pathological crying was associated with left-sided destructive lesions and right-sided irritative lesions. Right-sided hemispherectomy was associated with euphoria, while there was insufficient data to comment on left-sided resections.

The evidence cited above suggests a partial hemispheric dissociation for emotional expression. The right hemisphere is more involved in the mediation of negative emotions, such as anxiety and sadness, while the left hemisphere serves a less critical role in emotional functions but tends towards positive emotional expression (Benson, 1973; Sackeim *et al.*, 1982).

The right hemisphere's dual roles in attention and emotion are intertwined (Mesulam *et al.*, 1976). Bear (1983) has proposed a model of two complementary corticovisual systems with independent limbic connections that includes a ventral, temporofrontal system and a second, dorsal–parietofrontal system (Fig. 53.1).

In this model, the *ventral system* is concerned with emotionally relevant responses to foveal input and sequential temporal relations. This system, which is essential for acquiring and storing visual–emotional associations, includes the inferotemporal visual association cortex, amygdala, hippocampus and orbital frontal cortex. The *dorsal system* is more concerned with peripheral spatial vision, simultaneously surveying the different environmental areas for drive-relevant stimuli (e.g. 'a lion is coming from the right side of space'). This system is essential for simultaneous, spatial surveillance with coding of position. The dorsal system includes the inferior parietal lobule, cingulate gyrus and dorsolateral frontal cortex.

The right hemisphere thus dominates in attentional, spatial and emo-

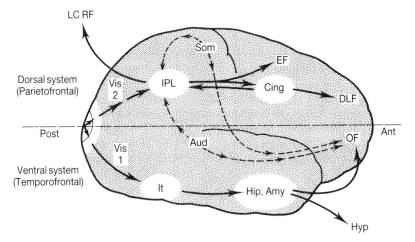

Fig. 53.1 Two cortical visuolimbic systems in monkey (and human?) right hemisphere. Analogous pathways for somatesthetic and auditory processing are probable. LC, locus ceruleus. RF, reticular formation. Vis 1, ventral visual pathway. Vis 2, dorsal visual pathway. IPL, inferior parietal lobe. It, inferotemporal visual cortex. Som, somatesthetic pathway. Aud, auditory pathway. Cing, cingulate gyrus. EF, frontal eye fields. DLF, dorsolateral frontal cortex. OF, orbital frontal cortex. Hip, hippocampus. Amy, amygdala. Hyp, hypothalamus. Ant, anterior. Post, posterior. Reproduced with permission from Bear, *Archives of Neurology*. xx

tional spheres (perhaps because the linguistic specialization of the human left hemisphere 'tied up' much of its circuitry for language and analytic functions). The dorsal corticovisual system surveys for drive-relevant stimuli in both the internal and external milieu, directs the arousal–affective response to stimuli, and maintains a spatial representation of the body and environment. The right ventral corticovisual system recognizes the emotional significance of non-verbal visual stimuli and helps direct the appropriate response. Although the visual system is the best studied, and is probably the most important in humans, analogous hemispheric relations presumably exist for other sensory modalities with regard to specialization.

References

Babinski J. Contribution à l'étude des troubles mentaux dans l'hemiplegie organique cerebrale (anosognosie). *Rev Neurol (Paris)* 1914; **27**: 845–8.

Bear DM. Hemispheric specialization and the neurology of emotion. *Arch Neurol* 1983; **40**: 195–202.

Benowitz LI, Bear DM, Mesulam M-M *et al*. Nonverbal sensitivity following lateralized cerebral injury. *J McLean Hosp* 1980; **3**: 146–67.

Benson DF. Psychiatric aspects of aphasia. *Br J Psychiat* 1973; **123**: 555–66.

Carmon A, Nachson I. Ear asymmetry in perception of emotional and nonverbal stimuli. *Acta Psychol* 1973; **37**: 351–7.

Dimond SJ, Farrington L. Emotional response to films shown to the right and left hemisphere of the brain measured by heart rate. *Acta Psychol* 1977; **241**: 255–60.

Dimond SJ, Farrington L, Johnson P. Differing emotional responses from right and left hemispheres. *Nature* 1976; **261**: 690–2.

Finklestein S, Benowitz LI, Baldessarini RJ, Arana G, Levine D, Woo E, Bear D, Moya K, Stoll AL. Mood, vegetative disturbance, and dexamethasone suppression test after stroke. *Ann Neurol* 1982; **12**: 463–8.

Gainnoti G. Emotional behavior and hemispheric side of the lesion. *Cortex* 1972; **8**: 41–5.

Gasparrini WG, Satz P, Heilman K *et al.* Hemispheric asymmetries of affective processing as determined by the Minnesota Multiphasic Personality Inventory. *J Neurol Neurosurg Psychiat* 1978; **41**: 470–3.

Goldstein, K. *Language and Language Disturbances.* New York: Grune and Stratton, 1948.

Heilman KM, Scholes R, Watson RT. Auditory affective agnosia. *J Neurol Neurosurg Psychiat* 1974; **38**: 69–72.

Ley RG, Bryden MP. Hemispheric differences in processing emotions and faces. *Brain Lang* 1979; **7**: 127–38.

Mesulam M-M, Waxman SG, Geschwind N, Sabin TD. Acute confusional states with right middle cerebral artery infarctions. *J Neurol Neurosurg Psychiat* 1976; **39**: 84–9.

Rizzolatti G, Umilta C, Berlucchi G. Opposite superiorities of the right and left cerebral hemispheres in discriminative reaction time to physiognomical and alphabetical material. *Brain* 1971; **94**: 431–42.

Robinson RG, Kubos KL, Starr LB, Rao K, Price TR. Mood disorders in stroke patients: importance of location of lesion. *Brain* 1984; **107**: 81–93.

Ross ED, Mesulam M-M. Dominant language functions of the right hemisphere? Prosody and emotional gesturing. *Arch Neurol* 1979; **36**: 144–8.

Rossi GF, Rosadini G. Experimental analysis of cerebral dominance in man. In: *Brain Mechanisms Underlying Speech and Language* (Millikan CH, Darley FL, eds). New York: Grune and Stratton, 1967, pp. 167–84.

Sackeim HA, Greenberg MS, Weiman AL, Gur RC, Hungerbuhler JP, Geschwind N. Hemispheric asymmetry in the expression of positive and negative emotions. *Arch Neurol* 1982; **39**: 210–8.

Sackeim HA, Gur RC, Savoy MC. Emotions are expressed more intensely on the left side of the face. *Science* 1978; **202**: 424–35.

Serafetinides EA, Hoare RD, Driver MV. Intracarotid sodium amylobarbitone and cerebral dominance for speech and consciousness. *Brain* 1965; **88**: 107–30.

Starkstein SE, Robinson RG, Honig MA, Parikh RM, Joselyn J, Price TR. Mood changes after right-hemisphere lesions. *Br J Psychiat* 1989; **155**: 79–85.

Terzian H. Behavioral and EEG effects of intracarotid sodium amytal injections. *Acta Neurochir* 1964; **12**: 230–40.

Tucker DM, Watson RT, Heilman KM. Discrimination and evocation of affectively intoned speech in patients with right parietal disease. *Neurology* 1977; **27**: 947–50.

8
Frontal Lobe Disorders

54. *Prefrontal lesions cause prominent personality changes without loss of general intelligence, motor, sensory or memory functions – a disorder known as 'frontal lobe syndrome'*

The frontal lobes are enormous (Fig. 54.1), comprising approximately a third of the cerebral hemispheres. The motor areas lie posteriorly and have well-defined functions. The prefrontal area consists of paralimbic (anterior cingulate and posterior orbitofrontal) and high-order association cortex (dorsolateral convexity and anteromedial surface) and forms the bulk of the frontal lobe, but its functions are mysterious. This area is considered 'silent' because unilateral, and occasionally bilateral, destruction of a large cortical volume often produces no detectable neurological signs or symptoms. Why is the area of human brain which differs the most from that of the great apes missed so little?

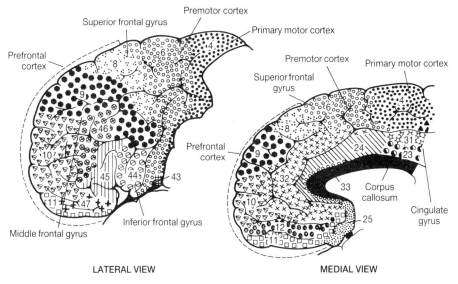

Fig. 54.1 The frontal lobe.

The paradox of the prefrontal lobes persists. Following dominant frontal lobe resections anterior to the motor strip and Broca's area, patients may have normal memory and an intelligence quotient over 150! (Hebb, 1939; Black, 1976). When prefrontal lesions are bilateral, behavioral changes may be difficult to measure, but families, friends and employers tell you the person is no longer the same. For example, patients may drive past stop signs, fail to show concern when a kettle is boiling over, become slovenly and unkempt, joke about someone's physical deformity in front of them, become violent after minor provocation and quickly return to their previous calm state, urinate on the street, or leave a baby unattended to watch TV. In the frontal lobe syndrome, there is a dissociation between the results achieved on neuropsychological tests and the ability to apply tested abilities (Eslinger and Damasio, 1985): the patients do fairly well on standardized tests, but fail at life.

The essential features of the frontal lobe syndrome are (1) disinhibition and impulsivity of thought, affect and action; (2) diminished capacity to sustain attention; (3) lack of spontaneity and initiative; (4) inability to respond appropriately to complex social situations; and (5) inability to foresee, plan, organize and execute complex behavior. Other features of this syndrome include blunted and labile affect, perseveration, impersistence, confabulation and loss of manners and social graces. The personality, affective, cognitive and motor changes that occur in the frontal lobe syndrome are summarized in Table 54.1.

Phineus Gage is a paradigmatic case of the frontal lobe syndrome (Harlow, 1868). This energetic, reliable and effective foreman accidentally blasted a pointed tamping iron more than three feet long and one inch wide through his frontal lobes. He survived. Prior to the accident Gage was warm and caring, well-mannered and highly productive. The 'new' Gage was described as 'fitful, irreverant, indulging at times in the grossest profanity, manifesting but little deference for his fellows, impatient of restraint or advice when it conflicts with his desires, at times pertinaciously obstinate – yet capricious and vacillating, devising many plans of operation, which are no sooner arranged than they are abandoned in turn for others'.

As in most behavioral syndromes, the clinical picture varies among patients. Individual features depend on the nature and time course of the pathological process; the lateralization, localization and extent of involvement among subcortical and callosal fibers; and the secondary effects of increased intracranial pressure. Although intellectual and memory functions are usually spared with prefrontal lesions, tumors may compress adjacent brain areas and raise intracranial pressure, causing dementia (Hecaen, 1964).

Kleist (1934) first suggested that components of the frontal lobe syndrome may be related to specific regional involvement. Expanding on Kleist's observations, more recent studies have found that orbital lesions cause disinhibition, failure to appreciate the consequences of one's actions,

Table 54.1   Behavioral changes after bilateral prefrontal lesions.

Personality and affect
Lack of concern and interest
Loss of will power (abulia)
Blunted or labile affect
Depression
Euphoria, hypomania, grandiosity
Facetiousness, lack of tact (Witzelsucht)
Disinhibition and impulsivity
Irritability and aggressivity

Cognitive
Impaired attention, frontal neglect
Impaired abstract thought (concrete proverb interpretations)
Poor judgment, especially in real life versus hypothetic setting
Poor insight into complex situations
Inability to plan and perform sequential behaviors
Perseveration, inability to shift thought processes
Impaired problem solving and creativity
Memory normal, but 'absent-mindedness' and confabulation may occur

Motor
Lack of spontaneity
Lack of initiative
Motor neglect
Motor perseveration
Catatonia
Incontinence

and euphoria that is often replaced by dysphoria. Lesions of the dorso-lateral convexity produce apathy, aspontaneity, and impoverished and stereotyped thought processes (Milner, 1963; Girgis, 1971; Blumer and Benson, 1975; Stuss and Benson, 1984). Grafman *et al.* (1986) found that patients with penetrating wounds in the right orbitofrontal region are prone to anxiety and depression, whereas those with left dorsofrontal injury display more anger and hostility. However, these anatomic subsyndromes are neither pure nor consistent. For example, depression is most common after left frontal cortical and subcortical strokes (Robinson *et al.*, 1983; Starkstein *et al.*, 1987).

Patients with the 'classic' frontal syndrome usually have bilateral lesions that encompass both orbital and lateral cortex, although unilateral frontal lesions also cause neurobehavioral changes. The most prominent features of left prefrontal injury are a subtle loss of executive and planning functions, depression and – when supplementary or premotor areas are also affected – transcortical motor aphasia and impairment of rapid, skilled manual movements. Following right prefrontal injury, patients may exhibit left-sided extinction and neglect, blunted or labile affect, impersistence, disinhibition, confabulation and the alien hand sign.

Finally, involvement of the frontal lobes – either directly or indirectly – in multi-infarct dementia and degenerative disorders (e.g. Parkinson's disease, progressive supranuclear palsy and Alzheimer's disease) may give rise to many of the behavioral changes often attributed to these subcortical or diffuse disorders.

References

Black FW. Cognitive deficits in patients with unilateral war-related lesions. *J Clin Psychol* 1976; **32**: 366–72.

Blumer D, Benson DF. Personality changes with frontal and temporal lobe lesions. In: *Psychiatric Aspects of Neurologic Disease* (Benson DF, Blumer D, eds). New York: Grune and Stratton, 1975, pp. 151–70.

Eslinger PJ, Damasio AR. Severe disturbance of higher cognition after bilateral frontal lobe ablation: Patient EVR. *Neurology* 1985; **35**: 1731–41.

Girgis M. The orbital surface of the frontal lobe of the brain and mental disorders. *Acta Psychiat Scand Suppl* 1971; **221**: 7–58.

Grafman J, Vance SC, Weingartner H, Salazar AM, Amin D. The effects of lateralized frontal lesions on mood regulation. *Brain* 1986; **109**: 1127–48.

Harlow JM. Recovery from the passage of an iron bar through the head. *Mass Med Soc Pub* 1868; **2**: 327–46.

Hebb DO. Intelligence in man after large removal of cerebral tissue: report of four left frontal lobe cases. *J Gen Psychol* 1939; **21**: 73–87.

Hecaen H. Mental symptoms associated with tumors of the frontal lobe. In: *The Frontal Granular Cortex and Behavior* (Warren J, Akert K, eds). New York: McGraw-Hill, 1964.

Kleist K. *Gehirnpathologie*. Leipzig: Barth, 1934.

Milner B. Effects of different brain lesions on card sorting. *Arch Neurol* 1963; **9**: 91–100.

Robinson RG, Starr LB, Kubos KL, Price TR. A two-year longitudinal study of post-stroke mood disorders: Findings during the initial evaluation. *Stroke* 1983; **14**: 736–41.

Starkstein SE, Robinson RG, Price TR. Comparison of cortical and subcortical lesions in the production of poststroke mood disorders. *Brain* 1987; **110**: 1045–59.

Stuss DT, Benson DF. Neuropsychological studies of the frontal lobes. *Psychol Bull* 1984; **95**: 3–28.

55.   *The inability to plan and execute multistepped behaviors is the hallmark of prefrontal lesions*

We forget how many steps are needed to execute even simple tasks. To make spaghetti, one must find the spaghetti and pot, fill the pot with water, turn the stove on, put the pot on the stove, allow the water to boil, put the spaghetti in the pot, note the time, get out the sauce and another small pot, and so on. Superimpose upon that sequence the telephone ringing, a television show in the background and a child running through the house. What is trivial to the intact brain becomes insurmountable to a patient with frontal lesions. We need to plan behavior in relation to the environment, start it and switch actions within a task. All these steps are problematic in frontal lobe disease.

Patients with frontal lobe disorders have difficulty organizing their actions or a body of information into a meaningful sequence. They manage simple one- or two-step commands but fail at more elaborate or demanding tasks. This behavioral deficit is not usually assessed by standard bedside mental status tests, but it can be evaluated by asking the patient, spouse or significant others about activities of daily living (e.g. 'Are there problems?' or 'Do things get started but not completed?'). Alternatively, one can ask the patient to describe how he would perform various tasks, such as planning a vacation, preparing spaghetti and meatballs, or changing a tire.

Grafman (1989) argues that managerial knowledge units are the predominant type of information unit represented in the human frontal lobe. These units are overlearned sequences of events or 'scripts' that are retrieved automatically and have a chronological sequence with a beginning and an end. Managerial knowledge units are analagous to software programs that are written and modified by the brain through experience. These programs allow us to put certain functions on 'autopilot,' so that we can make spaghetti while talking on the telephone and focus our attention on the conversation. Patients with prefrontal lesions lose their scripts and therefore have to pause to recall the next line, during this pause they may completely lose their train of thought if another stimulus comes into consciousness and causes the original script to be abandoned.

Tests of sequential motor and visual patterns are also useful for assessing frontal lobe functions (Luria, 1970). In the reciprocal coordination test, the patient is instructed to hold one hand open with the palm down and the other in a fist. He is then asked to switch the positions of the two hands simultaneously. With premotor lesions, the patient cannot perform this task quickly or smoothly. A more sensitive test of frontal lobe functions is the alternating, sequential motor test, in which the patient is instructed to mimic the examiner in a series of hand movements. The patient repetitively makes the sequence of three movements on her thigh or a countertop. The three hand positions are (1) hand open with palm down, (2) a fist and (3) hand open with palm up. After one or two demonstrations by the examiner, the patient is asked to perform the movements. Normal individuals may make an occasional error during the first several trials, but quickly perform the sequence accurately. Patients with prefrontal lesions usually fail at this task; they often make perseverative errors by repeating the same movement over and over, or they have difficulty and give up. The visual pattern completion task is a third simplified test of sequential behavior and pattern recognition. The patient is shown a pattern on a sheet of white paper (Fig. 55.1) and asked to copy the pattern and then continue the

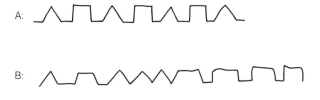

Visual Completion Test
Part A: Examiner's Original
Part B: Copy made by patient with frontal lesion

Fig. 55.1 The visual completion test in a patient with bilateral prefrontal lesions.

sequence. Directions should be repeated or clarified if needed; normal persons should perform these tasks without difficulty, whereas patients with frontal lesions perseverate (Strub and Black, 1985).

The Wisconsin Card Sorting Test requires subjects to 'shift their cognitive sets' and often yields abnormal results in patients with frontal lesions (Milner, 1963). In this test, patients are shown cards with figures that vary in form, number and color. Patients are asked to sort the cards and are told if their choice is correct. First, the criterion for sorting is color, and after 10 consecutive cards are arranged by color, the criterion is shifted to the number of figures. Normal individuals quickly learn the new criterion, but patients with frontal lesions 'get stuck' in one mode of thinking and cannot shift.

The *perseverative* quality of patients with frontal lobe disorders is another hallmark of their behavioral syndrome. They are comfortable with simple repetitive tasks but fail with novel, abstract problems. Perseverative responses may cause confusion when patients are tested and are often mistaken for impaired comprehension, praxis, visuospatial and other cognitive functions. However, perseveration is by no means pathognomonic of frontal disease. Sandson and Albert (1987) defined three forms of perseverative behavior: (1) recurrent: characterized by repetition of a previous response to a subsequent stimulus and associated with aphasia; (2) stuck-in-set: an inability to shift cognitive set that is associated with dopamine deficiency; and (3) continuous: the excessive prolongation of an ongoing activity, which is associated with right hemisphere damage.

Concrete thinking or the *lack of abstraction* is found in patients with frontal, as well as more posteriorly situated, lesions (Rylander, 1943; Tueber, 1964; Hecaen and Albert, 1975). Abstract thought is often tested with proverb interpretation. The problem with this test is that it is often culturally biased, and a patient who is familiar with selected proverbs is at a distinct advantage. A well-to-do psychiatry resident asked an alcoholic ghetto patient the meaning of the phrase, 'People in glass houses shouldn't throw stones'. The patient appeared puzzled and, after some hesitation, replied that they could break a window. The resident instructed the students that this was a classic concrete response, indicating frontal lobe disease. A medical student from a background similar to that of the patient asked, 'Yo, what does it mean, what goes around comes around?' Without hesitation, the patient responded, 'Well, if you mess with somebody, you better look out, because either they'll come looking for you or one of their friends will'. Cultural and linguistic biases are not restricted to the proverb interpretation test but can affect the results on many mental status and neuropsychological tests. Nevertheless, proverbs can be helpful in assessing abstract thought. Useful proverbs include 'Don't put the cart before the horse' and 'Don't cry over spilt milk'. Verbal abstraction can be tested with similarities. Ask the patient to state how two objects are alike, for example, an apple and orange (fruit is the best answer), belt and shoe, train and bus, and so on. Abstract thought is important for everyday life and allows one to make the connections between different events, detect subtle shades of meaning, surmise the underlying motivations for the actions of others, and enjoy a good joke.

References

Grafman J. Plans, actions, and mental sets: Managerial knowledge units in the frontal lobes. In: *Integrating Theory and Practice in Neuropsychology* (Perecman E, ed.). Hillsdale, NJ: Lawrence Erlbaum Associates, 1989, pp. 93–138.

Hecaen H, Albert M. Disorders of mental functioning related to frontal lobe pathology. In: *Psychiatric Aspects of Neurologic Diseases* (Benson DF, Blumer D, eds). New York: Grune and Stratton, 1975, pp. 137–49.

Luria AR. *Traumatic Aphasia*. The Hague: Moulton and Company, 1970.

Milner B. Effects of different brain lesions on card sorting. *Arch Neurol* 1963; **9**: 91–100.

Rylander G. *Mental Changes After Excision of Cerebral Tissue*. Copenhagen: Ejnar Munksgaards Forlag, 1943.

Sandson J, Albert ML. Perseveration in behavioral neurology. *Neurology* 1987; **37**: 1736–41.

Strub RL, Black FW. *The Mental Status Examination in Neurology*. Philadelphia: FA Davis Company, 1985, p. 19.

Tueber HL. The riddle of frontal lobe function in man. In: *The Frontal Granular Cortex and Behavior* (Warren J, Akert K, eds). New York: McGraw-Hill, 1964, pp. 410–44.

56.   *Prefrontal lesions impair judgment and attention*

Bedside and standardized psychological tests of brain function are artificial and may not contribute to understanding how the patient functions outside the examination room. One's intelligence and memory capacities do not necessarily correlate with success in life. Survival in the wild and success in a complex, changing world also demand several other, less easily defined faculties, including mental flexibility, adaptability and quickness, and ability to creatively solve novel problems, obey social rules and judge the behavioral relevance of environmental events. These faculties, in turn, rely on the healthy functioning of the prefrontal areas.

Patients with bifrontal lesions have bad judgment, resulting from numerous deficits that affect the planning and carrying out of multistepped behaviors, adaptation to new situations and understanding and reacting to social cues. Because of these deficits, and, in some cases, an additional lack of awareness, understanding, sensitivity and communicative skills, they often develop family problems, such as poor relations with their spouse or children. They are also frequently fired from work because they offend co-workers or can no longer 'do the job'. These unfortunate complications are well illustrated by the following case, which illustrates the dissociation between how well a patient with bifrontal lesions may appear during an initial visit, or on intelligence and memory tests, and how poorly they perform in real life:

> A 45-year-old man with bilateral prefrontal strokes was found to have a normal neurological examination, except for slightly flattened affect, lack of spontaneity and mental slowness, and increased left-sided motor tone. Neuropsychological testing revealed normal intelligence and memory. He was demoted at his managerial job because of ineffective work habits. His wife was forced to hire a babysitter to be home with the two- and five-year-old children and with the husband, because he was unable to adequately supervise the children and often lost his temper. One night his wife returned home to find the children playing with matches, unattended on the first floor, while her husband taught the babysitter basic geometry on the second floor. He had bad judgment!

The seemingly diffuse effects of bilateral prefrontal lesions – such as abulia, emotional indifference, and failure to plan and execute complex, sequential behaviors seen in frontal lobe syndrome – result in part from the inability to sustain attention.

In fact, an *attentional deficit* is a fundamental component of the frontal lobe syndrome; affected patients are slow, aspontaneous and uninterested. Ferrier (1876) reported that anterior prefrontal lesions impaired attention and curiosity in monkeys, who 'remained apathetic, responding only to the sensations and impressions of the moment, or varying their listlessness with restlessness. While not actually deprived of intelligence, they had lost, to all appearance, the faculty of attentive and intelligent observation'. Keen observation, recognition of positive and negative social and environmental cues, and the ability to adapt rapidly to new stimuli and problems all depend, in part, on frontal attentional mechanisms. Loss of these functions renders people ineffectual and vulnerable on the streets of the real world.

Attentional deficits are often obvious in patients with frontal lesions. At bedside testing, patients may fail to answer questions because of inattention and are easily distracted by irrelevant environmental stimuli (Luria,

1969; Duncan, 1986). Divided attention, the capacity to attend to several simultaneous stimuli or mental processes, is often disrupted by frontal lesions.

Unilateral neglect of contralateral stimuli occurs after either left or right frontal lesions (Heilman and Valenstein, 1972; Damasio *et al.*, 1980; Stein and Volpe, 1983). Right frontal lesions are more likely than left frontal lesions to produce contralateral visual or auditory neglect, a lateralization similar to that found in parietal neglect (Heilman and Valenstein, 1972; Woods and Knight, 1986). Neglect may result from anterior, posterior, medial or dorsolateral frontal lesions. The strong projections from the dorsolateral frontal cortex to the medial anterior cingulate and supplementary motor areas probably account for the attentional deficits following lesions in any of these frontal areas. Furthermore, interconnections between parietal area 7 (destroyed in classic cases of parietal neglect) and both frontal heteromodal and paralimbic cortex suggest that disruption of the attentional circuit at several nodal points produces similar findings. However, long-lasting unilateral neglect is more common after parietal, rather than frontal, lesions.

References

Damasio A, Damasio H, Chui HC. Neglect following damage to frontal lobe or basal ganglia. *Neuropsychologia* 1980; **18**: 123–31.

Duncan J. Disorganization of behavior after frontal lobe damage. *Cog Neuropsychol* 1986; **3**: 271–90.

Ferrier D. *Functions of the Brain*. London: Smith, Elder and Company, 1876, pp. 231–2.

Heilman KM, Valenstein E. Frontal lobe neglect in man. *Neurology* 1972; **22**: 660–4.

Luria AR. Frontal lobe syndromes. In: *Handbook of Clinical Neurology* (volume 2) (Vinken PJ, Bruyn GW, eds). New York: Elsevier–North Holland, 1969, pp. 725–57.

Stein S, Volpe BT. Classical 'parietal' neglect syndrome after subcortical right frontal lobe infarction. *Neurology* 1983; **33**: 797–9.

Woods DL, Knight RT. Electrophysiologic evidence of increased distractibility after dorsolateral prefrontal lesions. *Neurology* 1986; **36**: 212–16.

57. *Abulia – poverty of thought, action and emotion – is common with large midline and bilateral dorsofrontal lesions*

Abulia is characterized by loss of spontaneity and will power. It is easy to miss abulia: will power is difficult to measure, and spontaneity is easily missed as a behavioral sign, partly because there is considerable variation among individuals. Children are hyperactive and overly spontaneous; the elderly are slow, make few extraneous movements, and are generally aspontaneous.

When you walk into the room, the abulic patient lies there, silent and motionless. He sees you enter, understands who you are, comprehends your questions, hesitates, seems to ignore you, or gives yes–no answers to your questions. This patient is the intern's dream – he offers no complaints, asks no questions and gives one-word answers.

In some cases, abulia is extreme. Like bumps on a log, severely abulic patients do not speak unless spoken to; they do not move unless very hungry or ready to void. Even when ready to urinate, they may be incontinent because they are unable to energize themselves to go to the bathroom or do not care about the consequences of voiding in the bed or chair. In some patients, this apathy or aspontaneity is confused with depression, catatonia or laziness (Hunter *et al.*, 1968; Thompson, 1970; Carlson, 1977; Ruff and Russakoff, 1980; Ron, 1989).

Tidal waves of emotional and motoric behavior may emerge from the tranquil sea of abulia. A patient who is usually placid, apathetic and disinterested may be provoked by a trivial stimulus to brief rage or irritability and hyperactivity, only to return to aspontaneous, fixture-like behavior and to act as if nothing had happened (Weigert and Bear, 1988). The 45-year-old manager described in Maxim 56, set off by an annoying insult from his wife, attempted to kill her. He strangled her and beat her with a telephone until she screamed to him 'Do you want your kids to have no mother?' The beating paused and she fled. He later recalled the incident without any emotion, matter-of-factly saying he 'got mad and overreacted', but didn't understand 'why she was making such a big deal about it'!

Central nervous system lesions involving the reticular activating system or frontal lobes often reduce behavior globally (Table 27.2). Normal initiation of verbal and motor behavior depends upon ascending reticular-activating, limbic, striatal and frontal systems. Extensive lesions of the ascending reticular-activating system in the brainstem or its rostral fibers in the cerebrum cause coma or akinetic mutism, depending on the nature, rate and extent of the pathological process. Limbic lesions disrupt the emotional activation of behavior. Bilateral frontal, and less often, striatal lesions cause abulia, with its characteristic impoverished thought, action and emotion.

Mild abulia is often present in patients with unilateral frontal lesions. For example, transcortical motor aphasia resulting from supplementary motor area lesions is characterized by diminished initiation of speech, as well as impaired articulation and fluency in spontaneous speech. Also, patients who undergo unilateral prefrontal lobectomy for tumor removal appear normal but, on careful observation, are less spontaneous.

The assessment of abulia begins with appreciation of spontaneous motor and verbal behavior. Secondly, delayed response to a question or command is another sensitive, although non-specific, indicator. When a patient with abulia is asked to count backwards from 20, they often do so only after repeated requests, reach 17 or 15, and stop without further prompting. Another simple bedside test for abulia is to have the patient say 'yes' everytime you move their finger. Again, patients will correctly identify the first several movements and then cease responding. Finally, abulia may also be assessed by the random 'A' test for sustained attention (vigilance). A patient can be tested verbally by asking her to raise her right hand every time you say the letter A in a series of random letters, or with the paper and pencil letter cancellation test which asks the patient to put a line through all of the A's on a sheet of paper with letters randomly displayed. Again, abulic patients correctly respond to the first few stimuli (with prompting) and then fail to persist in the task. The written test is also useful for assessing unilateral neglect (Maxim 63). Impersistence and abulia are related deficits.

In assessing patients with frontal lesions one must be careful to distinguish perseveration (Maxim 55) from abulia. Perseveration is the repetition of the same verbal or motor response to different stimuli or persistence of a response long after the inciting stimulus is removed. Patients with frontal lesions are unable to disengage from a cognitive set and shift sets – they perseverate. On the random 'A' test, a patient might correctly raise her hand with the first 'A', but perseverate and again raise her hand with the next, non-target letter (e.g. 'G'). In contrast, abulic patients do not start, or fail to continue with, the test. In some patients with frontal lesions, both abulia and perseveration may occur.

References

Carlson RJ. Frontal lobe lesions masquerading as psychiatric disturbances. *Can Psychiat Assoc J* 1977; **22**: 315–18.

Hunter R, Blackwood W, Bull J. Three cases of frontal lobe meningioma presenting psychiatrically. *Br Med J* 1968; **3**: 9–16.

Ron MA. Psychiatric manifestations of frontal lobe tumours. *Br J Psychiat* 1989; **155**: 735–8.

Ruff RL, Russakoff LM. Catatonia with frontal lobe atrophy. *J Neurol Neurosurg Psychiat* 1980; **43**: 185–7.

Thompson G. Cerebral lesions simulating schizophrenia: three case reports. *Biol Psychiat* 1970; **2**: 59–64.

Weigert WA, Bear DM. An approach to the neurology of aggression. *J Psychiat Res.* 1988; **22**: 85–98.

9
Temporal Lobe Disorders

58. *The temporal lobes are important in memory, emotional, auditory, olfactory and certain visual functions*

In most lower mammals, vision is less important than smell or hearing. As a result, the temporal lobe evolved to integrate olfactory and auditory sensory perception, memory (most important in lower animals for smell) and emotion (often triggered by smells, sounds and sights). Similarly, the limbic system (Maxim 61) evolved in close relation to the olfactory system, although this connection is vestigial in higher mammals. For example, dolphins have a highly developed limbic system but no olfaction and, in humans, emotional responses are most often elicited by (1) visual stimuli that are sequentially processed by occipital visual association and infero-

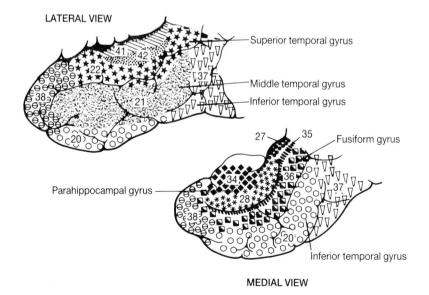

Fig. 58.1 The temporal lobe.

Table 58.1 Behavioral features and anatomic correlates of
temporal lobe lesions.

Behavioral change	Area involved	Reference
Left		
Wernicke's aphasia	Wernicke's area	Geschwind (1967)
Anomic aphasia	Wernicke's area; inferolateral temporal	Benson (1979, 1988)
Transcortical sensory aphasia	Temporo-occipital junction	Rubens (1983); Alexander (1989)
Verbal amnesia	Hippocampus; lateral temporal	Milner (1967); Ojemann (1985)
Euphoria, indifference, paranoia, agitation	Wernicke's area	Benson (1973); Fisher (1970)
Aggression	Limbic, Wernicke's area	Fisher (1970); Taylor (1969); Lishman (1966)
Delirium	Posterior limbic, fusiform gyrus	Devinsky (1988); Fisher (1986)
Synesthesia	?Auditory association	Vike (1984)
Right		
Visuospatial amnesia	Hippocampus	Milner (1968); Jones-Gotman (1986)
Receptive amusia	Auditory association; ? Wernicke's homologue	Mazzuchi (1982); Wertheim (1969)
Delirium, paranoia, agitation, psychosis	Temporoparietal	Mesulam (1976); Caplan (1986); Levine (1982 ; 1989)
Bilateral		
Amnesia (verbal and visuospatial)	Hippocampus;? lateral temporal cortex	Scoville (1957); Ojemann (1985)
Kluver–Bucy syndrome	Amygdala and anterior hippocampus; ? anterolateral convexity	Kluver and Bucy (1939); Lilly (1983)
Delirium, paranoia, agitation, aggression	Posterior hippocampus; fusiform and lingual gyri	Symonds (1957) Medina (1977)
Cortical deafness	Heschl's gyrus	Earnest (1977)
Auditory agnosia*	Auditory association cortex	Vignolo (1982)

*May occur with unilateral lesions (verbal – left; non-verbal auditory agnosia – right).
?-Localization remains unproven.

temporal visual areas en route to temporal lobe limbic regions; or (2) conceptual ideas, such as 'Joe beat up your father', that rely on Wernicke's area for meaning.

The temporal lobe can be simplistically divided into a phylogenetically older, medial portion and a newer, lateral portion. The *medial, limbic and paralambic, temporal lobe* receives olfactory input, regulates emotional state, and crystalizes memory formation. Within this medial portion, the primary olfactory sensory area lies in the periamygdaloid and prepiriform areas; the secondary olfactory sensory area is located in the entorrhinal area of the parahippocampal gyrus. Limbic portions of the temporal lobe (e.g. amygdala and hippocampus) are essential for emotional regulation (Maxim 61). These limbic areas have connections with paralimbic and neocortical areas, as well as hypothalamic regions. Therefore, they serve as a bridge for communication between the intellect and the animal drives. The hippocampus and adjacent paralimbic areas are also critical for the formation of short-term memories (Maxim 24). The posterior medial temporal paralimbic areas in the fusiform and lingual gyri contain higher order visual association cortex. Bilateral lesions in these areas cause prosopagnosia, the inability to recognize face and other specific members of a visual class (e.g. specific types of cars) (Maxim 47).

The *lateral, neocortical, temporal lobe* is a processing station for all auditory stimuli (e.g. spoken language, music; Maxim 59) and specific, emotionally relevant, visual stimuli that are then fed into medial, limbic temporal areas. The resulting emotional stimuli trigger autonomic, affective and behavioral responses based on hard-wired instinct and past memory.

Temporal lobe lesions produce a wide range of behavioral changes and deficits depending on the side, rate and extent of the pathological process. Table 58.1 summarizes the principal features and anatomic correlates of temporal lobe disorders.

References

Alexander MP, Hiltbrunner B, Fischer RS. Distributed anatomy of transcortical sensory aphasia. *Arch Neurol* 1989; **46**: 885–92.

Benson DF. Psychiatric aspects of aphasia. *Br J Psychiat* 1973; **123**: 555.

Benson DF. Neurologic correlates of anomia. In: *Studies in Neurolinguistics* (volume 4) (Whitaker H, Whitaker HA, eds). New York: Academic Press, 1979, pp. 292–328.

Benson DF. Anomia in aphasia. *Aphasiology* 1988; **2**: 229–36.

Caplan LR, Kelly M, Kaase CS *et al*. Infarcts of the inferior division of the right middle cerebral artery: Mirror image of Wernicke's aphasia. *Neurology* 1986; **36**: 1015–20.

Devinsky O, Bear D, Volpe BT. Confusional states following posterior cerebral artery infarction. *Arch Neurol* 1988; **45**: 160–3.

Earnest MP, Monroe PA, Yarnell PR. Cortical deafness: demonstration of the pathologic anatomy by CT scan. *Neurology* 1977; **27**: 1172–5.

Fisher CM. Anger associated with dysphasia. *Trans Am Neurol Assoc* 1970; **95**: 240–2.

Fisher CM. Unusual vascular events in the territory of the posterior cerebral artery. *Can J Neurol Sci* 1986; **13**: 1–7.

Geschwind N. Wernicke's contribution to the study of aphasia. *Cortex* 1967; **3**: 449–63.

Jones-Gotman M. Memory for designs: The hippocampal contribution. *Neuropsychologia* 1986; **25**: 193–203.

Kluver H, Bucy PC. Preliminary analysis of functions of the temporal lobes in monkeys. *Arch Neurol Psychiat* 1939; **42**: 979–1000.

Levine DN, Finkelstein S. Delayed psychosis after right temporoparietal stroke or trauma: Relation to epilepsy. *Neurology* 1982; **32**: 267–73.

Levine DN, Grek A. The anatomic basis of delusions after right cerebral infarction. *Neurology* 1984; **34**: 577–82.

Lilly R, Cummings JL, Benson DF, Frankel M. The human Kluver–Bucy syndrome. *Neurology* 1983; **33**: 1141–5.

Lishman WA. Psychiatric disability after head injury: the significance of brain damage. *Proc Roy Soc Med* 1966; **59**; 261.

Mazzuchi A, Marchini C, Budai R, Parma M. A case of receptive amusia with prominent timbre preception defect. *J Neurol Neurosurg Psychiat* 1982; **45**: 644–7.

Medina JL, Chokroverty S, Rubino FA. Syndrome of agitated delirium and visual impairment: A manifestation of medial temporo-occipital infarction. *J Neurol Neurosurg Psychiat* 1977; **40**: 861–4.

Mesulam M-M, Waxman SG, Geschwind N *et al*. Acute confusional states with right middle cerebral infarctions. *J Neurol Neurosurg Psychiat* 1976; **39**: 84–9.

Milner B. Brain mechanisms suggested by studies of the temporal lobes. In: *Brain Mechanisms Underlying Speech and Language* (Darley F, ed.). New York: Grune and Stratton, 1967, pp. 122–45.

Milner B. Visual recognition and recall after right temporal-lobe excision in man. *Neuropsychologia* 1968; **6**: 191–209.

Ojemann G, Dodrill C. Verbal memory deficits after left temporal lobectomy for epilepsy. *J Neurosurg* 1985; **62**: 101–7.

Rubens AB, Kertesz A. The localization of lesions in transcortical aphasias. In: *Localization in Neuropsychology* (Kertesz A, ed.). Orlando, FL: Academic Press, 1983, pp. 245–68.

Scoville W, Milner B. Loss of recent memory after bilateral hippocampal lesions. *J Neurol Neurosurg Psychiat* 1957; **20**: 11–21.

Symonds C, MacKenzie I. Bilateral loss of vision from cerebral infarction. *Brain* 1957; **80**: 415–55.

Taylor DC. Aggression and epilepsy. *J Psychosom Res* 1969; **13**: 229–36.

Vignolo LA. Auditory agnosia. *Phil Trans Roy Soc London* 1982; **298**: 8212.

Vike J, Jabbari B, Maitland CG. Auditory – visual synesthesia. *Arch Neurol* 1984; **41**: 680–1.

Wertheim N. The amusias. In: *Handbook of Clinical Neurology* (volume 4) (Vinken PJ, Bruyn GW, eds). Amsterdam: Elsevier Science Publishing, 1969, pp. 195–206.

59. The temporal lobes receive and process auditory input and are critical for language and musical comprehension

The *primary auditory cortex* (Heschl's gyrus; Brodmann's area 41) is situated on the transverse temporal gyrus, buried in the sylvian fissure. This area receives auditory input from the medial geniculate body. In primates, the primary auditory cortex is organized tonotopically by sound frequency (Brodal, 1981). Each of the brain's hemispheres receives input from both ears, with some predominance of contralateral input. Because the ascending auditory projections are bilateral, unilateral lesions in the primary auditory cortex produce minimal hearing loss.

Auditory association cortex (Brodmann's area 42) is lateral to the primary cortex and extends to the convexity of the superior temporal gyrus. This area receives fibers from area 41 and is involved in higher order processing of auditory input.

Wernicke's area (Brodmann's area 22) is a *higher order auditory association cortex* situated on the posterolateral portion of the left superior temporal gyrus. This area is vital for language comprehension (Maxim 29). Electrical stimulation of Wernicke's area causes speech arrest and comprehension deficits (Penfield and Jasper, 1954; Lesser *et al.*, 1986).

Lüders *et al.* (1987) reported a *basal temporal speech area* located in the basal, medial portion of the left inferior temporal gyrus. Electrical stimulation of this area impairs comprehension in some, but not all, patients with medically refractory partial seizures (Lüders *et al.*, 1987). The role of this area in normal auditory and language comprehension remains uncertain, since patients with chronic seizure disorders beginning in childhood may have anomalous patterns of hemispheric specialization and localization of cognitive functions. For example, the organization of language systems may differ in patients with chronic epilepsy, as suggested by the increased incidence of right-hemisphere language dominance in right-handed epilepsy patients (Rausch and Walsh, 1984). Finally, removal of the basal temporal speech area for control of seizures does not produce a persistent language disorder.

Cortical deafness is a rare disorder resulting from bilateral damage to Heschl's gyri or the auditory radiations from the medial geniculate body (Earnest *et al*, 1977).

Electrical stimulation of Heschl's gyrus elicits unformed auditory sensations – ringing, clicking, buzzing and humming sounds – that are often localized to the contralateral ear (Penfield and Jasper, 1954). More complex auditory hallucinations, including voices and music, may be evoked by stimulation of temporal association or limbic areas (Halgren *et al.*, 1978; Gloor *et al.*, 1982).

Auditory agnosia is an inability to appreciate the meaning of sounds despite normal perception of pure tones (Vignolo, 1969). Non-verbal and verbal forms of auditory agnosia may occur independently or together.

Non-verbal auditory agnosia refers to impaired recognition or understanding of non-linguistic sounds, such as those produced by a siren, a barking dog or music. Such patients usually have right hemisphere or bilateral lesions of auditory association cortex.

Verbal auditory agnosia, or pure word deafness, is the inability to comprehend spoken language despite preservation of reading, writing and non-verbal sound comprehension. The lesion is either in the dominant hemisphere – destroying Heschl's gyrus and neighboring, white-matter fibers between the contralateral temporal lobe and the auditory association cortex – or in the primary and/or auditory association cortex of both hemispheres (Weisenburg and McBride, 1964; Coslett *et al.*, 1984; Buchman *et al.*, 1986).

The cerebral mechanisms responsible for *musical appreciation* are incompletely understood, but auditory association cortex is probably critical for this function. *Instrumental amusia* is the acquired loss of ability to play an instrument, which does not result from weakness. *Musical agraphia* is the inability to write music (Benton, 1977). *Musical alexia* is the inability to read music, and *musical amnesia* is the inability to recall or identify familiar melodies (Benton, 1977; Brust, 1980).

Expressive and receptive amusia are more commonly encountered impairments of musical appreciation. Expressive, or vocal, amusia refers to acquired loss of the ability to sing, whistle or hum a tune, and usually results from right frontotemporal lesions. Receptive amusia is the defective perception of music despite normal pure-tone perception, and is most often linked with right temporal lesions (Botez and Wertheim, 1959; Benton, 1977; McFarland and Fortin, 1982). Milner (1962) found that ability to judge tone quality and recall tones is more impaired after right anterior temporal lobectomy than when the same procedure is performed on the left hemisphere. In addition, when different melodies are simultaneously presented to both ears, perception is more accurate from the left ear, which feeds preferentially to the right auditory cortex (Bever and Chiarello, 1974). While expressive and receptive amusia most often result from lesions of the right temporal lobe (Wertheim, 1969; Critchley and Henson, 1977), this lateralization is weaker in professional musicians, who use left temporal auditory association cortex for analysis of melody (Bever and Chiarello, 1974). Appreciation of musical rhythm and pitch is probably subserved by auditory association cortex in both temporal lobes.

Auditory hallucinations and illusions occur in a wide variety of pathological processes. Simple, unformed auditory hallucinations are reported by patients with lesions of the middle ear, auditory nerve, brainstem and primary auditory cortex; migraine; salicylate intoxication; and with simple partial seizures arising in the temporal lobe. Complex, formed auditory hallucinations occur in schizophrenia, psychotic depression, cocaine and amphetamine psychoses, alcoholic hallucinosis, delirium, simple partial seizures arising in the temporal lobe, brainstem disease and bilateral middle ear or auditory nerve lesions (Victor and Hope, 1958; Schneider, 1959; Sacks, 1970; Wells, 1985; Cascino and Adams, 1986; Devinsky *et al.*, 1991). Also, auditory hallucinations and illusions, as well as loss of hearing, occur with somatization and conversion disorders (Fitzgerald and Wells, 1977; Modai *et al.*, 1980; American Psychiatric Association, 1987).

Schizophrenia is the most common cause of prolonged (i.e. more than 5 minutes), formed auditory hallucinations in clear consciousness. Schneider (1959) described several typical forms of schizophrenic auditory hallucinations: voices commenting on the patient's actions, voices discussing the patient in the third person, and voices repeating the patient's thoughts.

Alcoholic hallucinosis is characterized by the abrupt or gradual onset of auditory (and occasionally transient, visual) hallucinations with relatively clear consciousness (Victor and Hope, 1958). These prolonged auditory hallucinations may be persecutory, are often accompanied by paranoid ideation, and they occur while the subject is drinking or has recently been drinking (Surawicz, 1980). While most patients recover within hours or days, the disorder persists in some for weeks and months (Wells, 1985). Benzodiazepines are helpful in treating hallucinations if they develop during withdrawal, while neuroleptics are helpful in chronic cases (Stoudemire, 1987).

Simple partial seizures that arise in the temporal lobe can cause both unformed and formed auditory hallucinations (Devinsky and Luciano, 1991). These hallucinations are almost always recognized as unreal, are paroxysmal in onset and offset, and usually last less than three minutes.

Migrainous auditory hallucinations typically consist of hissing, rumbling or growling noises (Sacks, 1970). Both epileptic and migrainous auditory hallucinations are often associated with distortion, or partial loss, of hearing.

Destructive lesions in the auditory end-organs, nerves or brainstem nuclei or pathways may give rise to *auditory release hallucinations* (Cascino and Adams, 1986). These hallucinations may be formed or unformed, and they tend to be more prolonged than epileptic hallucinations.

Auditory illusions are perceptual distortions of sounds. These phenomena can occur with all of the same pathological processes associated with auditory hallucinations.

References

American Psychiatric Association. *Diagnostic and Statistical Manual of Mental Disorders* (3rd edition, revised). Washington, DC: American Psychiatric Association Press, 1987.

Benton AL. The amusias. In: *Music and the Brain* (Critchley M, Henson RA, eds). Oxford: Heinemann Medical Books, 1977.

Bever TG, Chiarello RJ. Cerebral dominance in musicians and nonmusicians. *Science* 1974; **185**: 537–9.

Botez MI, Wertheim N. Expressive aphasia and amusia following right frontal lesion in a right-handed patient. *Brain* 1959; **82**: 186–202.

Brodal A. *Neurological Anatomy* (3rd edition). Oxford, New York: Oxford University Press, 1981, 623–9.

Brust JCM. Music and language: musical alexia and agraphia. *Brain* 1980; **103**: 367–92.

Buchman AS, Garron DC, Trost-Cardamone JE, Wichter MD, Schwartz M. Word deafness: one hundred years later. *J Neurol Neurosurg Psychiat* 1986; **49**: 489–99.

Cascino GD, Adams RD. Brainstem auditory hallucinosis. *Neurology* 1986; **36**: 1042–7.

Coslett HB, Brashear HR, Heilman KM. Pure word deafness after bilateral primary auditory cortex infarcts. *Neurology* 1984; **34**: 347–52.

Critchley M, Henson RA, eds. *Music and the Brain*. Oxford: Heinemann Medical Books, 1977.

Devinsky O, Luciano D. Psychic phenomena in partial seizures. *Sem Neurol* 1991; **11**: 100–9.

Earnest MP, Monroe PA, Yarnell PR. Cortical deafness: demonstration of the pathologic anatomy by CT scan. *Neurology* 1977; **27**: 1172–5.

Fitzgerald PA, Wells CE. Hallucinations as a conversion reaction. *Dis Neurol Syst* 1977; **38**: 381–3.

Gloor P, Olivier A, Quesney LF, Andermann F, Horowitz S. The role of the limbic system in experiential phenomena of temporal lobe epilepsy. *Ann Neurol* 1982; **12**: 129–44.

Halgren E, Walter RD, Cherlow DG, Crandall PH. Mental phenomena evoked by electrical stimulation of the human hippocampal formation and amygdala. *Brain* 1978; **101**: 83–117.

Lesser RP, Luders H, Morris HH, Dinner DS, Klem G, Hahn J, Harrison M. Electrical stimulation of Wernicke's area interferes with comprehension. *Neurology* 1986; **36**: 658–63.

Lüders H, Lesser RP, Dinner DS, Morris HH, Hahn JF, Friedman L, Skipper G, Wyllie E, Friedman D. Commentary: Chronic intracranial recording and stimulation with subdural electrodes. In: *Surgical Treatment of the Epilepsies* (Engel J, ed.). New York: Raven Press, 1987, pp. 297–321.

McFarland HR, Fortin D. Amusia due to right temporoparietal infarct. *Arch Neurol* 1982; **39**: 725–7.

Milner B. Laterality effects in audition. In: *Interhemispheric Relations and Cerebral Dominance* (Mountcastle VB, ed.). Baltimore, MA: Johns Hopkins University Press, 1962, pp. 177–95.

Modai I, Sirota P, Cygielman G, Wijsenbeck, H. Conversive hallucinations. *J Nerv Ment Dis* 1980; **168**: 564–5.

Penfield W, Jasper H. *Epilepsy and the Functional Anatomy of the Human Brain*. Boston, MA: Little, Brown and Company, 1954.

Rausch R, Walsh GO. Right-hemisphere language dominance in right-handed epileptic patients. *Arch Neurol* 1984; **41**: 1077–80.

Sacks OW. *Migraine: Evolution of a Common Disorder*. Berkley, CA: University of California Press, 1970, p. 85.

Schneider K. *Clinical Psychopathology* (Hamilton M, transl.). New York: Grune and Stratton, 1959.

Stoudemire GA. Selected organic mental disorders. In: *Textbook of Neuropsychiatry* (Hales RE, Yudofsky SC, eds). Washington, DC: American Psychiatric Association Press, 1987, pp. 125–40.

Surawicz FG. Alcoholic hallucinosis: a missed diagnosis: differential diagnosis and management. *Can J Psychiat* 1980; **25**: 57–63.

Victor M, Hope JM. The phenomenon of auditory hallucinations in chronic alcoholism. *J Nerv Ment Dis* 1958; **126**: 451–81.

Vignolo LA. Auditory agnosia: A review and report of recent evidence. In: *Contributions to Clinical Neuropsychology* (Benton AL, ed.). Chicago, IL: Aldine Publishers, 1969.

Weisenburg TS, McBride KL. *Aphasia*. New York: Hafner Publications: 1964.

Wertheim N. The amusias. In: *Handbook of Clinical Neurology* (volume 4) (Vinken PJ, Bruyn GW, eds). New York: Elsevier, 1969, pp. 195–206.

Wells CE. Other organic brain syndromes. In: *Comprehensive Textbook of Psychiatry* (volume 1; 4th edition) (Kaplan HI, Sadock BJ, eds). Baltimore, MA: Williams & Wilkins, 1985, pp. 873–82.

60.   *Kluver–Bucy syndrome results from extensive bilateral anterior temporal lesions in monkeys and perhaps in humans*

Kluver and Bucy (1939) observed a dramatic behavioral syndrome following bilateral anterior temporal lobectomies in male rhesus monkeys characterized by (1) 'psychic blindness' (*visual agnosia*); (2) a marked tendency to examine all objects orally (*hyperorality*); (3) an irresistible impulse to attend and react to visual stimuli (*hypermetamorphosis*); (4) emotional changes (*loss of aggressive and fearful responses*), and (5) *hypersexuality* and change in sexual preference (increased heterosexual, homosexual and self-stimulatory behaviors). Later, they reported that the hyperorality was associated with hyperphagia and obesity (Bucy and Kluver, 1955). Kluver–Bucy syndrome (KBS) is clear evidence that the limbic system is required to attach emotional valence to environmental stimuli and to coordinate neocortical and hypothalamic activities.

   Brown and Schafer (1888) originally described KBS in a fierce monkey that would assault any person who teased or tried to handle him; following bilateral temporal lobectomy the monkey became docile and made no attempt to resist handling. Although the special senses appeared intact, he would approach objects repetitively, as if they were strange. In their words, 'He no longer clearly understands the meaning of the sounds, sights and other impressions that reach him. His food is devoured greedily, the head being dipped into the dish, instead of the food being conveyed to the mouth by the hands. He reacts to all kinds of noises, even slight ones – such as the rustling of a piece of paper – but shows no consequent evidence of alarm or agitation [and] displays tyrannizing proclivities towards his mate.' Brown and Schafer also observed that many of the syndromic behavioral traits, excepting tameness, resolved over several months and that this monkey became one of the brightest and most intelligent animals they had worked with. However, Bucy and Kluver (1955) later observed more persistent behavioral changes.

   Features of KBS have been reported in humans after bilateral temporal lobectomy (Terzian and Dalle Ore, 1955), herpes simplex encephalitis (Marlow *et al.*, 1975), head trauma (Hooshmand *et al.*, 1974), anoxia (Sandson *et al.*, 1988), Alzheimer's and Pick's diseases (Pilleri, 1966; Cummings and Duchen, 1981) and adrenoleukodystrophy (Powers *et al.*, 1980).

In humans, the KBS syndrome is often partial, with one or two of the five primary features predominating. Tameness, a prominent and enduring behavioral feature in monkeys, is often absent. Although indifference and flattened affect have been reported (Pilleri, 1966; Lilly *et al.*, 1983), aggressive and agitated behavior is not uncommon (Pilleri, 1966; Hooshmand *et al.*, 1974; Cummings and Duchen, 1981; Lilly *et al.*, 1983). Another interspecies difference involves fear responses following lesions: monkeys uniformly lose their fearfulness, while humans sometimes become paranoid.

This variance between monkeys and humans may result from differences in living conditions among monkeys, individual temperament and the extent of temporal lobe destruction. Experimental monkeys are caged and fiercely aggressive toward their captors, but free-living rhesus monkeys are not especially violent. Human personalities and behavior are subject to wide individual variation and, in humans with severe aggressive behavior, bilateral amygdalotomy markedly reduces aggression (Vaernet and Madsen, 1970; Kiloh *et al.*, 1974). Therefore, the effects of bilateral temporal lobectomy on aggressive behavior in humans and in monkeys may be similar if the baseline level of aggression is considered. Furthermore, in experimental animals, temporolimbic areas are completely resected; in humans, disease states destroy these areas incompletely and may cause irritative lesions in remaining tissue.

It is important to distinguish depression from the emotional changes of KBS. The experimental monkeys enjoyed playful activity and were hypersexual, behaviors inconsistent with typical human depression (Devinsky and Bear, 1983).

Humans with features of KBS usually do not display overt hypersexuality, but may make inappropriate sexual gestures and comments, or become hyposexual (Lilly *et al.*, 1983). Hyperorality is common and may be associated with bulimia and marked weight gain. It is of interest that human infants are hyperoral and have a tendency to place all objects in their mouths. Hyperorality may therefore represent a disinhibited or regressive behavior (Pilleri, 1966).

Many patients with bitemporal lesions have associated disorders, including aphasia, amnesia, dementia, auditory agnosia and partial seizures. Fluent aphasia is particularly common in these patients, and the accompanying comprehensional deficit makes evaluation of other cognitive functions difficult.

References

Brown S, Schafer EA. An investigation into the functions of the occipital and temporal lobes of the monkey's brain. *Phil Trans Roy Soc London* 1888; **179**: 303–27.

Bucy PC, Kluver H. An anatomic investigation of the temporal lobe in monkeys. *J Comp Neurol* 1955; **103**: 151–252.

Cummings JL, Duchen LW. Kluver–Bucy syndrome in Pick's disease: clinical and pathologic correlations. *Neurology* 1981; **31**: 1115–22.

Devinsky O, Bear D. Kluver–Bucy syndrome in Pick's disease. *Neurology* 1983; **33**: 957–8.

Hooshmand H, Sepdham T, Vries JK. Kluver–Bucy syndrome: successful treatment with carbamazepine. *JAMA* 1974; **229**: 1782.

Kiloh LG, Gye RS, Rushworth RG, Bell DS, White RT. Stereotactic amygdaloidiotomy for aggressive behavior. *J Neurol Neurosurg Psychiat* 1974; **37**: 437–44.

Kluver H, Bucy PC. Preliminary analysis of functions of the temporal lobes in monkeys. *Arch Neurol Psychiat* 1939; **42**: 979–1000.

Lilly R, Cummings JL, Benson DF, Frankel M. The human Kluver–Bucy syndrome. *Neurology* 1983; **33**: 1141–5.

Marlow WB, Mancall EL, Thomas JJ. Complete Kluver–Bucy syndrome in man. *Cortex* 1975; **11**: 53–9.

Pilleri G. The Kluver-Bucy syndrome in man. *Psychiat Neurol* 1966; **152**: 65–103.

Powers JM, Schaumburg HH, Gaffney CL. Kluver–Bucy syndrome caused by adrenoleukodystrophy. *Neurology* 1980; **30**; 1231–2.

Sandson TA, Lilly RB, Sodkol M. Kluver–Bucy syndrome associated with delayed post-anoxic leucoencephalopathy following carbon monoxide poisoning. *J Neurol Neurosurg Psychiat* 1988; **51**: 146–57.

Terzian H, Dalle Ore G. Syndrome of Kluver and Bucy reproduced in man by bilateral removal of the temporal lobes. *Neurology* 1955; **5**: 373–80.

Vaernet K, Madsen A. Stereotaxic amygdalotomy and basofrontal tractotomy in psychotics with aggressive behavior. *J Neurol Neurosurg Psychiat* 1970; **33**: 858–63.

61. *Medial temporal lobe lesions often affect emotion*

The limbic system regulates or strongly influences *emotion* and *motivation, instinct, social relations, attention* and *memory*. It contains four principal components: the amygdala, hippocampal formation, septum and cingulate gyrus. Brain regions that are sometimes considered as part of the limbic system, because they are integrally connected to limbic areas, include: the orbitofrontal cortex, dorsomedial and anterior thalamic nuclei, striatum (especially the nucleus accumbens), and the ventral tegmental area and periaqueductal gray matter of the brainstem.

The limbic system acts as the brain's mediator between the basic, drive-related demands of the hypothalamus (e.g. hunger, thirst, sex, aggression, defense) and the more conceptual, often externally based, needs of the association cortex. Limbic areas have strong interconnections with other parts of the limbic system, as well as the hypothalamus and association cortex. This phylogenetically ancient system has 'hard-wired' cells and circuitry that mediate instinctive responses as well as 'maleable or plastic' components that mediate learned responses.

Broca (1878) introduced the term 'limbic lobe' to denote a ring of gray matter separating the cortical mantle from deep structures. Papez (1937) suggested that these interconnected limbic structures formed a system for the regulation of emotion (Fig. 61.1). His theory was based partly on the observations that rabid patients have paroxysms of anxiety, fear and rage, and that the hippocampus bears the brunt of cerebral rabies infection. In Papez' formulation, the hippocampus functions as the brain's emotional center, and the fornix (or large fiber bundle connecting the hippocampus with the hypothalamus/mammillary bodies) transmits emotional states from the hippocampus to the hypothalamus, where they are translated into autonomic phenomena (e.g. tachycardia with fear). The hypothalamus/ mammillary bodies project via mammillothalamic fibers to the anterior thalamic nuclei, which in turn sends thalamocingulate fibers to the cingu- late gyrus. The cingulate gyrus is the limbic way-station to the neocortex, and the loop is closed by the cingulum, connecting the cingulate and amygdala/hippocampus.

Subsequently, observations from electrical stimulation and lesions in animals and humans have confirmed the importance of limbic areas in emotion. Although the concept of a limbic system that forms a functional unit has been strongly criticized, on the grounds that anatomic and physio- logical borderlines of 'limbic areas' are imprecise (Brodal, 1981), it continues to serve as a useful formulation for a group of structures that are related both neuroanatomically and functionally.

The medial temporal lobe contains two of the four principal components of the limbic system: the *amygdala* (anterior) and *hippocampus* (posterior). Electrical stimulation of the amygdala and hippocampal formation pro-

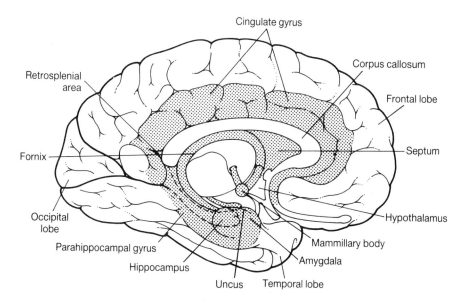

Fig. 61.1   The limbic system: medial surface of the brain.

duces feelings of anxiety, fear, depression, guilt, irritability, anger, pleasure and *déjà vu*, as well as visceral feelings. Such stimulation can also trigger auditory, visual and olfactory illusions and hallucinations (Halgren *et al.*, 1978; Gloor *et al.*, 1982). In primates, the amygdala appears to attach emotional valence to social stimuli, especially those concerning ambiguity, fear and attack (Kling, 1983). Furthermore, in depth electrode radio-telemetry–EEG studies of ambulatory monkeys, it was found that the amygdala is activated during sexual and aggressive contacts (Kling *et al.*, 1979). Bilateral amygdalectomy in monkeys interferes with affective vocalization (Jurgens, 1982) and results in a decline of dominance due to the loss of social skills and the inability to mount appropriate aggressive responses (Rosvold *et al.*, 1954). Amygdalar lesions are necessary – but not sufficient – for the full Kluver–Bucy syndrome (Maxim 60). In patients with structural lesions or seizure foci, amygdalar involvement may contribute to interictal personality and psychopathological changes and aggressive behavior. The human hippocampus has been functionally linked with memory, detection of novel stimuli and instinct.

The *cingulate gyrus* is divided into anterior and posterior halves. The anterior portion is interconnected with the amygdala and hippocampus and is important in emotion, personality and memory. The cingulate gyrus is also involved in modulation of autonomic responses, attention, motivation and vocalization, and other motor sequences (Pool and Ransohoff, 1949; Tow and Whitty, 1953; Pechtel *et al.*, 1958; Pribram *et al.*, 1962; Whitty and Lewin, 1970; Talairach *et al.*, 1973). Intentional lesions in the anterior

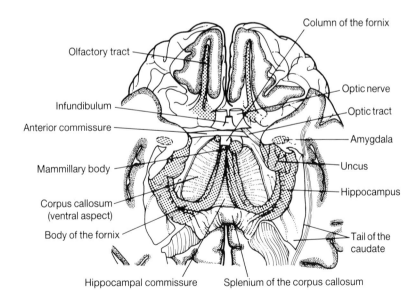

Fig. 61.2 The limbic system: inferior surface of the brain after partial dissection.

cingulate or cingulum (the fiber bundle from the cingulate to the amygdala and hippocampus) can reduce anxiety, obsessive–compulsive and depressive behaviors (Whitty *et al.*, 1952; Meyer *et al.*, 1973; Wilson and Chang, 1974). Although the procedure is usually well tolerated, patients may become easily fatigued, less meticulous in their habits, slower in thoughts and actions, show impaired judgment in social settings, display shallower affective responses, and lose previous interests such as reading literature or gardening (Tow and Whitty, 1953).

The *septum* includes the septal nucleus and substantia inominata. The inominata, or basal nucleus of Meynert, is the origin for cholinergic fibers that terminate throughout the neocortex and limbic system (Mesulam *et al.*, 1983). This cholinergic input is important in memory, and degeneration of this nucleus in Alzheimer's disease may partly account for the memory disorder (Maxim 17). Because lesions are rarely restricted to the small, septal area, knowledge of its behavioral relevance in humans is limited. However, septal tumors cause severe short-term memory impairment. In humans, electrical stimulation of the septum may elicit either rage or pleasureful, sexual sensations (Heath *et al.*, 1955; Gol, 1967). In animals, the septum is important in memory and learning and helps regulate aggressive and pleasant emotions, eating and drinking behavior, and desire to be with other animals (Brady and Nauta, 1953; Meyer *et al.*, 1978).

Patients with limbic tumors, strokes, trauma or infections may develop marked changes in emotion or psychiatric disturbance (Malamud, 1967; Williams, 1968; Glaser and Pincus, 1969; Levine and Finkelstein, 1982). Among patients with limbic lesions and prominent behavioral changes, epilepsy is common. Limbic seizure foci in patients without structural lesions have also been linked with a diverse spectrum of cognitive, personality and psychopathologic changes (Maxims 75, 76 and 79) (Slater and Beard, 1963; Bear and Fedio, 1977; Devinsky, 1991).

References

Bear DM, Fedio P. Quantitative analysis of interictal behavior in temporal lobe epilepsy. *Arch Neurol* 1977; **34**: 454–67.

Brady JV, Nauta WJH. Subcortical mechanisms in emotional behavior: affective changes following septal forebrain lesions in the albino rat. *J Comp Physiol Psychol* 1953; **46**: 339–46.

Broca P. Anatomic comparée circonvolutions cérébrales: Le grand lobe limbique et la scissure limbique dans la série des mammifères. *Rev Anthropol* 1878; ser 2; **1**: 384–498.

Brodal A. *Neurological Anatomy in Relation to Clinical Medicine*. Oxford, New York: Oxford University Press, 1981, p. 690.

Devinsky O. Interictal changes in behavior. In: *Epilepsy and Behavior* (Devinsky O, Theodore WH, eds). New York: Alan R Liss, 1991.

Glaser GH, Pincus JH. Limbic encephalitis. *J Nerv Ment Dis* 1969; **149**: 59–67.

Gloor P, Olivier A, Quesney LF, Andermann F, Horowitz S. The role of the limbic system in experimental phenomena of temporal lobe epilepsy. *Ann Neurol* 1982; **12**: 129–44.

Gol A. Relief of pain by electrical stimulation of the septal area. *J Neurol Sci* 1967; **5**: 115–20.

Halgren E, Walter RD, Cherlow DG, Crandall PH. Mental phenomena evoked by electrical stimulation of the human hippocampal formation and amygdala. *Brain* 1978; **101**: 83–117.

Heath RG, Monroe RR, Mickle WA. Stimulation of the amygdaloid nucleus in a schizophrenic patient. *Am J Psychiat* 1955; **111**: 862–3.

Jurgens U. Amygdalar vocalization pathways in the squirrel monkey. *Brain Res* 1982; **241**: 189–96.

Kling AS. Is there a psychopathology of the amygdala? *Contemp Psychiat* 1983; **2**: 14–16.

Kling AS, Steklis HD, Deutsch S. Radiotelemetered activity from the amygdala during social interactions in the monkey. *Exp Neurol* 1979; **66**: 8–96.

Levine DN, Finkelstein S. Delayed psychosis after right temporoparietal stroke or trauma: Relation to epilepsy. *Neurology* 1982; **32**: 267–73.

Malamud N. Psychiatric disorder with intracranial tumors of the limbic system. *Arch Neurol* 1967; **17**: 113–23.

Mesulam M-M, Mufson EJ, Levey AI, Wainer BH. Cholinergic innervation of cortex by the basal forebrain: Cytochemistry and cortical connections of the septal area, diagonal band nuclei, nucleus basalis (substantia innominata) and hypothalamus in the rhesus monkey. *J Comp Neurol* 1983; **214**: 170–97.

Meyer G, MacElhaney M, Martin W, MacGraw CP. Stereotaxic cingulotomy with results of acute stimulation and serial psychological testing. In: *Surgical Approaches in Psychiatry* (Laitinen LV, Livingston KE, eds). Lancaster: Medical and Technical Publications, 1973, pp. 38–58.

Meyer DR, Ruth RA, Lavond DG. The septal social cohesiveness effect: its robustness and main determinants. *Physiol Behav* 1978; **21**: 1027–9.

Papez JW. A proposed mechanism of emotion. *Arch Neurol Psychiat* 1937; **38**: 725–43.

Pechtel C, McAvoy T, Levitt M, Kling A, Masserman JH. The cingulates and behavior. *J Nerv Ment Dis* 1958; **126**: 148–51.

Pool JL, Ransohoff J. Autonomic effects on stimulating rostral portion of cingulate gyri in man. *J Neurophysiol* 1949; **12**: 385–92.

Pribram KH, Wilson WA, Connors J. Effects of lesions of the medial forebrain bundle on alternation behaviors of rhesus monkeys. *Exp Neurol* 1962; **6**: 36–47.

Rosvold HE, Mirsky AF, Pribram K. Influence of amygdalectomy on social behavior in monkeys. *J Comp Physiol Psychol* 1954; **47**: 173–8.

Slater E, Beard AW. The schizophrenia-like psychoses of epilepsy. *Br J Psychiat* 1963; **109**: 95–150.

Talairach J, Bancaud J, Geier S, Bordas-Ferrer M, Bonis A, Szikla G, Rusu M. The cingulate gyrus and human behavior. *Electroenceph Clin Neurophys* 1973; **34**: 45–52.

Tow PM, Whitty CWM. Personality changes after operations of the cingulate gyrus in man. *J Neurol Neurosurg Psychiat* 1953; **16**: 186–93.

Whitty CWM, Duffield JE, Tow PM, Cairns H. Anterior cingulectomy in the treatment of mental illness. *Lancet* 1952; **i**: 475–81.

Whitty CWM, Lewin WA. Korsakoff syndrome in the post-cingulectomy confusional state. *Brain* 1970; **83**: 648–53.

Williams D. Man's temporal lobe. *Brain* 1968; **91**: 639–54.

Wilson DH, Chang AE. Bilateral anterior cingulectomy for the relief of intractable pain (report of 28 patients). *Confin Neurol* 1974; **36**: 61–8.

10
Parietal Lobe Disorders

62. *The parietal lobes contain somatosensory cortex and multimodal association cortex that are vital for attention, language, praxis and spatial orientation*

The anterior parietal lobe contains the primary and secondary somatosensory cortices (Fig. 62.1). Cells in the *primary somatosensory area* (Brodmann's areas 3, 2 and 1) are arranged by body parts; functionally important parts, such as the hand, have a disproportionately large representation on the sensory homonculus. This primary sensory area receives input for tactile, pressure and position sensations and is essential for finer somatosensory discriminations, including two-point discrimination and graphesthesia.

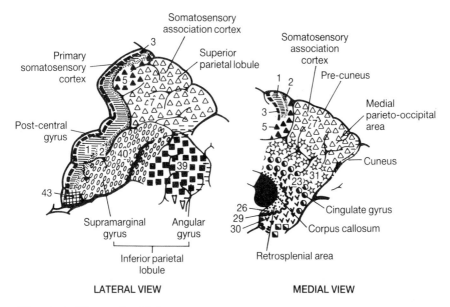

Fig. 62.1 The parietal lobe.

The *somatosensory association cortex* (Brodmann area 5) is located posterior to primary cortex within anterior portions of the superior and inferior parietal lobules. It contributes to (1) precise tactile localization; (2) appreciation of differences in size, shape, spatial relations and weight; (3) sensory feedback for fine motor actions; and (4) somatosensory memories (Critchley, 1953; Mountcastle, 1957; Mesulam, 1985). Lesions in this area cause deficits in somatosensory integration and in three-dimensional orientation of body parts relative to each other and the environment. The somesthetic association area contains cells that help integrate sensory information with movement, especially hand movements (Mountcastle *et al.*, 1975; Hyvarinen, 1982). Other higher order somesthetic cells detect patterns, sequences and directionality of movements, and they probably mediate the localization and 'hearing' of sound vibrations by deaf people. Lesions in primary and associative somatosensory cortex can cause appendicular ataxia similar to the ataxia induced by cerebellar lesions (Appenzeller and Hanson, 1966).

Parietal multimodal association cortex ('the association area of association areas') receives input from the motor association and modality-specific sensory-association cortices. In monkeys, the posterior part of the inferior parietal lobule (corresponding to the supramarginal and angular gyri in humans) is the only cortex that is connected exclusively with multimodal and paralimbic areas, or is 'supramodal' (Mesulam *et al.*, 1977). Geschwind (1965) postulated that the supramodal cortex of the supramarginal and angular gyri makes cross-modal (e.g. auditory–visual) associations and that this capacity is critical for language development. Indeed, the supramodal cortex in the left inferior parietal area evolved as a center for communications processing and integration of language and praxis functions. At the same time, however, a parallel center with similar 'wiring' evolved in the right inferior parietal area. This 'non-dominant' parietal cortex has gained dominance for another set of behavioral functions – attention and spatial orientation.

Left-sided lesions of the supramarginal and angular gyri cause dyscalculia, finger agnosia, left–right disorientation, agraphia (the four features of Gertsmann's syndrome; Maxim 64), alexia, anomia, conduction aphasia (Maxim 35), and ideomotor, ideational and constructional apraxia (Maxim 43). Neglect for right-sided stimuli may occur, but this is far less common than extinction of right-sided stimuli with double simultaneous stimulation. Spatial disorders after left parietal injury usually affect functions that include a linguistic component, such as left–right orientation, calculations and writing (Luria, 1973).

Right-sided lesions of the parietal multimodal association cortex can cause: extinction or neglect of varied left-sided internal or external stimuli, including the patient's own left side, left visual field or sounds on the left side (Maxim 63); delirium and topographical disorientation; dressing and constructional apraxia; anosognosia (the denial or inability to recognize bodily disease, most often left-sided hemiplegia); and allesthesia (the referral of a sensory stimulus on one body side to the other side) (Bender *et al.*, 1949).

The right parietal lobe is dominant for *spatial localization* of both auditory and visual stimuli (Kimura, 1969; DeRenzi *et al.*, 1971; Meerwaldt and Van Harskamp, 1982).

Topographical disorientation and loss of topographic memory follow right, or bilateral, parietal lesions. Patients typically get lost and have difficulty identifying familiar locations (Paterson and Zangwill, 1944; Critchley, 1953; Fisher, 1982). *Prosopagnosia* (Maxim 47) – inability to recognize faces – is often associated with topographic disorientation (Hecaen, 1962).

Patients with right parietal lesions often synthesize geographic information from two places into one, or believe they are in two places at once (Luria, 1973; Benson *et al.*, 1976; Ruff and Volpe, 1981). This phenomenon, called *reduplication for place*, is a form of topographic disorientation related to confabulation.

Constructional apraxia or *visuospatial agnosia* is impaired spatial manipulation of objects (Kleist, 1934). This disorder occurs with parietal lesions of either hemisphere, but is more common after right-sided injury, possibly because of associated unilateral spatial neglect (Arrigoni and DeRenzi, 1964; Black and Strub, 1976). The manifestations of constructional apraxia vary with side of lesion. Left-sided lesions may impair executive motor control; patients may create drawings that contain less detail, although improvement occurs with visual cueing (Warrington *et al.*, 1966). The constructional apraxia following right-sided lesions disrupts visual–spatial–motor integration and is more akin to agnosia for spatial perception (Whitty and Newcombe, 1965). *Dressing apraxia* is a type of constructional apraxia that impairs orientation and placement of clothes on one's body, and occurs exclusively with right hemisphere (usually parietal) lesions (Brain, 1941; Roth, 1949; McFie *et al.*, 1950).

Bilateral lesions of parietal multimodal association area cause *autopagnosia*, the inability to identify body parts (finger agnosia is a partial autopagnosia), *Balint's syndrome* of visuospatial disorientation and oculomotor apraxia (inability to foveate) and optic ataxia (Maxim 48). They also cause all of the lateralized deficits mentioned above, often in a more severe form.

References

Appenzeller O, Hanson JC. Parietal ataxia. *Arch Neurol* 1966; **15**: 264–9.

Arrigoni G, DeRenzi E. Constructional apraxia and hemispheric locus of lesion. *Cortex* 1964; **1**: 170–94.

Bender MB, Shapiro MF, Teuber HL. Allesthesia and disturbance of the body scheme. *Arch Neurol Psychiat* 1949; **62**: 222–31.

Benson DF, Gardner H, Meadows JC. Reduplicative paramnesia. *Neurology* 1976; **26**: 147–51.

Black FW, Strub RL. Constructional apraxia in patients with discrete missile wounds of the brain. *Cortex* 1976; **12**: 212–20.

Brain R. Visual disorientation with special reference to the lesions of the right hemisphere. *Brain* 1941; **64**: 244–72.

Critchley M. *The Parietal Lobes*. Sevenoaks: Edward Arnold, 1953.

DeRenzi E, Faglioni P, Scotti G. Judgment of spatial orientation in patients with focal brain damage. *J Neurol Neurosurg Psychiat* 1971; **34**: 489–95.

Fisher CM. Topographic disorientation. *Arch Neurol* 1982; **39**: 33–6.

Geschwind N. Disconnection syndromes in animals and man. *Brain* 1965; **88**: 585–644.

Hecaen H. Clinical symptomatology in right and left hemisphere lesions. In: *Interhemispheric Relations and Cerebral Dominance* (Mountcastle V, ed.). Baltimore, MA: Johns Hopkins Press, 1962.

Hyvarinen J. The parietal cortex of monkey and man. Berlin: Springer-Verlag, 1982.

Kimura D. Spatial localization in left and right visual fields. *Can J Psychol* 1969; **23**: 445–58.

Kleist K. Gehirnpathologie. Liepzig: Barth, 1934.

Luria AR. *The Working Brain*. New York: Basic Books, 1973.

McFie J, Piercy MF, Zangwill OL. Visual spatial agnosia associated with lesions of the right cerebral hemisphere. *Brain* 1950; **73**: 167–90.

Meerwaldt JD, Van Harskamp F. Spatial orientation in right-hemisphere infarction. *J Neurol Neurosurg Psychiat* 1982; **45**: 586–90.

Mesulam M-M, ed. Patterns in behavioral neuroanatomy: Association areas, the limbic system, and hemispheric specialization. *Principles of Behavioral Neurology*. Philadelphia: FA Davis Company, 1985, pp. 1–70.

Mesulam M-M, Van Hoesen GW, Panday DN, Geschwind N. Limbic and sensory connections of the inferior parietal lobule (Area PG) in the rhesus monkey: A study with a new method for horseradish peroxidase histochemistry. *Brain Res* 1977; **136**: 393–414.

Mountcastle VB. Modalities and topographic properties of single neurons of cat's sensory cortex. *J Neurophysiol* 1957; **20**: 408–34.

Mountcastle VB, Lynch JC, Georgopoulos A. Posterior parietal association cortex of the monkey. *J Neurophysiol* 1975; **38**: 871–908.

Paterson A, Zangwill OL. Disorders of visual space perception associated with lesions of the right hemisphere. *Brain* 1944; **67**: 331–58.

Roth M. Disorders of body image caused by lesions of the right parietal lobe. *Brain* 1949; **72**: 89–111.

Ruff RL, Volpe BT. Environmental reduplication associated with right frontal and parietal lobe injury. *J Neurol Neurosurg Psychiat* 1981; **44**: 382–6.

Warrington EK, James M, Kingbourne M. Drawing disability in relation to laterality of cerebral lesion. *Brain* 1966; **89**: 53–82.

Whitty CWM, Newcombe F. Disabilities associated with lesions in the posterior parietal region of the non-dominant hemisphere. *Neuropyschologia* 1965; **3**: 175–85.

63.   *Unilateral neglect and denial syndromes usually result from right parietal lesions*

Unilateral neglect or inattention is impairment of the ability to orient toward, perceive or act on stimuli from one side, despite preserved primary motor and sensory functions. The deficit varies in severity from a minor form, detectable only with double simultaneous stimulation, to a devastating neglect of all left-sided stimuli, including the left side of one's body.

The severe form of left-sided unilateral neglect often complicates the acute stage of a right middle cerebral artery infarction involving the posterior two-thirds of the right parietal lobe. The head and eyes are turned toward the right and patients may fail to bring the eyes left of the midline on command, although leftward eye movements are normal with the doll's eyes maneuver (passive head movements). Therefore, the defect is not oculomotor weakness but failure to direct gaze toward the left. Visual testing often reveals a dense, left, homonymous-field cut, which may be due to either involvement of the visual radiations or visual neglect. To distinguish visual neglect from hemianopia, the left hemifield should be tested in a dark room with a small penlight: patients with neglect will then detect the left-sided visual stimulus. Unilateral left-sided neglect may affect any combination of visual, tactile or auditory stimuli. When asked to draw a clock, they may place all or most of the numbers on the right side (Fig. 61.1). In some patients, left-sided visual neglect causes spatial alexia (Behrmann *et al.*, 1990).

In patients with left-sided neglect, there is often a change in the personality or affect that is best appreciated by relatives and is characterized by indifference, irritability, silliness and mild euphoria. Overt mania probably occur when the lesion extends to the basal region of the right temporal lobe (Starkstein *et al.*, 1990).

Patients with acute right parietal lesions may deny or fail to recognize their own deficit, a symptom termed *anosognosia* by Babinski (1914). For example, a patient may be unaware of left hemiparesis. When the examiner raises the patient's left arm and presents it to her intact, right visual field, the patient may be unable to identify the body part as her own, commenting that it is the examiner's arm. When she is shown that the examiner has two arms in addition to the presented arm, she may laugh, say it's a trick, or comment, 'Who knows – maybe it's mine?' Gerstmann (1942) reported a patient with anosognosia who believed that 'another person was in bed with her, a little Negro girl, whose arm had slipped into (her) sleeve'.

Anosognosia is one of the disorders of body schema, which are summarized in Table 63.1. We all possess an awareness, that is often peripheral to consciousness, of our body and the spatial relations of body parts to each other and to the environment. The body schema is formed from prior and current sensory information, particularly somatosensory data (Frederiks, 1969). The parietal lobe controls the body schema, and the right parietal lobe has a dominant role in this function (Oldfield and Zangwill, 1942–3; Roth, 1949).

Confabulation, the unintentional filling in or fabrication of information, usually in response to direct questioning, is common among patients with anosognosia. In this setting, confabulation probably results from disconnection of left hemisphere language areas from right hemisphere perceptual areas. The left hemisphere doesn't know whose arm it really is and

Table 63.1 Disorders of body schema.

Disorder	Clinical Features
Hemiasomatognosia	*Conscious type*: patient reports loss of perception of body half or part; occurs with left- or right-sided lesions, may be more common with subcortical lesions *Nonconscious type (neglect)*: patient is unaware of body half or part (e.g. may shave only right side of face); usually occurs with right parietal lesions
Autopagnosia	Inability to correctly name or localize body parts (e.g. finger agnosia); usually occurs with lesions in or near the dominant posteroinferior parietal region
Anosognosia for left hemiplegia	Patient is unaware of left hemiparesis; includes *verbal* (explicit verbal denial of paralysis) and *non-verbal* (behavioral neglect, e.g. failing to attempt to compensate for paralysis); usually occurs with right parietal lesions
Macrosomatognosia	Perception that a body part is enlarged; occurs with destructive or irritative lesions in either temporal or parietal lobes
Microsomatognosia	Perception that a body part is abnormally small; occurs with destructive or irritative lesions in either temporal or parietal lobes
Autoscopy	Perception of seeing one's double or an out-of-body experience in which one's consciousness leaves the body and views oneself from another vantage point; occurs with destructive or irritative lesions in either temporal or parietal lobes
Phantom limb phenomena	Perception of a body schema which has been amputated or for which sensation has been lost; occurs after amputation, and with sensory lesions in the peripheral and central nervous systems
Asymbolia for pain	Failure to exhibit the normal behavioral and subjective reactions to painful stimuli; results from acquired dominant hemisphere lesions

uses whatever thread it has to weave a response. Even if our concept of the body schema is localized in the right hemisphere, it remains a mystery, however, why the analytical left hemisphere cannot figure out whose arm it really is!

In contrast to the catastrophic depressive reaction that often occurs with left hemisphere strokes and right hemiplegia, patients with acute right frontoparietal insults may be aware of, but unconcerned about, their left hemiplegia and speak of it as though it were affecting someone else. However, some patients with anosognosia develop a delusional denial and may become paranoid, agitated and fearful concerning their left side (Bisiach and Berti, 1987; Critchley, 1953). Unilateral neglect and denial of left-sided deficits often have adverse effects on the patient's rehabilitation (Denes *et al.*, 1982).

Allesthesia, perception of a stimulus at a position remote from stimulus location, usually occurs with right parietal lesions and may be related to neglect. Most often, a left-sided stimulus is incorrectly identified as coming from the right side.

The most sensitive test to demonstrate unilateral neglect is the simultaneous presentation of bilateral stimuli (Critchley, 1953). For example, a patient may recognize a tactile stimulus on the left hand but only identify the right-sided stimulus when touched on both hands simultaneously. This deficit, known as extinction, may also occur with visual or auditory stimuli. Visual neglect can also be effectively demonstrated by asking the patient to bisect a horizontal line; patients with left-sided visual neglect cut the line off to the right of center. Alternatively, the Cancellation Test may be employed by asking the patient to draw a perpendicular line through a set of randomly oriented lines on a sheet of paper (Albert, 1973). In this test, patients with left-sided neglect only draw on lines located on the page's right side (Schenkenberg *et al.*, 1980). Sequential numbering of lines on the Cancellation Test improves performance, which suggests that strategies to motivate the patient toward visuospatial searching may help reduce neglect (Ishiai *et al.*, 1990). Other forms of the Cancellation Test require the patient to draw a line through a specific target stimulus such as the letter 'A' (Weintraub and Mesulam, 1985).

The importance of the right parietal lobe in attentional dominance also extends to internal space. Patients with right parietal lesions may fail to attend to such internal events as angina or abdominal discomfort. Thus, the finding of severe left-sided neglect should alert the physician to be extra vigilant regarding general medical problems, such as a deep venous thrombosis.

Unilateral neglect also occurs with lesions in the left parietal lobe, right prefrontal area, cingulate gyrus, striatum, posterior internal capsule and thalamus (Denny-Brown *et al.*, 1952; Heilman and Valenstein, 1972; Watson and Heilman, 1979; Damasio *et al.*, 1980; Watson *et al.*, 1981; Healton *et al.*, 1982; Hier *et al.*, 1983; Stein and Volpe, 1983; Ferro and Kertesz, 1984; Ferro *et al.*, 1987; Ogden, 1987). Neglect is usually milder and more transient when due to lesions outside the right parietal lobe (Ferro *et al.*, 1987). Right anterior choroidal artery strokes are a common cause of subcortical neglect; infarction of the posterior limb of the internal capsule disconnects sensory input from the left body to the right parietal lobe (Viader *et al.*, 1985; Ferro *et al.*, 1987). Although strokes most commonly cause unilateral neglect, it can follow any structural lesion, or even seizures (Heilman and Howell, 1980).

Left hemispatial motor neglect results from right-sided frontal, parietal, or striatal lesions (Watson *et al.*, 1978; Valenstein and Heilman, 1981; Heilman *et al.*, 1983, 1985a; Meador *et al.*, 1986). In this syndrome, initiation and execution of left-extremity movements is impaired – a condition that worsens when movements are attempted in the left hemispace. Patients often exhibit hypokinesia, bradykinesia and hypometria (reduced movement amplitude). Motor neglect may involve oculomotor, as well as appendicular, musculature.

As earlier noted, unilateral neglect is more frequent, more severe and more persistent after right hemispheric lesions (Gainotti *et al.*, 1972; Denes *et al.*, 1982). In patients with left hemisphere lesions, the intact right hemisphere is usually able effectively to attend to both halves of space. The simplest explanation for this observation is that the right hemisphere is dominant for directed attention and surveys stimuli from both sides, while the left hemisphere attends only to right-sided stimuli.

The anatomy of neglect suggests that attention is mediated by a neural network that includes the posterior parietal and prefrontal association cortices, cingulate gyrus, striatum and thalamus (Mesulam, 1981). An attentional deficit appears to be the principal mechanism of unilateral neglect. However, alternative or contributing mechanisms include impairment of (1) sensory integration, or amorphosynthesis (Denny-Brown *et al.*, 1952); (2) arousal, due to interruption of ascending reticular activity system fibers (Heilman and Watson, 1977); (3) unilateral memory (Heilman *et al.*, 1985b); (4) topographical representation (Bisiach *et al.*, 1979); and (5) inhibition, resulting in overattentiveness to contralateral space (Kinsbourne, 1970; Posner *et al.*, 1984).

Many of the structures in the attentional network receive dopaminergic innervation. This observation – supported by animal experiments which demonstrate dopaminergic modulation of neglect – led Fleet *et al.* (1987) to test bromocriptine, a dopaminergic agonist, in humans with unilateral neglect. Their preliminary investigation suggests this drug may be helpful in treating patients with neglect.

References

Albert ML. A simple test of visual neglect. *Neurology* 1973; **23**: 658–64.

Babinski J. Contribution a l'etude des troubles mentaux dans l'hemiplegie organique cerebrale (anosognosie). *Rev Neurol* 1914; **27**: 845–7.

Behrmann M, Moscovitch M, Black SE, Mozer M. Perceptual and conceptual mechanisms in neglect dyslexia. *Brain* 1990; **113**: 1163–83.

Bisiach E, Berti A. Dyschiria. An attempt at its systemic explanation. In: *Neurophysiological and Neuropsychological Aspects of Spatial Neglect* (Jeannerod M, ed.) Amsterdam: North-Holland, 1987.

Bisiach E, Luzzatti C, Perani D. Unilateral neglect, representational schema and consciousness. *Brain* 1979; **102**: 609–18.

Critchley M. *The Parietal Lobes*. Sevenoaks: Edward Arnold, 1953.

Damasio AR, Damasio H, Chui HC. Neglect following damage to frontal lobe or basal ganglia. *Neuropsychologia* 1980; **18**: 123–32.

Denes G, Semenza C, Stoppa E, Lis A. Unilateral spatial neglect and recovery from hemiplegia. *Brain* 1982; **105**: 543–52.

Denny-Brown D, Meyers JS, Horenstein S. The significance of perceptual rivalry resulting from parietal lobe lesion. *Brain* 1952; **74**: 433–71.

Ferro JM, Kertesz A. Posterior internal capsule infarction associated with neglect. *Arch Neurol* 1984; **41**: 422–4.

Ferro JM, Kertesz A, Black SE. Subcortical neglect: Quantitation, anatomy, and recovery. *Neurology* 1987; **37**: 1487–92.

Fleet WS, Valenstein E, Watson RT, Heilman KM. Dopamine agonist therapy for neglect in humans. *Neurology* 1987; **37**: 1765–70.

Frederiks JAM. Disorders of the body schema. In: *Handbook of Clinical Neurology* (volume 4) *Disorders of Speech, Perception, and Symbolic Behavior* (Vinken PJ, Bruyn GW, eds). New York: Elsevier Publishers, 1969, pp. 207–40.

Gainotti G, Messerli P, Tissot R. Quantitative analysis of unilateral spatial neglect in relation to laterality of cerebral lesions. *J Neurol Neurosurg Psychiat* 1972; **35**: 545–50.

Gertsmann J. Problem of imperception of disease and of impaired body territories with organic lesions. *Arch Neurol Psychiat* 1942; **48**: 890–913.

Healton EB, Navarro C, Bressman S, Brust JCM. Subcortical neglect. *Neurology* 1982; **32**: 776–78.

Heilman KM, Bowers D, Coslett HB, Whelan H, Watson RT. Directional hypokinesia: Prolonged reaction times for leftward movements in patients with right hemisphere lesions and neglect. *Neurology* 1985a; **35**: 855–9.

Heilman KM, Bowers D, Watson RT. Performance on hemispatial pointing task by patients with neglect syndrome. *Neurology* 1983; **33**: 661–4.

Heilman KM, Howell GJ. Seizure-induced neglect. *J Neurol Neurosurg Psychiat* 1980; **43**: 1035–40.

Heilman KM, Valenstein E. Frontal lobe neglect in man. *Neurology* 1972; **22**: 660–4.

Heilman KM, Watson RT. Mechanisms underlying the unilateral neglect syndrome. *Adv Neurol* 1977; **18**: 93–105.

Heilman KM, Watson RT, Valenstein E. Neglect and related disorders. In: *Clinical Neuropsychology* (Heilman KM, Valenstein E, eds). Oxford, New York: Oxford University Press, 1985b, pp. 243–93.

Hier DB, Mondlock JR, Caplan LR. Behavioral abnormalities after right hemisphere stroke. *Neurology* 1983; **33**: 337–44.

Ishiai S, Sugishita M, Odajima N, Yaginuma M, Gono S, Kamaya T. Improvement of unilateral spatial neglect with numbering. *Neurology* 1990; **40**: 1395–8.

Kinsbourne M. A model for the mechanism for unilateral neglect of space. *Trans Am Neurol Assoc* 1970; **95**: 143–6.

Meador KJ, Watson RT, Bowers D, Heilman KM. Hypometria with hemispatial and limb motor neglect. *Brain* 1986; **109**: 293–305.

Mesulam M-M. A cortical network for directed attention and unilateral neglect. *Ann Neurol* 1981; **10**: 309–25.

Ogden JA. The 'neglected' left hemisphere and its contributions to visuo-spatial neglect. In: *Neurophysiological and Neuropsychological Aspects of Spatial Neglect* (Jeannerod M, ed.). Amsterdam: North-Holland, 1987.

Oldfield RC, Zangwill OL. Head's concept of the body schema and its application in contemporary British psychology. *Br J Psychol* 1942–3; **32–33**: 267–86, 58–64, 113–29, 143–9.

Posner MI, Walker JA, Friedrich FJ, Rafal RD. Effects of parietal injury on covert orienting of attention. *J Neurosci* 1984; **4**: 1863–74.

Roth M. Disorders of body image caused by lesions of the right parietal lobe. *Brain* 1949; **72**: 89–111.

Schenkenberg T, Bradford DC, Ajax ET. Line bisection and unilateral visual neglect in patients with neurologic impairment. *Neurology* 1980; **30**: 509–17.

Starkstein SE, Mayberg HS, Berthier ML, Fedoroff P, Price TR, Dannals RF, Wagner HN, Leiguarda R, Robinson RG. Mania after brain injury: Neuroradiologic and metabolic findings. *Ann Neurol* 1990; **27**: 652–9.

Stein S, Volpe BT. Classical 'parietal' neglect syndrome after subcortical right frontal lobe infarction. *Neurology* 1983; **33**: 797–9.

Valenstein E, Heilman KM. Unilateral hypokinesia and motor extinction. *Neurology* 1981; **31**: 445–558.

Viader F, Cambier J, Masson Decroix JP. Subcortical neglect: Intentional or attentional. *Arch Neurol* 1985; **44**: 423–4.

Watson RT, Heilman KM. Thalamic neglect. *Neurology* 1979; **29**: 690–4.

Watson RT, Miller BD, Heilman KM. Nonsensory neglect. *Ann Neurol* 1978; **3**: 505–8.

Watson RT, Valenstein E, Heilman KM. Thalamic neglect. The possible role of the medial thalamus and nucleus reticularis thalami in behavior. *Arch Neurol* 1981; **38**: 501–7.

Weintraub S, Mesulam M-M. Mental state assessment of young and elderly adults in behavioral neurology. In: *Principles of Behavioral Neurology* (Mesulam M-M, ed.). Philadelphia: FA Davis Company, 1985, pp 71–123.

64.   Gerstmann's syndrome results from damage to the left posterioinferior parietal lobe and is characterized by the tetrad of agraphia, dyscalculia, finger agnosia and right–left disorientation

Gerstmann (1930, 1940) first described this clinical–anatomical syndrome, localizing the associated lesion to the left angular gyrus and its transition to the second occipital convolution.

Just as the primary and association somatosensory areas have a disproportionately large representation for the hand, the posterioinferior parietal association cortex has a special relationship to the hand. Ontogenetically, children use their hands and fingers extensively in counting, exploring the world, naming objects as they point towards them and in learning to perform complex motor tasks (praxis). Although humans are visual animals, they also rely on fine movements and coordination. Cross-modal associations between visual and tactile sensations and motor programs are a hard-wired capacity of the parietal association cortex.

In Gerstmann's syndrome, damage to this cortex causes *finger agnosia*— the inability to recognize, identify, differentiate, name, select, indicate and orient individual fingers either from oneself's hands or those of another person (Gerstmann, 1957). Finger agnosia is often a partial defect, with the patient identifying fingers inconsistently. For example, the patient may correctly recognize his thumb and little finger but not identify his index, middle or ring fingers, or any of the examiner's fingers. Comprehension deficit and loss of visual or somatosensory input may interfere with finger recognition and must be excluded before finger agnosia is diagnosed. The observation that children first count with their fingers suggests that the association of finger agnosia and dyscalculia may be a vestige of cognitive development. Finger agnosia is a partial autopagnosia (Maxim 63; Table 63.1).

Dyscalculia is an acquired loss of arithmetic skills. Primary dyscalculia, as seen in Gerstmann's syndrome, is a pure arithmetic disorder and is not due to language, writing or spatial disorders. Patients are unable to calculate mentally or with pen and paper. In addition to making errors with reading and interpreting signs, such as '+' and '×', these subjects also fail to perform simple functions such as addition, borrowing and carrying numbers (Boller and Grafman, 1983). Knowledge of baseline arithmetic skills is required to detect impairment. In addition, errors on the serial sevens subtraction test should not be the criterion for diagnosing primary dyscalculia, since more than half of normal adults make at least one error on this test (Smith, 1967). Many of my 'normal' patients get '100–7 = 93' quickly, but then hesitate with '93–7,' and finally answer '84'. Dyscalculia may also be associated with aphasia and with right hemispheric lesions that cause constructional apraxia, visuospatial disorders and unilateral neglect (Benson and Denckla, 1969; Ferro and Silveira Botelho, 1980; Dahmen *et al.*, 1982; Grafman *et al.*, 1982).

Right–left disorientation is the inability to name or point to the right and left sides of objects, including body parts of the patient or examiner. Again, comprehension disorder must be excluded to diagnose right–left disorientation (Maxim 29). Crossed commands such as 'Touch your left thumb to your right ear' are more difficult than uncrossed commands, such as 'Show me your left hand' or 'Touch your left ear'. It is a common practice to combine tests of right–left disorientation and finger agnosia (e.g. 'Show me your left little finger'), but care must be taken to distinguish these disorders because they often occur independently. Right–left disorientation is rare with right hemisphere lesions (Gerstmann, 1930; McFie and Zangwill, 1960).

Agraphia is the acquired loss of writing skills (Maxim 41).

There is considerable controversy surrounding the specificity and even the existence of Gerstmann's syndrome (Benton, 1961, 1977; Critchley, 1966; Poeck and Orgass, 1966; Geschwind and Strub, 1975). Sceptics have argued that the degree of intercorrelation between the four components is low, making the existence of a syndrome dubious. However, Geschwind and Strub (1975) put forth a persuasive counterargument:

> It is of no importance whether the intercorrelation is low or whether it is no higher than the correlation of any component with other deficits. Depending on the frequency of acoustic neuromas in the population studied, the correlation of nystagmus with deafness would be higher than, lower than, or equal to the correlation of nystagmus with a Horner's syndrome or a left X (vagus nerve) paralysis. The intercorrelations of components with each other or their correlations with other deficits are thus irrelevant. What is relevant is the predictive ability of the entire complex of components. The predictive value of the Gerstmann syndrome is simply stated: When all four components are present, it predicts with a high degree of accuracy the presence of a left parietal lesion.

Additional clinical observations leave little doubt that the correlation of the clinical tetrad with left posterioinferior parietal lesions is valid, assuming that a confusional state and increased intracranial pressure are excluded (Heimberger *et al.*, 1964; Roeltgen *et al.*, 1983; Morris *et al.*, 1984).

Developmental Gerstmann's syndrome occurs in children, occurring with or without dyslexia (Kinsbourne and Warrington, 1963; Kinsbourne, 1968; Benson and Geschwind, 1970). Children may have the classic tetrad plus constructional apraxia, or they may have isolated components. Verbal IQ among such children is often significantly higher than performance IQ.

References

Benson DF, Denckla MB. Verbal paraphasia as a cause of calculation disturbances. *Arch Neurol* 1969; **21**: 96–102.

Benson DF, Geschwind N. Developmental Gerstmann syndrome. *Neurology* 1970; **20**: 293–8.

Benton AL. The fiction of the 'Gertsmann syndrome'. *J Neurol Neurosurg Psychiat* 1961; **24**: 176–81.

Benton AL. Reflections on the Gertsmann syndrome. *Brain Lang* 1977; **4**: 45–62.

Boller F, Grafman J. Acalculia: Historical development and current significance. *Brain Cognition* 1983; **2**: 205–23.

Critchley M. The enigma of the Gerstmann syndrome. *Brain* 1966; **89**: 183–98.

Dahmen W, Hartje W, Bussing A, Sturm W. Disorders of calculation in aphasic patients–spatial and verbal components. *Neuropsychologia* 1982; **20**: 145–53.

Ferro JM, Silveira Botelho MA. Alexia for arithmetic signs: a cause of disturbed calculation. *Cortex* 1980; **16**: 175–80.

Gerstmann J. Zür symptomatologie der herderkrankungen in der ubergangsregion der unteren parietal- und mittleren okzipitalhirnwindung. *Dtsch Z Nervenheilk* 1930; **116**: 46–9.

Gerstmann J. Syndrome of finger agnosia, disorientation for right and left, agraphia and acaculia. *Arch Neurol Psychiat* 1940; **44**: 398–408.

Gerstmann J. Some notes on the Gertsmann syndrome. *Neurology* 1957; **7**: 866–9.

Geschwind N, Strub RL. Gerstmann syndrome without aphasia: a reply to Poeck and Orgass. *Cortex* 1975; **11**: 296–8.

Grafman J, Passafiume D, Faglioni P, Boller F. Calculation disturbances in adults with focal hemispheric damage. *Cortex* 1982; **18**: 37–49.

Heimberger RF, DeMyer W, Reitan RM. Implications of Gerstmann's syndrome. *J Neurol Neurosurg Psychiat* 1964; **27**: 52–7.

Kinsbourne M. Developmental Gerstmann syndrome. *Pediat Clin N Am* 1968; **15**: 771–8.

Kinsbourne M, Warrington E. The developmental Gerstmann syndrome. *Arch Neurol* 1963; **8**: 490–501.

McFie J, Zangwill O. Visual-constructive disabilities associated with lesions of the left cerebral hemisphere. *Brain* 1960; **83**: 243–60.

Morris HH, Luders H, Lesser RP, Dinner DS, Hahn J. Transient neuropsychological abnormalities (including Gerstmann's syndrome) during cortical stimulation. *Neurology* 1984; **34**: 877–83.

Poeck K, Orgass B. Gerstmann's syndrome and aphasia. *Cortex* 1966; **2**: 421–37.

Roeltgen DP, Sevush S, Heilmann KM. Pure Gerstmann's syndrome from a focal lesion. *Arch Neurol* 1983; **40**: 46–7.

Smith A. The serial sevens subtraction test. *Arch Neurol* 1967; **17**: 77–80.

11
Vascular, Infectious, Inflammatory and Neoplastic Brain Disorders

65. Embolic, thrombotic and hemorrhagic strokes produce characteristic clinical syndromes

Stroke has been one of the great teachers of behavioral neurology. Many of the classic neurobehavioral syndromes – aphasia, apraxia, alexia without agraphia, cortical blindness, left-sided neglect, anosognosia and peduncular hallucinosis – were originally described in patients with strokes. Cerebral infarction and hemorrhage usually occur in distinct arterial distributions, giving rise to characteristic syndromes based on the areas and anatomical volume involved. Unlike tumors, demyelinating and infectious processes that more diffusely insult the brain – often with increased pressure, edema, compression of surrounding structures, and disseminated or multifocal lesions – stroke produces focal lesions. Although edema and compression occur acutely in stroke, after four or five days, liquefaction and cavitation begin and the lesion is stable within several weeks (McCormick, 1983).

Understanding the clinical changes caused by strokes depends on a knowledge of the cerebral circulation. The *circle of Willis* is an anastomotic connection of cerebral vessels that conforms to the 'textbook' appearance in only half of all persons. Variations in the posterior half are most common. The collateral supply and variations in the circle are not important in health, but become essential when one of the vessels is occluded.

Thrombotic and embolic strokes

The *internal carotid artery* (ICA) gives rise to the ophthalmic, anterior choroidal, middle cerebral arteries and anterior cerebral arteries. In some people, the posterior cerebral artery (PCA) receives its major supply from the carotid, not the basilar artery. Internal carotid occlusion may be clinically silent, especially if the process is slowly progressive and the collateral supply is effective. Sudden occlusion of the ICA may cause a syndrome similar to middle cerebral artery occlusion with variable involvement of the anterior cerebral artery (and occasionally PCA) territory. Cerebral edema may be extensive, causing midline shift, stupor or coma. In many cases, the maximal ischemic injury occurs at the most distal ICA territory, encompassing a curved area along the superolateral convexity from frontal to occipital lobes. These patients experience sensorimotor deficits in the *leg*, *arm* and *face*, and homonymous hemianopsia. Dominant side occlusions cause mutism, aphasia, apathy and depression, whereas left-sided neglect, anosognosia, apathy and euphoria follow infarctions of the right, non-dominant hemisphere (Bogousslavsky and Regli, 1986; Mohr and Pessin, 1986).

Occlusion of the *middle cerebral artery* (MCA) produces a characteristic picture dominated by sensorimotor deficits in the contralateral *face and arm that are more severe than those in the leg (in contrast to ICA infarcts, which usually cause more leg weakness)*, homonymous hemianopia, global aphasia (dominant) and left-sided neglect, anosognosia and delirium (non-dominant). The MCA (Fig. 65.1) supplies most of the lateral cerebral convexities through its two major divisions: superior (frontoparietal) and inferior (temporal). Proximal penetrating branches supply the basal ganglia, corona radiata and posterior limb of the internal capsule. Embolism is the most common cause of occlusion of the MCA or its main divisions, whereas thrombosis is usually implicated with occlusion of the penetrators.

The *anterior cerebral artery* (ACA) supplies the medial surface of the frontal and parietal lobes and its territory extends to the superior surface of the lateral convexity (Fig. 65.2). Huebner's artery is a proximal branch of the

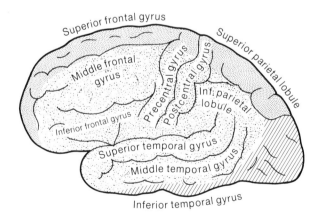

Fig. 65.1 Lateral surface of the left cerebral hemisphere showing areas supplied by the cerebral arteries. ▨ is the anterior cerebral artery, ▢ is the middle cerebral artery and ▨ is the posterior cerebral artery.

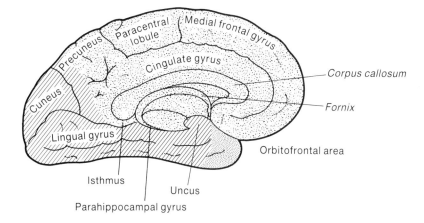

Fig. 65.2 Medial surface of the left cerebral hemisphere showing the areas supplied by the cerebral arteries. ⬚ is the anterior cerebral artery, ⬚ is the middle cerebral artery and ▨ is the posterior cerebral artery.

ACA supplying the head of the caudate, the anterior limb of the internal capsule, and the anterior globus pallidus. Occlusion of the ACA causes contralateral sensorimotor deficits that involve the *leg more than the arm with little or no facial involvement*. These deficits can include forced grasping and groping; paratonic rigidity; urinary incontinence; mental and psychomotor slowing; lack of spontaneity; perseveration; transcortical motor aphasia following lesions that damage the dominant supplementary motor area or its connection with Broca's area (Maxim 31); sympathetic apraxia for left-sided limbs following dominant frontal callosal involvement (Maxim 43); or left-sided neglect after lesions of the non-dominant frontal lobe (Maxim 63) (Critchley, 1930; Alexander and Schmidt, 1980; Brust, 1986). Infarction of the head of the caudate and rostral putamen usually result from occlusion of Huebner's artery or of direct, penetrating arteries off the ACA, and causes (in order of decreasing frequency): dysarthria, abulia, agitation and hyperactivity, left-sided neglect (right caudate) and mild aphasia (left caudate) (Caplan *et al.*, 1990). Behavioral deficits are most severe with bilateral ACA lesions, in which case akinetic mutism (Maxim 32) or a florid frontal lobe syndrome (Maxim 54) may occur.

The *anterior choroidal artery* arises from the ICA just proximal to the posterior communicating artery and supplies the posterior limb of the internal capsule, the geniculocalacarine visual radiations passing posterolaterally to the capsule, and the internal globus pallidus. Unilateral occlusion may cause contralateral sensorimotor deficit, dysarthria and homonymous hemianopsia (Graff-Radford *et al.*, 1985; Bogousslavsky *et al.*, 1986; Decroix *et al.*, 1986; Helgason *et al.*, 1986). *Left anterior choroidal artery infarction is virtually the only cause when the triad of right-sided hemiparesis, hemisensory loss and visual field defect occurs without aphasia.* Right anterior choroidal artery infarcts often cause left-sided neglect (Viader *et al.*, 1985; Ferro *et al.*, 1987). Bilateral infarction causes pseudobulbar mutism.

The *basilar artery* is formed by the union of the two vertebral arteries and supplies the pons. It divides into the PCAs that supply the thalamus, occipital lobes and posteromedial temporal lobes (including the hippocampus, parahippocampal and fusiform gyri). Occlusion near the bifurcation causes a complex picture that is sometimes known as *'top of the basilar'* *syndrome* and is characterized by somnolence, agitation, confusion, oculomotor disorders, skew deviation, memory loss, visual hallucinations and defects and, occasionally, hemiparesis (Victor *et al.*, 1961; Benson and Tomlinson, 1971; Benson *et al.*, 1974; Caplan, 1980). In the acute stages, unilateral PCA infarction causes homonymous hemianopsia, visual agnosia, achromatopsia, visual release hallucinations, palinopsia and visual illusions (Cogan, 1973; Brust and Behrens, 1977; Damasio, 1985). When the patient is aware of sudden visual loss, the cause is most often PCA infarction. However, lack of awareness of visual loss does not have localizing value. Movement disorders, including tremor, cerebellar ataxia and choreoathetosis, may develop weeks or months after PCA infarction (Fisher, 1986).

In addition to the deficits previously mentioned, left-sided PCA infarcts cause alexia with or without agraphia, anomia that is most severe for colors, transcortical sensory aphasia, verbal memory impairment and confusion (Victor *et al.*, 1961; Geschwind and Fusillo, 1966; Benson *et al.*, 1974; Kertesz *et al.*, 1982; Alexander and Albert, 1983; Devinsky *et al.*, 1988). Bilateral PCA infarcts cause confusion; cortical blindness and denial of cortical blindness (Anton's syndrome); and visual agnosias, including prosopagnosia (Maxims 46 and 47). In some patients, proximal PCA involvement results in components of the *thalamic syndrome of Dejerine and Roussy*. This thalamic syndrome results from lesions in the ventral posterior nucleus and is associated with loss or impairment of all contralateral sensory modalities. Spontaneous pain is the most disabling feature of the syndrome and is, at best, only partly ameliorated by narcotics, tricyclics or carbamazepine.

Lacunar infarcts result from occlusion of small, penetrating arteries less than 200 μm in diameter, which branch off large intracerebral arteries (e.g. lenticulostriate arteries come off the middle cerebral). Patients are usually hypertensive and may be asymptomatic or present with one of the classic lacunar syndromes: pure motor hemiparesis, pure sensory stroke, clumsy hand dysarthria or ataxic hemiparesis.

Binswanger's subcortical encephalopathy is a vascular cause of dementia associated with multiple white matter lacunes or infarcts located in the border zones between penetrating cortical and lenticulostriate arteries. These patients typically have a stuttering, stepwise course that includes pseudobulbar palsy and focal motor and sensory changes (Maxim 18) (Nichols and Mohr, 1986).

Hemorrhagic strokes

Cerebral hemorrhage often displaces rather than destroys brain parenchyma. The relative parenchymal sparing with cerebral hemorrhage is associated with a better prognosis for recovery than after ischemic infarcts, assuming the patient survives the initial insult. Extravasated blood forms a circular or oval mass that compresses and displaces, but does not typically destroy, the tissue. However, cerebral hemorrhage is more often associated with acutely increased intracranial pressure, herniation and mortality than ischemic stroke. Non-traumatic intracranial hemorrhage is most often due to hypertension, but also occurs with ruptured saccular (berry) aneurysms and arteriovenous malformations, primary and metastatic brain tumors, amyloid angiopathy, hemorrhagic disorders, septic emboli and vasculitis. Primary intracerebral hemorrhage occurs in five main sites: (1) the putamen-internal capsule (50 percent); (2) central white matter (lobar); (3) thalamus, (4) cerebellar hemisphere; and (5) pons. Massive hemorrhages are often fatal. Patients present with a depressed level of consciousness (50 percent) or headache (50 percent) (Caplan and Mohr, 1978). Focal neurological features vary with lesion site (Table 65.1).

Intracerebral hemorrhage associated with anticoagulant use often occurs in hypertensive patients during the first six months of therapy (Kase *et al.*, 1985). The hemorrhage usually occurs in the cerebellum, lobar white matter and basal ganglia, and has a high mortality.

Amyloid angiopathy is increasingly recognized as a cause of lobar hematomas in elderly patients, many of whom are normotensive. The hemorrhage in these cases is more peripheral than with hypertensive central white matter hemorrhage, and it often extends into the gray matter. The hemorrhage may also spread to the subarachnoid space and, less often, the subdural space or ventricular cavities. Amyloid is found in the leptomeningeal and cortical arteries and arterioles (Haberland, 1964; Okazaki *et al.*, 1979; Cosgrove *et al.*, 1985). Patients may present with stupor or coma, and focal deficits, such as hemiparesis, hemianopsia, left-sided neglect and aphasia. The prognosis is often poor because of the patient's age and neurological deficit.

Many patients with amyloid angiopathy develop dementia (independent or resulting from the hemorrhagic strokes) and multiple lobar hematomas (Gudmundsson *et al.*, 1972; Cosgrove *et al.*, 1985). Both clinically and pathologically, this dementia is similar to Alzheimer's disease. Senile plaques and neurofibrillary tangles are found in both neocortical and limbic areas in more than 50 percent of cases.

The behavioral features of cerebral hemorrhage are not distinctive since they overlap with those of ischemic stroke and other lesions. However, *the association of sudden focal neurological deficits with depressed levels of consciousness, nausea or vomiting, or new onset of hypertension suggests a hemorrhage with increased intracranial pressure.* The importance of recognizing an intrace-

Table 65.1   Hypertensive intracerebral hemorrhage.

Location	Neurological features
Putamen and internal capsule	Hemiparesis (anterior capsule lesions are mild and resolve; posterior lesions are severe and persistent)
	Hemisensory loss (less than motor loss)
	Aphasia: global (repetition returns earlier than with cortical lesions), nonfluent, or fluent
	Hemianopsia
	Gaze preference (toward lesion)
Thalamus	Hemisensory loss predominates
	Mild hemiparesis
	Contralateral ataxia, clumsiness, chorea
	Aphasia (most often relatively normal speech followed by paraphasias, fading voice volume, perseveration)
	Oculomotor abnormalities: (defective vertical gaze, downward and inward ocular deviation, gaze preference away from lesion or wrong-way eyes, skew
	Small, poorly reactive pupils
	Confusion, vivid hallucinations, amnesia
White matter	Frontal: abulia with or without weakness
	Temporal: visual and speech changes
	Occipital: visual and behavioral changes
	Parietal: somatosensory deficits, left-sided neglect
	Small slit hemorrhages: seizures, transient neurological deficit
Pons	Coma
	Small reactive pupils
	Quadriplegia
	Loss of horizontal eye movements
Cerebellum	Headache, vomiting, dizziness
	Ataxia
	Depressed consciousness
	Small, reactive pupils
	Sixth nerve palsy
Intraventricular	Headache, vomiting, stiff neck
	Confusion
	Depressed consciousness

rebral hemorrhage cannot be overestimated since antiplatelet, anticoagulant or thrombolytic therapy may be lethal to these patients.

References

Alexander MP, Albert ML. The anatomical basis agnosia. In: *Localization in Neuropsychology* (Kertesz A, ed.). Orlando, FL: Academic Press Inc., 1983.

Alexander MP, Schmitt MA. The aphasia syndrome of stroke in the left anterior cerebral artery territory. *Arch Neurol* 1980; **37**: 97–100.

Benson DF, Marsden CD, Meadows JC. The amnesic syndrome of posterior cerebral artery occlusion. *Acta Neurol Scand* 1974; **50**: 133–45.

Benson DF, Tomlinson EB. Hemiplegic syndrome of the posterior cerebral artery. *Stroke* 1971; **2**: 559–64.

Bogousslavsky J, Regli F. Borderzone infarctions distal to the internal carotid artery occlusion: Prognostic implications. *Ann Neurol* 1986; **20**: 346–50.

Bogousslavsky J, Regli F, Delaloye B, Delaloye-Bischoff A, Uske A, Despland PA. Hemiataxie et deficit sensitif ipsilateral. Infarctus du territoire de l'artere choroidienne anterieure. Diaschisis cerebelleux croise. *Rev Neurol* 1986; **142**: 671–6.

Brust JCM. Anterior cerebral artery. In: *Stroke* (Barnett HJM, Mohr JP, Stein BM, Yatsu FM, eds), Edinburgh: Churchill Livingstone, 1986.

Brust JCM, Behrens MM. 'Release hallucinations' as the major symptom of posterior cerebral artery occlusion. *Ann Neurol* 1977; **2**: 432–6.

Caplan LR. 'Top of the basilar' syndrome. *Neurology* 1980; **30**: 72–9.

Caplan LR, Mohr JP. Intracerebral hemorrhage: an update. *Geriatrics* 1978; **33**: 42–52.

Caplan LR, Schmahmann JD, Kase CS, Feldmann E, Baquis G, Greenberg JP, Gorelick PB, Helgason C, Hier DB. Caudate infarcts. *Arch Neurol* 1990; **47**: 133–43.

Cogan DG. Visual hallucinations as release phenomena. *Albrecht Graefes Arch Klin Exp Ophthal* 1973; **188**: 139–50.

Cosgrove GR. Leblanc R, Meagher-Villemure K, Ethier R. Cerebral amyloid angiopathy. *Neurology* 1985; **35**: 625–31.

Critchley M. The anterior cerebral artery, and its syndromes. *Brain* 1930; **53**: 120–64.

Damasio AR. Disorders of complex visual processing. In: *Principles of Behavioral Neurology* (Mesulam MM, ed.). Philadelphia: FA Davis, 1985, pp. 259–88.

Decroix JP, Graveleau P, Masson M, Cambier J. Infarction in the territory of the anterior choroidal artery: a clinical and computerized tomographic study of 16 cases. *Brain* 1986; **109**: 1071–85.

Devinsky O, Bear D, Volpe BT. Confusional states following posterior cerebral artery infarction. *Arch Neurol* 1988; **45**: 160–3.

Ferro JM, Kertesz A, Black SE. Subcortical neglect: Quantitation, anatomy, and recovery. *Neurology* 1987; **37**: 1487–92.

Fisher CM. Unusual vascular events in the territory of the posterior cerebral artery. *Can J Neurol Sci* 1986; **13**: 1–7.

Geschwind N, Fusillo M. Color-naming defects in association with alexia. *Arch Neurol* 1966; **15**: 137–46.

Graf-Radford NR, Damasio H, Yamada T, Eslinger PJ, Damasio AR. Non-hemorrhagic thalamic infarction: clinical, neuropsychological, and electrophysiological findings in four anatomical groups defined by computerized tomography. *Brain* 1985; **108**: 485–516.

Haberland C. Primary systemic amyloidosis: cerebral involvement and senile plaque formation. *J Neuropathol Exp Neurol* 1964; **23**: 135–50.

Helgason C, Caplan LR, Goodwin J, Hedges T. Anterior choroidal artery territory infarction: report of three cases and review. *Arch Neurol* 1986; **43**: 681–6.

Kase CS, Robinson RK, Stein RW, DeWitt LD, Hier DB, Harp DL, Williams JP, Caplan LR, Mohr JP. Anticoagulant-related intracerebral hemorrhage. *Neurology* 1985; **35**: 943–8.

Kertesz A, Sheppard A, Mackenzie R. Localisation in transcortical sensory aphasia. *Arch Neurol* 1982; **39**: 475–8.

McCormick WF. Vascular diseases. In: *Neuropathology* (Schochet SS, ed.) In: *The Clinical Neurosciences* (5 volumes) (Rosenberg RN, ed.). New York: Churchill Livingstone, 1983, pp. 35–84.

Mohr JP, Pessin MS. Extracranial carotid artery disease. In: *Stroke* (Barnett HJM, Mohr JP, Stein BM, Yatsu FM, eds). New York: Churchill Livingstone, 1986, Chapter 21.

Nichols FT, Mohr JP. Binswanger's subacute arteriosclerotic encephalopathy. In: *Stroke* (volume 2) (Barnett HJM Mohr JP, Stein BM, Yatsu FM, eds). New York: Churchill Livingstone, 1986, pp. 878–85.

Okazaki H, Reagan TJ, Campbell RJ. Clinicopathologic studies of primary cerebral amyloid angiopathy. *Mayo Clin Proc* 1979; **54**: 22–31.

Viader F, Cambier J, Masson M, Decroix J-P. Subcortical neglect: Intentional or attentional. *Arch Neurol* 1985; **42**: 423–4.

Victor M, Angenvine JB, Mancall EL *et al.* Memory loss with lesions of hippocampal formation. *Arch Neurol* 1961; **5**: 26–45.

66.   *Border zone infarcts may be unilateral or bilateral*

Border zone infarction is ischemic injury to brain tissue that lies between the territory of two or more cerebral arteries. The outer (distal) reaches of the arterial territory will suffer more ischemia than the proximal territory. For example, consider a town that lies at the terminus of two railroad lines, yet relies on them for food. In times of severe food shortage, the trains would unload their precious cargo before they reached the last stop; the unfortunate inhabitants of this town would starve.

Unilateral border zone infarcts occur in patients with highly stenotic vascular lesions or diffuse atherosclerosis, especially after such systemic hypotension as follows surgery or myocardial infarction. These unilateral infarcts can involve any pair of arteries, with the junctions of the superficial territories of the anterior-middle and middle-posterior cerebral arterial trees being the most common (Bogousslavsky and Regli, 1986). Less often, the infarction occurs between the superficial and deep branches of the middle cerebral artery (MCA). Emboli may also cause border zone infarcts (Torvik and Skullerud, 1982; Bogousslavsky and Regli, 1986). Regardless of the cause, symptoms are usually maximal at onset or progress over a brief period. Syncope for several minutes at onset occurs in a third of cases, with non-epileptic, focal limb shaking occurring in 10 percent of cases. Patients with unilateral border zone infarctions have a significantly increased mortality rate when compared to patients with thrombotic or embolic infarction.

Bogousslavsky and Regli (1986) identified distinctive clinical syndromes corresponding to the vascular distributions affected by border zone infarction. In *anterior border zone infarcts* (Fig. 66.1), paralysis is most severe in the leg, less severe in the arm, and spares the face. A non-cortical sensory loss, chiefly affecting the leg and reducing perception of light touch, vibration, pain and temperature, occurs in half of cases. With lesions of the dominant hemisphere, initial mutism is often followed by transcortical motor aphasia. Unilateral infarcts of the non-dominant anterior watershed often produce transient apathy or euphoria. In *posterior infarcts* (Fig. 66.2) the most common symptoms are hemianopia involving predominantly the contralateral superior quadrant and a cortical sensory loss with impaired

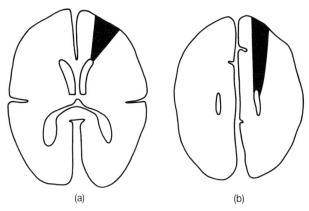

(a)   (b)

Fig. 66.1   Anterior watershed territory (between the superficial territory of the anterior and middle cerebral artery). (a) Inferior wt. (b) Superior wt. After Bogousslavsky and Regli xx.

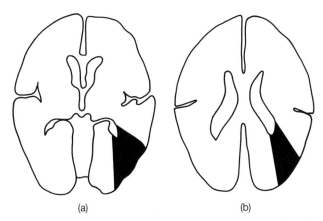

(a)   (b)

Fig. 66.2   Posterior watershed territory (between the superficial territory of the middle and posterior cerebral artery). (a) Inferior wt. (b) Superior wt. After Bogousslavsky and Regli xx.

graphesthesia, two-point discrimination, stereognosis and baragnosis. After left-sided posterior border zone lesions, common symptoms include anomia, transcortical sensory aphasia and depression. With non-dominant lesions, left-sided neglect and anosognosia are common. In *subcortical infarcts* (Fig. 66.3), common symptoms are non-cortical sensory loss and hemiparesis, which usually affects the face and arm more than the leg; non-fluent aphasia occurs when such lesions involve the dominant hemisphere.

Bilateral border zone infarcts occur in patients with systemic hypotension or hypoxia and with normal cerebral vasculature. Therefore, cerebral areas lying between arterial territories in both hemispheres become ischemic. These infarcts cause confusion, bilateral upper extremity weakness and sensory loss, cortical blindness, transcortical sensory aphasia, inability to make voluntary saccades and memory disorders (Gilman, 1965; Adams *et al.*, 1966; Tufo *et al.*, 1970; Howard *et al.*, 1987). As cortical blindness resolves, visual disorientation, dyslexia, agraphia and acalculia are often identified (Howard *et al.*, 1987). Less often, border zone infarctions cause isolation of the speech area (mixed transcortical sensorimotor aphasia) and tongue weakness, and may mimic a brainstem syndrome because of weakness of facial, tongue, laryngeal and pharyngeal musculature (Geschwind *et al.*, 1968; Fisher and McQuillen, 1981).

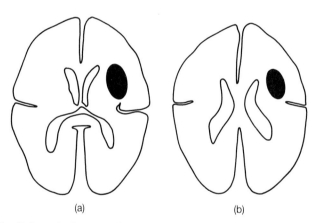

(a)   (b)

Fig. 66.3 Subcortical watershed territory (between the deep and superficial territory of the middle artery). (a) Inferior wt. (b) Superior wt. After Bogousslavsky and Regli xx.

References

Adams JH, Brierley JB, Connor RCR *et al.* The effects of systemic hypotension upon the human brain: Clinical and neuropathological observations in 11 cases. *Brain* 1966; **89**: 235–68.

Bogousslavsky J, Regli F. Unilateral watershed cerebral infarcts. *Neurology* 1986; **36**: 373–7.

Fisher M, McQuillen JB. Bilateral cortical border-zone infarction: A pseudo-brainstem stroke. *Arch Neurol* 1981; **38**: 62–3.

Geschwind N, Quadfasel FA, Segarra J. Isolation of the speech area. *Neuropsychologia* 1968; **6**: 327–40.

Gilman S. Cerebral disorders after open-heart surgery. *New Engl J Med* 1965; **272**: 489–98.

Howard R, Trend P, Ross R, Russell RW. Clinical features of ischemia in cerebral arterial border zones after periods of reduced cerebral blood flow. *Arch Neurol* 1987; **44**: 934–40.

Torvik A, Skullerud K. Watershed infarcts in the brain caused by microemboli. *Clin Neuropathol* 1982; **1**: 99–105.

Tufo HM, Ostfeld AM, Shekelle R. Central nervous system dysfunction following open heart surgery. *JAMA* 1970; **212**: 1333–40.

67.   *Infectious, inflammatory and autoimmune disorders often present with behavioral symptoms*

Alterations in behavior suggest brain dysfunction. Diseases that affect the brain in a multifocal or diffuse distribution, such as those reviewed in this maxim, produce unusual clinical pictures. Matching a set of clinical features such as age, sex, signs and symptoms with a disorder is the bread-and-butter of diagnostic medicine. However, the pigeon-hole approach, in which a patient must neatly fit a predetermined 'diagnostic hole', is a dangerous method of differential diagnosis. A common diagnostic pitfall is the assumption that emotional, bizarre and atypical cognitive disorders are psychiatric in nature, especially when exaggeration or 'emotional overlay' is superimposed on organic features.

Infectious disorders

All central nervous system (CNS) infections can disturb cognitive and emotional functions. Fever, headache and meningismus are the classic features of CNS infection, but may be absent early in the course of the illness. Any neurobehavioral disorder can result from an infection of the brain, which may secondarily cause venous, sinus, or arterial occlusions, as well as increased intracranial pressure. Table 67.1 summarizes the major CNS infections associated with behavioral disorders. This maxim will only review herpes simplex and human immunodeficiency virus encephalidites.

Herpes simplex encephalitis is the most common cause of fatal sporadic encephalitis (Meyer *et al.*, 1960; Whitley, 1988). However, a large medical center is unlikely to see more than two cases per year. The disease shows no age, sex or seasonal preference and is not transmissible (Price, 1986). The most common clinical features at presentation are (in order of decreasing frequency): fever, personality change, aphasia, hemiparesis and

Table 67.1 Principal CNS infections causing behavioral disorders.

Infectious process	Clinical features
Bacterial meningitis	Seizures, depressed LOC*
Bacterial encephalitis	
Legionnaire's	Delirium, brainstem syndrome
Mycoplasma pneumoniae	Delirium, brainstem syndrome
Listeria monocytogenes	Delirium, brainstem syndrome
Neurosyphilis	Memory, intellectual and behavioral changes predominate
Lyme disease	Irritability, memory and behavioral changes, depression, seizures
Tuberculous meningitis and tuberculomas	Delirium, depressed LOC, less often, focal symptoms
Brain abscess	Headache, depressed LOC, seizures, focal symptoms
Superior sagittal sinus thrombophlebitis	Headache, seizures, hemiplegia
Viral encephalitis	
Herpes simplex	See this Maxim
HIV	See this Maxim
Epstein–Barr virus	Mild delirium, seizures
Arthropod-borne rabies	Seizures, depressed LOC, anxiety, mania, dysarthria, seizures, psychosis
Fungal	
Cryptococcal meningitis	Delirium, dementia
Rickettsial	
Rocky Mountain spotted fever	Delirium, depressed LOC, (rash)
Protozoan	
Toxoplasmosis	Delirium, depressed LOC, seizures, focal symptoms
Malaria (falciparum)	Seizures, depressed LOC
Helminths	
Cysticercosis	Often asymptomatic; seizures
Trichinosis	Mild delirium

*LOC – level of consciousness

seizures (Whitley *et al.*, 1982). Behavioral changes result from infection of limbic and paralimbic areas of the temporal and frontal lobes, including the amygdala, hippocampus, parahippocampal gyrus, insula, orbitofrontal and cingulate gyri (Drachman and Adams, 1962; Hierons *et al.*, 1978). The behavioral changes vary across a wide spectrum, ranging from subtle alterations in mood, motivation and memory to hallucinations, delirium, psychosis, mania and aggression (Misra and Hay, 1971; Elian, 1975; Wilson, 1976). Simple (e.g. olfactory or gustatory hallucinations) and complex partial seizures are common and are often unreported or misdiagnosed. Misdiagnosis of herpes simplex encephalitis as a psychiatric disorder foils prompt, life-saving treatment with acyclovir.

The diagnosis of herpes simplex encephalitis requires a high index of suspicion. Fever – even one that is low-grade – in association with acute behavioral symptoms suggests the possibility of herpes encephalitis. Headache is often present, but is rarely prominent at presentation.

Laboratory studies are helpful in diagnosing this infection. The *EEG*, abnormal within 1 to 2 days of clinical onset in most cases, initially shows irregular theta and polymorphic delta slowing with a lateralized predominance over the involved frontotemporal region (Cobb, 1975; Ch'ien *et al.*, 1977). Rarely, the infection and EEG changes are maximal in the occipital lobes (Bergey *et al.*, 1982). Lateralized frontotemporal sharp waves appear and become periodic with a repetition rate of one every one to three seconds; they suggest, but are not pathognomonic, for herpes encephalitis (Westmoreland, 1987). These periodic waves usually appear between two and seven days after the onset of clinical symptoms, but may be delayed for as long as one month (Elian, 1975). Computed tomographic (CT) studies reveal low-intensity, non-enhancing areas, edema or scattered hemorrhage in the temporal and frontal lobes in up to 60 percent of cases. The EEG is usually abnormal before the CT (Smith *et al.*, 1975; Kaufamn *et al.*, 1979). Magnetic resonance imaging (MRI) reveals areas of increased signal on T2-weighted images due to increased water content, and preliminary studies suggest that MRI is superior to CT in detecting early changes in herpes encephalitis (Schroth *et al.*, 1987). Cerebrospinal fluid is characteristically under increased pressure, with a mildly increased protein concentration, and a lymphocytic pleocytosis of 10 to 400 cells per cm^3 (Whitley *et al.*, 1986). However, neutrophils may be abundant, or the CSF may be acellular (Schlageter *et al.*, 1984).

The survivors of herpes encephalitis are often left with severe memory, intellectual and behavioral disorders, including elements of the Kluver–Bucy syndrome (e.g. hyperorality, hypersexuality and visual angosia) (Marlowe *et al.*, 1975; Hierons *et al.*, 1978; Lilly *et al.*, 1983).

The *acquired immune deficiency disorder* (*AIDS*) results from infection with the human immunodeficiency virus (HIV), type 1. The central nervous system is a favored site for HIV infection. Acutely, there is often a mild meningoencephalitis. Subacute or chronic HIV encephalitis produces a slowly or rapidly progressing dementia accompanied by behavioral changes such as anxiety, irritability, depression and apathy, as well as weakness, hyperreflexia, ataxia and oculomotor disorders (Gabuzda and Hirsch, 1987; Brew *et al.*, 1988). The AIDS–dementia complex can be the major or sole presenting feature of AIDS (Navia and Price, 1987); it is present in a third of patients early in the course of AIDS and in two-thirds before death (Brew *et al.*, 1988). Non-HIV CNS infections are extremely common in AIDS patients; the most frequent are: toxoplasmosis, cytomegalovirus, meningovascular neurosyphilis, tuberculous meningitis and tuberculomas, cryptococcal meningitis and progressive multifocal leukoencephalopathy.

Inflammatory and autoimmune disorders

Sarcoidosis is a granulomatous, inflammatory disease of unknown etiology that involves the nervous system in 5 percent of patients (Siltzbach *et al.*, 1974; Delaney, 1977). Granulomata, inflammatory infiltrates or vasculitis can involve the peripheral nerves, cranial nerves and the central nervous system. Sarcoidosis has a predilection for the base of the brain, resulting in (1) visual disorders from optic nerve and chiasmal lesions, and (2) polyuria, polydypsia, somnolence, apathy, obesity and hormonal disorders from hypothalamic and pituitary lesions. Less common CNS manifestations of sarcoidosis include seizures, delirium, cognitive dysfunction, personality changes, depression and psychosis (Douglas and Maloney, 1973; Delaney, 1977). In addition, dementia can develop when the granulomas extend from the hypothalamus to adjacent subcortical areas, involve the brain diffusely, or when hydrocephalus occurs (Cordingley *et al.*, 1981; Thompson and Checkley, 1981; Hier *et al.*, 1983).

Multiple sclerosis is an autoimmune disorder in which a viral infection has been postulated to trigger aberrant immune response against CNS myelin. The mode of onset ranges from acute, apoplectic symptoms to non-specific complaints of fatigue, myalgias, arthralgias and weight loss that precede neurological symptoms by months or years. The classic neurological features of multiple sclerosis are weakness, numbness, ataxia, nystagmus, diplopia and optic or retrobulbar neuritis. Cognitive and behavioral symptoms are also prominent in multiple sclerosis. Depression, irritability, emotional lability, indifference, euphoria and exaggerated dramatic complaints (i.e. hysteria) are among the most common behavioral problems (Aring, 1965; Caplan and Nadelson, 1980; Dalos *et al.*, 1983). The presence of such non-specific complaints as fatigue; subjective complaints, such as numbness and paresthesia; and such behavioral changes as emotional lability and 'hysteria' can easily cause one to miss the diagnosis. Cognitive disorders occur in half of all patients with multiple sclerosis (Betrando *et al.*, 1983) and range from mild impairment of memory and judgment to aphasia and rapidly progressing dementia (Bergin, 1957; Koenig, 1968; Carroll *et al.*, 1984; Rao *et al.*, 1984).

The diagnosis of multiple sclerosis is made by the characteristic dissemination of CNS dysfunction over time (i.e. episodic) and space (i.e. multifocal). Magnetic resonance imaging (MRI) reveals multifocal areas of increased signal on T2-weighted images of the cerebral white matter in more than 80 percent of cases, with periventricular lesions predominating (Ormerod *et al.*, 1986; Stewart *et al.*, 1987). Evoked potentials are often abnormally prolonged or absent in patients with multiple sclerosis: visual evoked potentials are abnormal in 80 percent, brainstem auditory evoked potentials are abnormal in 50 percent, and somatosensory evoked potentials are abnormal in 70 percent of patients (Chiappa, 1990). Pathologically, there are disseminated plaques in the white matter of the spinal cord, brainstem, and cerebral hemispheres.

Glucocorticoids are often used in high-dose short-term regimens or in low to moderate dose long-term regimens. These drugs may have prominent behavioral side effects such as irritability, paranoia, depression, mania and psychosis. Patients with multiple sclerosis may be particularly prone to such complications, especially with chronic therapy.

Systemic lupus erythematosus (SLE) is accompanied by neurological signs and symptoms in three out of four patients (Johnson and Richardson, 1968; Devinsky *et al.*, 1988). Seizures, delirium, stupor or coma, depression, psychosis, hallucinations, paranoia, mania, dementia and focal large or small artery stroke syndromes are the most common CNS manifestations (Johnson and Richardson, 1968; Feinglass *et al.*, 1976; Devinsky *et al.*, 1988). Psychosis can result from CNS dysfunction induced by SLE, from glucocorticoid therapy, or from the interaction of both. If psychosis develops shortly after initiation of, or an increase in, glucocorticoid therapy, steroids are most probably the cause of psychosis, and they should be tapered. If the systemic disease requires active treatment, another immunosuppressive agent should be employed.

Misdiagnosis of CNS lupus as primary psychiatric disease is common; this usually occurs when neuropsychiatric symptoms are the presenting features, but also occurs when SLE has been previously diagnosed. As with multiple sclerosis, the congruence of vague symptoms such as fatigue and diffuse aches, subjective symptoms such as numbness and pain, affective disorders, and dramatization of symptoms leads one down the wrong path towards the diagnosis of conversion disorder.

The pathogenesis of neuropsychiatric symptoms in SLE remains poorly defined. Although vasculitis has been widely assumed to cause CNS symptoms, pathological studies have shown that CNS vasculitis is rare (Johnson and Richardson, 1968; Devinsky *et al.*, 1988). Occlusion of small blood vessels by platelet–fibrin thrombi and proliferative changes is the most pathological finding. Cardiac emboli from Libman–Sacks endocarditis is another important cause of stroke in SLE (Devinsky *et al.*, 1988). Antiphospholipid antibodies (e.g. lupus anticoagulant and anticardiolipin antibodies) may predispose to small vessel occlusion, development of Libman–Sacks endocarditis, thrombotic thrombocytopenic purpura and the resultant neuropsychiatric disorders in many patients with SLE (Devinsky *et al.*, 1988; Levine and Welch, 1989; Levine *et al.*, 1990). Anticoagulation and antiplatelet agents, as well as immunosuppressive – anti-inflammatory therapy, may be effective for certain forms of CNS lupus. The role of antineuronal antibodies in the pathogenesis of neurobehavioral symptoms in lupus is uncertain.

References

Aring CD. Observations on multiple sclerosis and conversion hysteria. *Brain* 1965; **88**: 663–74.

Bergey GK, Coyle PK, Kaumholz A, Niedermeyer E. Herpes simplex encphalitis with occipital localization. *Arch Neurol* 1982; **39**: 312–13.

Bergin JD. Rapidly progressive dementia in disseminated sclerosis. *J Neurol Neurosurg Psychiat* 1957; **20**: 285–92.

Betrando P, Maffei C, Ghezzi A. A study of neuropsychological alterations in multiple sclerosis. *Acta Psychiat Belg* 1983; **83**: 13–21.

Brew B, Sidtis J, Petito CK, Price RW. The neurologic complications of AIDS and human immunodeficiency virus infection. In: *Advances in Contemporary Neurology* (Plum F, ed.). Philadelphia: FA Davis Company, 1988.

Caplan LR, Nadelson T. Multiple sclerosis and hysteria. *JAMA* 1980; **243**: 2418–21.

Carroll M, Gates R, Rodlan F. Memory impairment in multiple sclerosis. *Neuropsychologia* 1984; **22**: 297–302.

Chiappa KH. *Evoked Potentials in Clinical Medicine* (2nd edition). New York: Raven Press, 1990, p. 408.

Ch'ien LT, Boehm RM, Robinson H, Liu C, Frenkel LD. Characteristic early electroencephalographic changes in herpes simplex encephalitis. Clinical and virologic studies. *Arch Neurol* 1977; **34**: 361–4.

Cobb WA. Electroencephalographic changes in viral encephalitis. In: *Viral Diseases of the Central Nervous System* (Illis LS, ed.). Baltimore, MA: Williams & Wilkins, 1975, pp. 76–89.

Cordingley G, Navarro C, Brust JCM, Healton EB. Sarcoidosis presenting as senile dementia. *Neurology* 1981; **31**: 1148–51.

Dalos NP, Robins PV, Brooks BR *et al.* Disease activity and emotional state in multiple sclerosis. *Ann Neurol* 1983; **13**: 573–8.

Delaney P. Neurological manifestations in sarcoidosis. *Ann Int Med* 1977; **87**: 336–45.

Devinsky O, Petito CK, Alonso D. Clinical and pathological features of systemic lupus erythematosis. *Ann Neurol* 1988; **23**: 380–4.

Douglas AC, Maloney AFJ. Sarcoidosis of the central nervous system. *J Neurol Neurosurg Psychiat* 1973; **36**: 1024–33.

Drachman DA, Adams RD. Herpes simplex and acute inclusion-body encephalitis. *Arch Neurol* 1962; **7**: 45–63.

Elian M. Herpes simplex encephalitis. Prognosis and longterm follow-up. *Arch Neurol* 1975; **32**: 39–43.

Feinglass EJ, Arnett FC, Dorsch CA *et al.* Neuropsychiatric manifestations of systemic lupus erythematosus. *Medicine* 1976; **55**: 323–39.

Gabuzda D, Hirsch MS. Neurologic manifestations of infection with human immunodeficiency virus: Clinical features and pathogenesis. *Ann Int Med* 1987; **107**: 383–91.

Hier DB, Thomas CT, Shindler AG. A case of subcortical dementia due to sarcoidosis of the hypothalamus and fornices. *Brain Cogn* 1983; **2**: 189–98.

Hierons R, Janota I, Corsellis JAN. The late effects of necrotizing encephalitis of the temporal lobes and limbic areas: a clinicopathological study of 10 cases. *Psychol Med* 1978; **8**: 21–42.

Johnson RT, Richardson EP. The neurologic manifestations of systemic lupus erythematosus. *Medicine* 1968; **47**: 337–68.

Kaufman DM, Zimmerman RD, Leeds NE. Computed tomography in herpes simplex encephalitis. *Neurology* 1979; **29**: 1392–6.

Koenig H. Dementia associated with the benign form of multiple sclerosis. *Trans Am Neurol Assoc* 1968; **93**: 227–8.

Levine SR, Welch KMA. Antiphospholipid antibodies. *Ann Neurol* 1989; **26**: 386–9.

Levine SR, Deegan MJ, Futrell N, Welch KMA. Cerebrovascular and neurologic disease associated with antiphospholipid antibodies: 48 cases. *Neurology* 1990; **40**: 1181–9.

Lilly R, Cummings JL, Benson DF, Frankel M. The human Kluver – Bucy syndrome. *Neurology* 1983; **33**: 1141–5.

Marlowe WB, Mancall EL, Thomas TJ. Complete Kluver – Bucy syndrome in man. *Cortex* 1975; **11**: 53–9.

Meyer HM, Johnson RT, Crawford JP, Dascomb HE, Rogers NG. Central nervous system syndromes of 'viral' etiology: a study of 713 cases. *Am J Med* 1960; **29**: 334–42.

Misra PC, Hay GG. Encephalitis presenting as acute schizophrenia. *Br Med J* 1971; **1**: 532–3.

Navia BA, Price RW. The acquired immunodeficiency syndrome dementia complex as the presenting or sole manifestation of human immunodeficiency virus infection. *Arch Neurol* 1987; **44**: 65–9.

Ormerod IEC, McDonald WI, DuBoulay GH *et al*. Disseminated lesions at presentation in patients with optic neuritis. *J Neurol Neurosurg Psychiat* 1986; **49**: 124–7.

Price RW. Neurobiology of human herpesvirus infections. *CRC Crit Rev Clin Neurobiol* 1986; **2**: 61–123.

Rao SM, Hammeke TA, McQuillen MP, Khatri BO, Lloyd D. Memory disturbance in chronic progressive multiple sclerosis. *Arch Neurol* 1984; **41**: 625–41.

Schlageter N, Jubelt B, Vick NA. Herpes simplex encephalitis without CSF leukocytosis. *Arch Neurol* 1984; **41**: 1007–8.

Schroth G, Gawehn J, Thron A, Vallbracht A, Voigt K. Early diagnosis of herpes simplex encephalitis by MRI. *Neurology* 1987; **37**: 179–83.

Siltzbach LE, James DG, Neville E *et al*. Course and prognosis of sarcoidosis around the world. *Am J Med* 1974; **57**: 847–52.

Smith JB, Westmoreland BF, Reagan TJ. A distinctive clinical EEG profile in herpes simplex encephalitis. *Mayo Clin Proc* 1975; **50**: 469–74.

Stewart JM, Houser GW, Baker HL. Magnetic resonance imaging and clinical relationships in multiple sclerosis. *Mayo Clin Proc* 1987; **62**: 174–84.

Thompson C, Checkley S. Short term memory deficit in patient with central sarcoidosis. *Br J Psychiat* 1981; **139**: 161–1.

Westmoreland BF. The EEG in cerebral inflammatory processes. In: *Electroencephalography* (Niedermeyer E, Lopes da Silva F, eds). Baltimore, MA: Urban & Schwarzenberg, 1987, pp. 259–73.

Whitley RJ. The frustrations of treating herpes simplex virus infections of the central nervous system. *JAMA* 1988; **259**: 1067.

Whitley RJ, Alford CA, Hirsch MS *et al* and the NIAID collaborative antiviral study group. Vidarabine versus acyclovir therapy in herpes simplex encephalitis. *N Engl J Med* 1986; **314**: 144–9.

Whitley RJ, Soong SJ, Linnenman C, Liu C, Pazin G, Alford CA. Herpes simplex encephalitis. *JAMA* 1982; **247**: 317–20.

Wilson LG. Viral encephalopathy mimicking functional psychosis. *Am J Psychiat* 1976; **133**: 165–70.

68.   *Cerebral tumors cause behavioral deficits through local and diffuse effects*

Truly benign brain tumors are rare. Even histologically benign tumors may be lethal when they grow and compress vital structures. The cranial vault is filled with brain, blood and cerebrospinal fluid – it has a limited capacity. After the fontanelles close, there is no room for additional, space-occupying masses.

In general, the signs and symptoms of a brain tumor depend on the patient's age; the tumor's location, rate of growth, invasion and compression of cerebral tissue and blood vessels; and the presence and extent of edema and increased intracranial pressure.

Headache, seizures, sensorimotor deficits and behavioral changes are the most common presenting manifestations of brain tumors. However, the tumor headache may be difficult to distinguish from benign headaches. Any patient who develops a new headache type should be carefully examined and a computed tomographic (CT) or magnetic resonance imaging (MRI) scan should be obtained if an intracranial mass is suspected. Danger signs of a brain tumor headache are awakening from sleep in the middle of the night or morning with the headache, exacerbation with positional changes or Valsava maneuver, and consistent localization of the head pain.

Approximately one-third of patients with brain tumors develop seizures. These are focal seizures, but they often generalize secondarily to tonic–clonic convulsions without any reported aura. Frontal and temporal tumors are most likely to present with seizures.

Somatosensory, visual and motor deficits are common in patients with tumors. These deficits typically develop and progress slowly, and the involved cerebral area does not conform to vascular distributions. However, 5 to 15 percent of patients with brain tumors present acute apoplectic or transient signs and symptoms, and may be misdiagnosed with a stroke (Groch *et al.*, 1960; Weisberg and Nice, 1977; Ross, 1983). Furthermore, strokes may present with slowly progressive symptoms (Clarke and Harris, 1958; Carter, 1960; Fisher and Pearlman, 1967; Melamed *et al.*, 1975).

Behavioral changes are perhaps the most common and most subtle effects of cerebral tumors. Because brain tumors cause behavioral changes through direct and remote effects, any neurobehavioral disorder may result from brain tumors. Family members and employers may report a loss of spontaneity, initiative and motivation, overall slowing of behavior (psychomotor retardation), 'mental dullness', forgetfulness, difficulty in finding names (anomia), uncharacteristic depression, irritability or moodiness, and a deterioration in social graces. Lethargy and confusion are also common features of brain tumors. There are no pathognomic behavioral features of brain tumors, but whenever a change in behavior is associated with a new headache disorder, a brain tumor should be considered.

Brain tumors are classified by their histology and location. Pituitary adenomas, meningiomas, craniopharyngiomas and pinealomas are among the most common 'benign' brain tumors.

Pituitary adenomas often cause behavioral effects through their hormonal products (e.g. ACTH – Cushing's disease; prolactin – amenorrhea, impotence) but when they extend beyond the sella turcica, they may compress the optic chiasm, hypothalamus and medial temporal lobes.

Meningiomas usually arise from the arachnoid layer of the meninges (i.e. intracranial but outside the cerebrum) and compress the brain without invading. Rarely, meningiomas are found within the cerebral ventricles.

Craniopharyngiomas are congenital tumors that usually develop from cell rests above the sella turcica. These tumors typically present in childhood with compression of the hypothalamus, pituitary and visual pathways, and often cause increased intracranial pressure and headache (Hoff and Patterson, 1972). Presenting symptoms include mental changes in more than a third of cases (Petito *et al.*, 1976). Computed tomography almost always shows calcium, while MRI scans most clearly demonstrate the tumor mass.

Pinealomas produce symptoms by compressing adjacent structures. When such pressure affects the midbrain tectum, it causes paresis of upgaze and impairment of convergence and the pupillary light reflex (Parinaud's syndrome); when the hypothalamus is involved, precocious puberty and labile emotions may result; obliteration of the cerebral aqueduct can occur and causes hydrocephalus (Donat *et al.*, 1978; Jooma and Kendall, 1983).

The most common malignant brain tumors are gliomas and metastases. *Astrocytomas* are the most common glioma. Low-grade ('benign') astrocytomas often evolve into anaplastic astrocytomas and glioblastomas multiforme (Shapiro, 1982; Laws *et al.*, 1984). *Oligodendrogliomas* are slow-growing tumors that often contain calcium and typically present with headache or seizures (Weir and Elvidge, 1968; Ludwig *et al.*, 1986). Personality changes, dementia and psychosis may develop in patients with oligodendrogliomas. Gliomas are intracerebral and usually infiltrate well beyond the area of abnormal brain visualized by the surgeon or neuroimaging study. *Metastases* are usually well-circumscribed, but are often multifocal (Posner and Chernik, 1978; Cairncross and Posner, 1983).

The location of brain tumors frequently plays a critical role in patient symptoms.

Frontal tumors cause contralateral hemiparesis, focal and generalized seizures, personality cognitive and emotional changes (Chapter 8), and – when located in the dominant hemisphere – non-fluent aphasia. Midline frontal tumors cause prominent disinhibition, abulia and depression, as well as incontinence, ataxia, and gegenhalten (paratonic rigidity). Subfrontal tumors may compress the olfactory nerve to cause unilateral anosmia.

Temporal tumors, like frontal tumors, often present with focal and secondarily generalized seizures, and personality and emotional changes. Temporal lobe seizures produce an astounding array of symptoms: olfactory (usually an unpleasant smell), gustatory, auditory, visual or vertiginous hallucinations and illusions, as well as autonomic and psychic (e.g. dreamy state, *déjà vu*, depersonalization) symptoms. Temporal lobe tumors may also cause a contralateral superior quadrantanopsia, amnesia and – when in the dominant hemisphere – fluent aphasia. In addition, patients with temporal tumors may develop psychosis (Malamud, 1967).

Sensory symptoms are the most prominent features of *parietal tumors*. Impaired sensation mainly affects higher, discriminatory functions such as two-point discrimination and position sensation, while pain and temperature sensation are usually unaffected. Tactile hallucinations from focal sensory seizures are common. Dominant parietal tumors cause non-fluent aphasia, apraxia and features of Gerstmann's syndrome (Maxim 64). Nondominant parietal tumors cause contralateral neglect, dressing apraxia, topographic disorientation and impairment of visuospatial functions (Maxim 63).

Occipital tumors produce visual changes: quadrantaopsia, hemisanopsia, hallucinations and illusions. Visual hallucinations resulting from occipital tumors are likely to be unformed, while those with temporal tumors are more often formed (Maxim 45).

Striatal and diencephalic tumors cause complex disorders of movement (e.g. dystonia, tremor, alterations in tone) and behavior (e.g. sleepiness, emotionality, depression, contralateral neglect) (Cairns, 1952; Arseni, 1958; McKissock and Paine, 1958; Cheek and Taveras, 1966; Hirose *et al.*, 1975; Bernstein *et al.*, 1984).

Hypothalamic tumors can produce polarized behavioral symptoms: hyperphagia or anorexia, compulsive or no fluid intake, aggression and agitiation or abulia. These tumors also cause profound hormonal changes, memory impairment, precocious puberty and gelastic (laughing) seizures (Lascelles and Lewis, 1972; Berkovic *et al.*, 1988).

From the previous discussion, one might anticipate that the neuroanatomy of the tumor site could be accurately predicted from a detailed neurological history and examination. Unfortunately, attempts at precise localization usually fail, because remote effects of brain tumors become interlaced with local effects. Although compression, shift of the midline, increased intracranial pressure and edema are the most obvious causes of contralateral or remote symptoms, there are other cases in which these factors are absent and localization remains poor. For example, anomia is a classic false-localizing sign that occurs with both right frontal and left temporoparietal tumors. Other classic false-localizing signs such as sixth and third nerve palsies, ipsilateral hemiparesis (compression of the opposite cerebral peduncle against the tentorium), bilateral increased deep tendon reflexes and extensor plantar responses, and 'hypopituitarism', usually result from increased intracranial pressure, hydrocephalus or herniation.

References

Arseni C. Tumors of the basal ganglia. Their surgical treatment. *Arch Neurol Psychiat* 1958; **80**: 18–24.

Berkovic SF, Andermann F, Melanson D, Ethier RE, Feindel W, Gloor P. Hypothalamic hamartomas and ictal laughter. *Ann Neurol* 1988; **23**: 429–39.

Bernstein M, Hoffman HJ, Halliday WC, Hendrick B, Humphreys RP. Thalamic tumors in children: Long-term follow-up and treatment guidelines. *J Neurosurg* 1984; **61**: 649–56.

Cairncross JG, Posner JB. The management of brain metastases. In: *Oncology of the Nervous System* (Walker MD, ed.). Boston, MA: Martinus Nijhoff Publishers, 1983, pp. 341–77.

Cairns H. Disturbances of consciousness with lesions of the brainstem and diencephalon. *Brain* 1952; **75**: 110–45.

Carter AB. Ingravescent cerebral infarction. *Q J Med* 1960; **29**: 611–25.

Cheek WR, Taveras JM. Thalamic tumors. *J Neurosurg* 1966; **24**: 505–13.

Clarke E, Harris P. Thrombosis of the internal carotid artery simulating an intracranial space occupying lesion. *Lancet* 1958; **i**: 1085–9.

Donat JF, Okaxaki H, Gomez MR, Reagan TJ, Baker HL, Laws ER. Pineal tumors: A 53-year experience. *Arch Neurol* 1978; **35**: 736–40.

Fisher CM, Pearlman A. The non-sudden onset of cerebral embolism. *Neurology* 1967; **17**: 1025–32.

Groch SN, Hurwitz LJ, Wright IS. Intracranial lesions simulating cerebral thrombosis. *JAMA* 1960; **172**: 1469–72.

Hirose G, Lombroso CT, Eisenberg H. Thalamic tumors in childhood: Clinical, laboratory, and therapeutic considerations. *Arch Neurol* 1975; **32**: 740–4.

Hoff JT, Patterson RH. Craniopharyngiomas in children and adults. *J Neurosurg* 1972; **36**: 299–302.

Jooma R, Kendall BE. Diagnosis and management of pineal tumors. *J Neurosurg* 1983; **58**: 654–65.

Lascelles PT, Lewis PD. Hypopdipsia and hypernatraemia associated with hypothalamic and suprasellar lesions. *Brain* 1972; **95**: 249–64.

Laws ER, Taylor WF, Clifton MB, Okazaki H. Neurosurgical management of low-grade astrocytoma of the cerebral hemispheres. *J Neurosurg* 1984; **61**: 665–73.

Ludwig CL, Smith MT, Godfrey AD, Armbrustmacher VW. A clinicopathological study of 323 patients with oligodendrogliomas. *Ann Neurol* 1986; **19**: 15–21.

Malamud N. Psychiatric disorder with intracranial tumors of the limbic system. *Arch Neurol* 1967; **17**: 113–23.

McKissock W, Paine KWE. Primary tumours of the thalamus. *Brain* 1958; **81**: 41–63.

Melamed E, Lavy S, Reches A *et al.* Chronic subdural hematoma simulating transient cerebral ischemic attacks. *J Neurosurg* 1975; **42**: 101–3.

Petito CK, DeGirolami U, Earle KM. Craniopharyngiomas: A clinical and pathological review. *Cancer* 1976; **37**: 1944–52.

Posner JB, Chernik NL. Intracranial metastases from systemic cancer. *Adv Neurol* 1978; **19**: 579–92.

Ross RT. Transient tumor attacks. *Arch Neurol* 1983; **40**: 633–6.

Shapiro WR. Treatment of neuroectodermal brain tumors. *Ann Neurol* 1982; **12**: 231–7.

Weir B, Elvidge AR. Oligodendrogliomas: An analysis of 63 cases. *J Neurosurg* 1968; **29**: 500–5.

Weisberg LA, Nice CN. Intracranial tumors simulating the presentation of cerebrovascular syndromes. *Am J Med* 1977; **63**: 517–24.

12
Head Trauma

69. *The severity of head injury can be estimated by the duration of post-traumatic amnesia*

The duration of post-traumatic amnesia is defined by the interval between injury and recovery of continuous memory function (Russell, 1932). This interval begins with the period of unconsciousness and delirium and extends until such time that the patient can once again store and retrieve new information in long-term memory (Symonds and Russell, 1943). Most patients are able to identify the time that normal continuous memory recovered, although corroboration from medical staff or family is often helpful (Schachter and Crovitz, 1977). While post-traumatic amnesia often follows brief loss of consciousness and confusion, it may also be the only sequelae of head trauma. For example, football players may suffer a blow to the head and continue the game with near-normal performance, but be unable to recall any part of the game that followed the blow.

Retrograde amnesia is the inability to retrieve memories of events experienced prior to head injury (Squire *et al.*, 1975). In general, retrograde amnesia is briefer and easier to quantify than post-traumatic amnesia. Malingerers often exaggerate the severity of their injury by describing events surrounding the impact with embellishment. However, truly injured patients with moderate-to-severe head trauma usually cannot recall the impact because of retrograde amnesia. Because the effects of retrograde amnesia tend to shrink over time, re-questioning the patient about the accident may provide new information. Prolonged retrograde amnesia, lasting more than 12 hours, that follows minor head injury suggests psychogenic factors. In most cases, however, emotional factors related to the accident do not contribute to retrograde amnesia, as demonstrated by thiopental interview (Russell and Nathan, 1946).

Although the duration of lost consciousness, confusion and post-traumatic amnesia all correlate with severity of injury, the post-traumatic amnesia is less likely to be influenced by secondary complications and is, therefore, a more reliable indicator of injury severity. The duration of post-traumatic amnesia correlates with neurological sequelae, including weakness, aphasia, epilepsy, chronic memory and intellectual impairment;

psychiatric sequelae, such as personality changes, disinhibition, euphoria or impaired judgment; and time until the patient returns to work (Russell and Smith, 1961; Smith, 1961; Jennett, 1962; Lishman, 1968; Steadman and Graham, 1970). Lishman (1978) estimated that when post-traumatic amnesia is less than one hour, return to work is within a month; with amnesia less than a day, return to work is within two months; with amnesia less than a week, return to work is within four months; and with post-traumatic amnesia longer than a week, return to work may be delayed for a year or more. The correlation between duration of post-traumatic amnesia and severity of intellectual and psychiatric disability is valid for both closed head trauma and penetrating wounds to the head (Lishman, 1968; Salazar *et al.*, 1986).

References

Jennett WB. *Epilepsy after Blunt Head Injuries*. Oxford: Heinemann Medical Books, 1962.

Lishman WA. Brain damage in relation to psychiatric disability after head injury. *Br J Psychiat* 1968; **114**: 373–410.

Russell WR. Cerebral involvement in head injury. *Brain* 1932; **55**: 549–603.

Russell WR, Nathan PW. Traumatic amnesia. *Brain* 1946; **69**: 280–300.

Russell WR, Smith A. Post-traumatic amnesia in closed head injury. *Arch Neurol* 1961; **5**: 4–17.

Salazar AM, Grafman JH, Vance SC, Weingartner H, Dillon JD, Ludlow CL. Consciousness and amnesia after penetrating head injury: neurology and anatomy. *Neurology* 1986; **36**: 178–87.

Schachter DL, Crovitz HF. Memory function after closed head injury: A review of the quantitative research. *Cortex* 1977; **13**: 150–76.

Smith A. Duration of impaired consciousness as an index of severity in closed head injuries: a review. *Dis Nerv Syst* 1961; **22**: 69–74.

Squire LR, Slater PC, Chace PM. Retrograde amnesia. *Science* 1975; **187**: 77–9.

Steadman JH, Graham JG. Head injuries: an analysis and follow-up study. *Proc Roy Soc Med* 1970; **63**: 23–8.

Symonds CP, Russell WR. Accidental head injuries. *Lancet* 1943; **i**: 7–10.

70. *Long-term deficits following concussion can result from organic, psychogenic and medico–legal factors*

Concussion is an acceleration–deceleration head injury that causes transient impairment of consciousness but does not result in macroscopic brain damage. 'Minor' or 'mild' head injury is often used synonomously with concussion, but are even more vague descriptors. The Glasgow Coma Scale (Maxim 4) is useful in grading moderate and severe head injuries, but is less helpful in evaluating patients with concussive injuries. Although computed tomography of the brain and gross neuropathological examination show no abnormalities after concussive injuries, microscopic examination or magnetic resonance imaging may reveal structural damage, especially to the anterior frontal and temporal regions (Oppenheimer, 1968; Adams *et al.*, 1980, 1981; Gandy *et al.*, 1984). Approximately 3 percent of patients diagnosed with mild head injury have focal neurological findings on initial examination, and another 3 percent deteriorate neurologically (Fischer *et al.*, 1981; Rimel *et al.*, 1981; Coloban *et al.*, 1986; Dacey *et al.*, 1986).

The postconcussive syndrome includes a diverse spectrum of clinical features that are multifactorial in origin (Table 70.1). Headache, dizziness, memory problems, malaise, tinnitus and nausea are the most common complaints in adults, while withdrawal and such behavioral problems as aggression, sleep disturbances and enuresis predominate in children (Dillon and Leopold, 1961; Elia, 1972; Alves *et al.*, 1986). Various etiologic factors contribute to the development and persistence of disorders after head injury (Table 70.2). Advanced age and history of prior head injury are important factors that predispose to greater intellectual and psychiatric morbidity (Russell, 1932; Adler, 1945; Rutherford, 1989; Gronwall, 1989).

Impairment of attention, vigilance, information processing capacity and memory are hallmarks of mild head injury, but these problems usually resolve after days or weeks (Gronwall, 1989; Ruff *et al.*, 1989). Interestingly, patients often complain of greater memory impairment one month after injury than on initial evaluation, although neuropsychological testing reveals an early deficit that improves, with attainment of control values, within one month (Ruff *et al.*, 1989).

Table 70.1   Common postconcussive symptoms.

Somatic
Headache
Dizziness
Vertigo
Blurred vision
Insomnia
Fatigability .
Noise sensitivity
Impaired taste/smell perception
Hallucinations
Cognitive impairment
Concentration
Recent memory
Remote memory
Thinking /planning
Affective
Irritability
Depression
Anxiety

Table 70.2   Factors related to behavioral disorders after head trauma.

Advanced age
Premorbid personality
Prior history of behavioral disorders
Family history of behavioral disorders
Supportive environment before and after injury
Emotional adjustment to injury
Injuries to loved ones during accident
Medical–legal compensation
Structural brain damage prior to injury
Area of brain injured
Extent of brain injury
Post-traumatic cognitive impairment
Post-traumatic epilepsy
Medications

Successful re-employment after head injury correlates with (1) consistent gainful employment prior to the trauma (i.e. ability, motivation and character); and (2) the presence of a spouse or 'significant other' that lives with the victim and helps support, guide and motivate.

The pathogenesis of the postconcussive syndrome remains hotly contested. The first point of contention pits those who champion organic causes against others who hold that the syndrome is purely psychogenic.

The repeated observation that postconcussive symptoms are more common after mild head trauma than in severe cases has led to the unscientific assumption that the complaints are entirely functional (Levin *et al.*, 1987). However, monozygotic and dizygotic twin studies in which only one twin was injured reveal that, although subtle intellectual deficits may result from mild head injury, many symptoms such as headache, dizziness and noise sensitivity may be more related to genetic constitution than the injury itself (Dencker, 1958, 1960). Family history of mental illness is associated with higher rates of psychiatric disability after head trauma (Symonds and Russell, 1943; Adler, 1945; Hillbom, 1960).

It is likely that both organic and psychogenic factors play varying roles depending on syndrome symptoms and stage of illness. For example, organic factors may predominate during the acute stage, accounting for stereotypical symptoms, such as headache and dizziness, and may later contribute to chronic disorders of attention and cognition. Psychogenic factors predominate during the chronic stage of the postconcussive syndrome, when neurotic and affective features such as anxiety, irritability, fatigability and sadness occur. Unfortunately, in some patients, depression develops when post-traumatic symptoms resolve (Merskey and Woodforde, 1972).

From a third perspective, some argue that greed is the most important factor in the postconcussive syndrome. But legal aspects of head injury are complex and often oversimplified. Once the issue of compensation is raised, the patient faces conflicting advice from family, friends and lawyers, and is subjected to both hostile and supportive medical reviews. Indeed, this process is often long and stressful.

It is probable that both conscious and unconscious factors related to compensation eventually color the clinical features. The low incidence of persistent problems following mild head injury that is sustained where compensation is not possible (e.g. home, sports) supports a contributing role by litigation (Miller, 1966, 1969). Also, the incidence of symptoms persisting one year after mild head injury is two to three times higher in patients with unsettled litigation (Rutherford, 1989). However, others have found no relation between post-traumatic symptoms and pending litigation (Merskey and Woodforde, 1972; McLean et al., 1984).

In the debate over the pathogenesis of postconcussive syndrome, organic, psychogenic and medico-legal factors are often presented as mutually exclusive bases. In reality, however, this syndrome is likely to result from the complex interaction of all three.

References

Adams JH, Graham DI, Murray LS, Scott G. Diffuse axonal injury due to nonmissile head injury in humans: An analysis of 45 cases. Ann Neurol 1981; 12: 557–63.

Adams JH, Graham DI, Scott G. Brain damage in fatal non-missile head injury. J Clin Pathol 1980; 33: 1132–45.

Adler A. Mental symptoms following head injury. Arch Neurol Psychiat 1945; 53: 34–43.

Alves WM, Coloban ART, O'Leary TJ, Rimel RW, Jane JA. Understanding post-traumatic symptoms after minor head injury. J Head Trauma Rehab 1986; 1: 1–12.

Coloban ART, Dacey RG, Alves W, Rimel RW, Jane JA. Neurologic and neurosurgical implications of mild head injury. J Head Trauma Rehab 1986; 1: 13–21.

Dacey RG, Alves WM, Rimel RW et al. Neurosurgical complications after apparently minor head injury. J Neurosurg 1986; 65: 203–10.

Dencker SJ. A follow-up study of 128 closed head injuries in twins using co-twins as controls. Acta Psychiat Neurol Scand 1958; 1–50 (Suppl 122).

Dencker SJ. Closed head injury in twins. Arch Gen Psychiat 1960; 2: 569–75.

Dillon H, Leopold RL. Children and the post-concussive syndrome. JAMA 1961; 14: 175–86.

Elia JC. The postconcussive syndrome. Indust Med 1972; 41: 23–31.

Fischer RP, Carlson J, Perry JF. Postconcussive hospital observation of alert patients in a primary trauma center. J Trauma 1981; 21: 920–4.

Gandy SE, Snow RB, Zimmerman RD, Deck MDF. Cranial nuclear magnetic resonance imaging in head trauma. Ann Neurol 1984; 16: 254–7.

Gronwall D. Cumulative and persisting effects of concussion on attention and cognition. In: Mild Head Injury (Levin HS, Eisenberg HM, Benton AL, eds). Oxford, New York: Oxford University Press, 1989, pp. 153–62.

Hillbom E. After-effects of brain-injuries. Acta Psychiatr Neurol Scand 1960: 1–195. (suppl 142).

Levin HS, Mattis S, Ruff RM et al. Neurobehavioral outcome following minor head injury. J Neurosurg 1987; 66: 234–43.

McLean A, Dikmen S, Temkin N, Wyler AR, Gale JL. Psychosocial functioning at one month after head injury. Neurosurgery 1984; 14: 393–9.

Merskey H, Woodforde JM. Psychiatric sequelae of minor head injury. *Brain* 1972; **95**: 521–8.

Miller H. Mental sequelae of head injury. *Proc Roy Soc Med* 1966; **39**: 257–61.

Miller H. Problems of medicolegal practice. In: *The Late Effects of Head Injury* (Walker AE, Caveness WF, Critchley M, eds). Springfield, IL: Charles C Thomas, 1969.

Oppenheimer DR. Microscopic lesions in the brain following head injury. *J Neurol Neurosurg Psychiat* 1968; **31**: 299–306.

Rimel RW, Giordani B, Barth JT, Boll TJ, Jane JA. Disability caused by minor head injury. *Neurosurg* 1981; **9**: 221–8.

Ruff RM, Levin HS, Mattis S, High WM, Marshall LF, Eisenberg HM, Tabaddor K. Recovery of memory after mild head injury: A three center study. In: *Mild Head Injury* (Levin HS, Eisenberg HM, Benton AL, eds). Oxford, New York: Oxford University Press, 1989, pp. 176–88.

Russell RWR. Cerebral involvement in head injury. *Brain* 1932; **55**: 549–603.

Rutherford WH. Postconcussive symptoms: Relationship to acute neurological indicies, individual differences, and circumstances of injury. In: *Mild Head Injury* (Levin HS, Eisenberg HM, Benton AL, eds). Oxford, New York: Oxford University Press, 1989, pp. 217–28.

Symonds CP, Russell WR. Accidental head injuries. *Lancet* 1943; **i**: 7–10.

71.   Post-traumatic psychiatric disorders result from organic, psychogenic and environmental factors

Behavioral consequences are among the most common and devastating effects of moderate-to-severe head trauma, but are difficult to quantify and treat. These disorders range from subtle personality changes to paranoid psychosis (Table 71.1). They may be detectable only to family members or immediately obvious to a stranger. Furthermore, the behavioral disorders may emerge or progress as the patient recovers motor and cognitive functions (Brooks and McKinlay, 1983; Fordyce *et al.*, 1983), and they frequently persist: one study found personality disorders in more than half of patients ten years after severe head trauma (Thomsen, 1984). The etiologic factors in post-traumatic behavioral disorders are summarized in Table 70.2.

Organic factors predominate when post-traumatic behavioral changes

Table 71.1   Psychiatric disorders after head trauma.

Personality change
Irritability–Aggressivity
Depression
Mania
Neurosis
Chronic postconcussive symptoms
Paranoia
Psychosis

develop. The frontal and temporal lobes are often injured by head trauma. Personality changes are most prominent after frontal injury and include lack of foresight and concern; loss of initative, spontaneity and social graces; disinhibition of sexual and aggressive impulses; inability to plan and judge; and affective lability (Chapter 8). Temporal lobe injury impairs memory as well as emotional control, and it can trigger depression, mania and psychosis (Chapter 9) (Lishman, 1968). Epilepsy may develop after frontal or temporal lobe injury and contribute to overall psychiatric morbidity (Hillbom, 1960; Levine and Finkelstein, 1982). In addition, hypothalamic and basal forebrain injury may disrupt control over emotions, spontaneity, motivation and drive-related (e.g. sexual and aggressive) behaviors and impair memory.

Irritability is common after head trauma and results mainly from frontal and temporal dysfunction. Patients are often placid in the hospital setting but when they return home, stressors (e.g. children, finances) unmask their impatience and temper. Family counseling, treatment of associated depression, or use of beta-blockers may be helpful.

Aggression following severe head trauma is not rare. It may occur with frontal, temporal or hypothalamic injury. Aggressive episodes are frequently explosive and are commonly precipitated by minor provocation or alcohol (Hooper et al., 1945). Important risk factors for aggression can include psychosocial adjustment, living environment following trauma and, less often, the premorbid personality.

Post-traumatic affective disorders are common and result from both organic and psychogenic factors. Depression is common after moderate-to-severe head trauma, affecting more than half of patients (McKinlay et al., 1981), while psychotic depression is rare (Parker, 1957; Lishman, 1987). Suicide is markedly increased after head injury, accounting for up to 14 percent of deaths (Lishman, 1987). Mania is less common than depression and may alternate with depression or occur in isolation. Manic episodes are characterized by irritable mood (rather than euphoria) and by assaultiveness (Shukla et al., 1987). Post-traumatic epilepsy may predispose to mania: while post-traumatic epilepsy develops in only 5 percent of patients after blunt head trauma,[1] 50 percent of those with mania also develop seizures (Jennett, 1962; Shukla et al., 1987).

Medications are the most overlooked organic cause of behavioral problems after head injury. Patients are often started on antihypertensive, antiepileptic, antianxiety, hypnotic or other drugs after hospitalization. The head-injured patient, like the elderly patient, is much more sensitive to the behavioral side effects of drugs. The following case illustrates this point:

> A 52-year-old woman was mugged and sustained severe head trauma. After a week-long coma and extensive rehabilitation, she was discharged from the rehabilitation center, nine months after injury. Eighteen months after injury,

---

[1] Post-traumatic epilepsy occurs in more than 30 percent of patients when the dura mater has been penetrated.

she was referred for evaluation because of episodic loss of consciousness. She was on carbamazepine 1300 mg/day (serum level 9 μ/ml) which had been progressively increased as episodes recurred. Her family complained she was no longer the same person as before the mugging. She was mentally slow, lethargic and slept 12–14 hours per day; her speech was slurred, and her short-term memory was markedly impaired. Although prolonged EEG recordings demonstrated no epileptiform activity, the history suggested post-traumatic epilepsy. She was tapered off of carbamazepine, and valproic acid was gradually increased to a dose of 1250 mg/day (level 70 μ/ml). She reawakened to her former self – many of her post-trauma cognitive and behavioral symptoms resolved and all were markedly improved. She has resumed her previous, stressful and demanding job as the senior accountant in a thriving a small business.

The message is not that carbamazepine is toxic. Rather, any drug given in the post-trauma setting has the potential for significant toxicity, even when blood levels fall in the so-called therapeutic range.

Psychogenic factors play a major role in the development of post-traumatic neurotic and anxiety disorders. These disorders may be severe, and they reflect a combination of constitutional factors, including premorbid personality, emotional reaction to injury and environment. In most cases, organic factors are less important. Post-traumatic anxiety and panic disorders are frequently confused with ictal fear episodes. However, psychogenic fear episodes are usually more prolonged, lasting more than five minutes, while ictal episodes typically end in less than three minutes. In addition, psychogenic episodes are not associated with episodic impairment of consciousness.

Psychogenic factors are also a major cause of post-traumatic depression. Patients react to their motor, cognitive and social losses with feelings of helplessness, hopelessness and worthlessness, withdrawing from their family and their passions. This reactive depression may be exacerbated by organic factors. As with all post-traumatic behavioral disorders, a multidisciplinary team approach – including psychiatrists, neurologists, therapists, nurses and social workers – is critical to identifying the relevant pathogenic factors.

The postconcussive syndrome is a complex disorder, in which neurophysiologic abnormalities predominate during the acute stage and psychogenic factors are important in 'maintaining' symptoms (Maxim 70). The most common symptoms are headache, dizziness, difficulty concentrating, emotional lability and sleepiness.

Premorbid personality has been alleged to determine the presence or form of post-traumatic behavioral disorders, but this connection has not been clearly demonstrated. Lishman (1987) found an association between emotional instability prior to head injury and development of post-traumatic psychiatric disorders. However, other investigators have found no relationship between premorbid personality and post-traumatic behavioral disorders (Rimel *et al.*, 1981; Barth *et al.*, 1983). In many cases, especially those with frontal or temporal lobe lesions, behavior is diametrically opposed to the pretrauma baseline (Harlow, 1868; Tobias, 1982).

Environmental stress is a major hurdle after head trauma. The real problems often begin when the patient is discharged home from the hospital or rehabilitation center (Thomsen, 1974). The structured and supportive environment, which placed so few demands, is replaced by cold reality. A deluge of what should be trivial stressors – children shouting at each other, the telephone ringing, inability to find a needed item quickly – can become overwhelming. These minor stresses are often accompanied by more significant ones such as loss of work, financial troubles, a family member's illness, new-found dependency, and adjustment to physical and emotional sequelae of the head trauma. The interaction of organic behavioral disorders and environmental stress can be devastating.

In the struggle to withstand and cope with this barrage of stressors, the relationships the patient shares with others – spouses and other close family members, friends and coworkers – are critical (Rosin, 1977). The family members must recognize the patient's problems as organic; it is essential that support is not withdrawn. Yet family members frequently have trouble coping with the 'new' person. The emotional and personality changes may allow spouses to feel 'that this is not the same person as before the injury, not the person I made my vows to'. There is an emotional collage of resentment, guilt, horror, loss and denial that all too often culminates in withdrawal and disengagement from the victim. This reaction from family members may, in turn, foment paranoia, dependency and depression in the patient. Family therapy is often extremely helpful in avoiding or reducing such consequences, which can devastate the victim of head trauma and those who are close to him.

References

Barth JT, Macciocchi SN, Giordani B, Rimel RW, Jane JA. Neuropsychological sequelae of minor head injury. *Neurosurgery* 1983; **13**: 529–33.

Brooks DN, McKinlay W. Personality and behavioral changes after severe blunt head injury – A relative's view. *J Neurol Neurosurg Psychiat* 1983; **46**: 336–44.

Fordyce DJ, Roueche JR, Prigitano GP. Enhanced emotional reactions in chronic head trauma patients. *J Neurol Neursurg Psychiat* 1983; **46**: 620–4.

Harlow J. Recovery from passage of an iron bar through the head. *Publ Mass Med Soc* 1868; **2**: 327–46.

Hillbom E. After-effects of brain-injuries. *Acta Psychiat Neurol Scand* 1960; 1–195 (Suppl 142).

Hooper RS, McGregor JM, Nathan PW. Explosive rage following head injury. *J Ment Sci* 1945; **91**: 458–71.

Jennett WB. Epilepsy after blunt head injuries. Oxford: Heinemann Medical Books, 1962.

Levine DN, Finkelstein S. Delayed psychosis after right temporoparietal stroke or trauma. *Neurology* 1982; **32**: 267–73.

Lishman WA. Brain damage in relation to psychiatric disability after head injury. *Br J Psychiat* 1968; **114**: 373–410.

Lishman WA. *Organic Psychiatry* (3rd edition). Oxford: Blackwell Scientific Publications, 1987, pp. 137–86.

McKinlay WW, Brooks DN, Bond MR, Martinage DP, Marshall MM. The short-term outcome of severe blunt head injury as reported by relatives of the injured person. *J Neurol Neurosurg Psychiat* 1981; **44**: 527–33.

Parker N. Manic-depressive psychosis following head injury. *Med J Aust* 1957; **2**: 20–2.

Rimel RW, Tiordani B, Barth JT, Boll TJ, Jane JA. Disability caused by minor head injury. *Neurosurgery* 1981; **9**: 221–8.

Rosin AJ. Reactions of families of brain-injured patients who remain in a vegetative state. *Scand J Rehab Med* 1977; **9**: 1–5.

Shukla S, Cook BL, Mukherjee S, Goodwin C, Miller MG. Mania following head trauma. *Am J Psychiat* 1987; **144**: 93–6.

Thomsen IV. Late outcome of very severe blunt head trauma: a 10–15 year second follow-up. *J Neurol Neurosurg Psychiat* 1984; **47**: 260–8.

Thomsen 1. The patient with severe head injury and his family. *Scand J Rehab Med* 1974; **6**: 180–3.

Tobias JS, Puria KB, Sheridan J. Rehabilitation of the severely brain-injured. *Scand J Rehab Med* 1982; **14**: 83–8.

72. The temporal tips and orbitofrontal areas are often contused in moderate-to-severe head trauma

Contusion is the most characteristic lesion after brain trauma. As with bruises in other parts of the body, mild acute cerebral contusion is associated with leakage of erythrocytes around small vessels. In more severe contusions, there is often gross intraparenchymal hemorrhage, edema, disruption of the *pia mater*, and subarachnoid, subdural or epidural hemorrhage. Contusions immediately beneath an area of head trauma are *coup contusions*. Those roughly opposite the site of direct trauma are *contre-coup contusions*. Other forms of contusion include (1) herniation, which usually results when structures shift intracranial compartments; for example, when the amygdala and hippocampus are bruised against firm tentorium as they are displaced from the middle to the posterior cranial fossa (i.e. uncal herniation); (2) gliding, which is most often seen along the superomedial surfaces of the frontal and parietal lobes; and (3) fracture, which, as the name suggests, is found beneath fractures. In addition to contusion, cerebral injury can also occur with sudden rotation of the head (and brain) (Table 72.1).

Figure 72.1 shows the sites with predilection for cerebral contusion. In general, contusions are most likely to occur at the crowns of gyri and at cerebral surfaces adjacent to bony ridges and firm dural membranes. Common sites include the temporal tips, orbitofrontal regions, medial cerebral hemispheres, the occipital pole and brainstem. The temporal tips and orbitofrontal areas are often contused irrespective of where the head was struck (Adams *et al.*, 1980).

Table 72.1 Mechanisms of neural injury in head trauma.

Mechanism	Features
Skull fracture	
Linear fracture	Cranial nerve injuries
	Epidural hematoma
Basilar fractures	Often difficult to detect
	Cranial nerve injuries*
	Pituitary insufficiency
	CSF leak
Depressed fracture	Focal injury
	Intracranial hematoma
	Meningitis
	Post-traumatic epilepsy
Hematoma	Occur with or without skull fracture
	Epidural, subdural, intracerebral – all may occur acutely or be delayed
Herniation	Usually due to hematomas and edema
	Subfalcian (cingulate), tentorial (uncal), central, and tonsillar forms
Contusion	Coup injury: bruise of brain underlying direct trauma
	Contrecoup injury: bruise of contralateral brain near bony prominences
Rotation–shearing injuries	Neocortical, subcortical, and brainstem damage
	Arterial and venous tears
	Diffuse axonal injury
Edema	Focal or diffuse
Hypoxic–ischemic injury	Results from elevated intracranial pressure and disruption of autoregulation

*Anosmia is common and is associated with damage to the cribiform plate and CSF leaks.

During the acute stage, cerebral contusions are almost always accompanied by cerebral edema. The edema may be maximal in an area of focal injury, multifocal or diffuse. Contusions, hemorrhages, localized and diffuse edema, and herniation contribute to early fatalities after head trauma. Osmotic agents (e.g. mannitol) and glucocorticoids are effective in reducing brain water content and edema to lower intracranial pressure.

In acute head trauma, recognition of contusion, intracranial hemorrhage and edema is critical for appropriate neurological and neurosurgical management. Computed tomography (CT) of the brain has replaced skull X-ray films and angiography as the imaging method of choice. Computed tomography is effective in identifying small intraparenchymal and moderate subdural hematomas and cerebral edema. Furthermore, CT is readily available and can be easily performed on seriously ill patients. Magnetic reso-

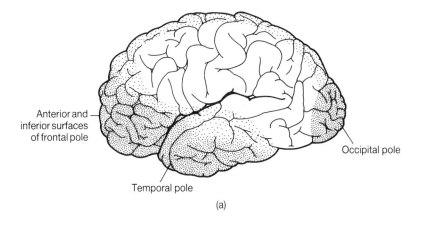

Anterior and
inferior surfaces
of frontal pole

Occipital pole

Temporal pole

(a)

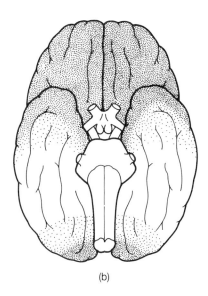

(b)

Fig. 72.1   Areas of the brain susceptible to injury. (a) Lateral view (b) Inferior
view

nance imaging (MRI) with T2-weighted images (proton density with
spin-spin; longer repetition time and echo delay) is more sensitive than
CT in detecting non-hemorrhagic contusions, edema and small subdural
hematomas (Gandy *et al.*, 1984). However, MRI may be less sensitive in
identifying small intracerebral bleeds and is much more difficult to obtain
than a CT while the patient is in the emergency room. Thus, while head
CT remains the imaging method of choice in acute head trauma, the lesions

seen on MRI scans may be helpful in defining the extent of injury and predicting subsequent cognitive deficits and behavioral disorders.

As cerebral contusions heal, erythrocytic and parenchymal debris is removed and the lesion organizes, forming a connective tissue and glial scar with meningeal discoloration and adhesions and demyelination of underlying white matter (Escourolle and Poirer, 1978). The shrunken area of scar tissue is often a focus for post-traumatic seizures.

References

Adams JH, Graham DI, Scott G. Brain damage in fatal non-missile head injury. *J Clin Pathol* 1980; **33**: 1132–45.

Escourolle R, Poirier J. Manual of Basic Neuropathology. (Rubinstein J, Translator). WB Saunders, Philadelphia, 1978.

Gandy SE, Snow RB, Zimmerman RD, Deck MDF. Cranial nuclear magnetic resonance imaging in head trauma. *Ann Neurol* 1984; **16**: 254–7.

73.   *Neurobehavioral complications of severe head trauma must be managed through a multidisciplinary approach*

The evaluation and treatment of head injury cannot be achieved by a single physician in isolation. There is a tendency to focus on those aspects of a case that are most comfortable. A neurologist will see the hemiparesis, but may miss the depression and marital conflicts that are tormenting the patient. Furthermore, severe head trauma alters mental function in ways that straddle the traditional boundaries between health care workers. Patients with severe head trauma should be treated by a team that includes neurologists, psychiatrists, neuropsychologists, rehabilitation physicians, physical therapists, occupational therapists, speech therapists, vocational counselors, nurses and social workers. The complete clinical picture may emerge clearly only after the input of all the parties is received.

The long-term sequelae of head trauma are determined by the presence of structural and psychological factors. Unfortunately, only gross lesions are visualized with existing neuroimaging methods and many neuropathological changes are only seen at the microscopic level. Physiological abnormalities that impair behavioral function may exist, undetected by current tools.

Language and motor deficits are the most obvious neurological deficits and quickly become the focus of attention, although other deficits may, in fact, cause comparable functional disability. Following bifrontal injury, for example, patients may have numerous disorders – including impulsivity, impaired judgment and planning, and loss of motivation and social graces – without motor, sensory or language deficits. Therefore, the neurobehavioral evaluation must be comprehensive and address psychosocial, as well as neurological and psychiatric disorders (Levin *et al.*, 1982). Depression is common after severe head injury and often results from a combination of psychosocial and organic factors. Depressed patients often require both antidepressant medications and psychotherapy.

During both the initial rehabilitation and long-term treatment phases, the team must focus on specific goals.

The rehabilitation process begins during the acute stage, even if the patient is unconscious. A passive range of motion exercises and, if possible, changes in body position on a tilt table or hospital bed to stimulate postural reflexes should be started early (Najenson *et al.*, 1974). As the patient awakens, he should be encouraged by the physical therapist to begin functional movements; splints or braces may be helpful. Early neuro-behavioral disorders include confusion, agitation and psychosis. Sedative or tranquilizing drugs may be needed to prevent self-injury. Many acute psychiatric disorders are best managed with an environment that is sup-portive and calm. The patient should be protected against extraneous noises and stimuli, and reorientation can be facilitated with a clock and calendar. Family and friends should be encouraged to visit frequently, thereby providing security and comfort. However, relatives may be pro-vocative and stress the patient; the rehabilitation team must be sensitive to this possibility.

The rehabilitation program is ultimately directed towards allowing the patient to return to a normal social and occupational level (Levin *et al.*, 1987). Patients benefit from individual psychotherapy supplemented by an environment that fosters a positive attitude and high self-esteem. Cognitive retraining (e.g. speech therapy and use of calculators) and vocational rehabilitation (e.g. work skills, social skills, manual tasks) help restore the patient to a more functional level. Group activities foster a supportive environment in which patients can share their frustrations, anxieties and accomplishments.

References

Levin HS, Benton AL, Grossmand RG. *Neurobehavioral Consequences of Closed Head Injury*. Oxford, New York: Oxford University Press, 1982.

Levin HS, Grafman J, Eisenberg HM. *Neurobehavioral Recovery from Head Injury*. Oxford, New York: Oxford University Press, 1987.

Najenson T, Mendelson L, Schechter I, Daviv C, Mintzaa N, Groswasser Z. Rehabilitation after severe head injury. *Scand J Rehab Med* 1974; **6**: 5–14.

13
Epilepsy

74. Most patients with epilepsy do not have psychiatric disorders

Throughout history, patients with epilepsy have had an undeservedly bad reputation based on lay fears and superstitions and, in part, on medical misinformation. In the 19th century, medical attention focused on those who were asylum-bound, leading to the misconception that psychopathology is ubiquitous among patients with epilepsy. This unfortunate generalization persisted. Sjobring (1944) opined that 'a mental change of a specific nature takes place in individuals suffering from epileptic seizures. They become torpid and circumstantial, "sticky" and adhesive, affectively tense and suffer from explosive outbursts of rage and anxiety'. Kinnier Wilson (1940) took a more lenient view: 'on epileptic temperament, inordinate stress has been laid. Life is difficult for these patients, and much that is attributed to temperament can with greater reason be assigned to chronic invalidism and unlucky circumstance'.

Interictal behavior is a topic of heated controversy. Does epilepsy cause psychopathology? If so, how often, and what types of deviant behavior result? Are certain forms of epilepsy, especially temporal lobe epilepsy, more likely to be associated with psychopathology or personality changes? Is it the epilepsy that causes the psychopathology or the associated central nervous system lesions, medications or psychosocial hardships?

Lost in the controversies and methodologic debates is the fact that many patients with epilepsy undergo neither cognitive nor behavioral deterioration and that the majority of these patients do not have psychiatric illness. Nevertheless, cognitive and behavioral changes do occur in some patients. Denial of these changes in order to 'protect' epilepsy from stigma denies patients the opportunity for effective treatment.

Psychiatric disorders reported to have an increased incidence among epilepsy patients include schizophrenic-like psychosis, depression (Maxim 75), personality disorders (Maxim 76), bipolar disorder, dissociative disorders, anxiety disorders and aggressive behavior (Maxim 78). Evidence supporting an association between epilepsy and these behaviors varies, and each association must be critically examined.

Psychosis is more prevalent among patients with epilepsy, and schizoprenic-like psychosis may be overrepresented in patients with seizure foci in the temporal lobe (Slater *et al.*, 1963; Bruens, 1971; Perez and Trimble, 1980; Parnas *et al.*, 1982; Ramani and Gumnit, 1982). There are no controlled epidemiologic studies of prevalence rates for psychosis in epilepsy and the validity of this relationship has been questioned (Stevens, 1975). In both retrospective and prospective studies, however, the prevalence rates of psychosis are increased among epilepsy patients when compared with the general population and to patients with other neurological and medical illness (Slater *et al.*, 1963; Lindsay *et al.*, 1979; Perez and Trimble, 1980; Whitman *et al.*, 1984). This increased prevalence, together with the finding that psychosis typically occurs *after* epilepsy in the vast majority of those patients with both disorders, suggests that the association is more than coincidental. Risk factors for psychosis among epilepsy patients may include left temporal seizure focus (Flor-Henry, 1969; Taylor, 1975; Sherwin, 1981), bilateral seizure foci (Kristensen and Sindrup, 1978a, b, 1979), structural pathology, (Taylor, 1975; Jensen and Larsen, 1979), and left-handedness (Taylor, 1975; Kristensen and Sindrup, 1978a). In contrast to patients with 'functional psychoses', who often have blunted affect, epilepsy patients with psychosis are more emotional.

An antagonistic relationship between epilepsy and psychosis may exist in certain cases. Poorly controlled epidemiologic studies supporting an antagonism were the basis for von Meduna's (1938) use of pentylenetetrazol therapy for schizophrenia. Although Landolt (1958) later observed the phenomenon of 'forced normalization', in which the improvement of interictal epileptiform activity correlated with the initiation or exacerbation of psychosis,[1] medical or surgical control of seizures rarely precipitates psychosis (Flor-Henry, 1969; Bruens, 1971; Kristensen and Sindrup, 1978a, b; Jensen and Larsen, 1979). The inconsistencies and contradictions in the literature on epilepsy and psychosis await resolution.

The evidence linking epilepsy with bipolar, anxiety and dissociative disorders is less compelling still. Epilepsy may coexist with these and other psychiatric disorders, but the existence of a pathophysiological role for epilepsy remains uncertain. In selected cases, epilepsy probably contributes to both ictal and interictal behavioral features that are identical to those seen in functional psychiatric disease. For example, Hermann and Chhabria (1981) reported two patients with ictal fear and interictal fear-related behaviors and paranoia, whose interictal behavior improved with effective antiepileptic drugs.

Lability of mood occurs in some epileptic patients and can resemble bipolar disorder (Mayer-Gross *et al.*, 1968). Anxiety disorders are more common among patients with epilepsy, although additional studies are needed to define the nature of this relationship (Currie *et al.*, 1971; Taylor, 1972; Trimble and Perez, 1980; Betts, 1981; Perini and Mendius, 1984). In

---

[1] Forced normalization has been reported in patients with either primary generalized and partial seizure disorders

several of my patients with prominent generalized anxiety disorder, effective surgical therapy for intractable temporal lobe seizures led to a resolution of the anxiety. Dissociative states and hypomania occur during and after partial seizures, but their association with interictal periods is less certain (Kenna and Sedman, 1965; Hurwitz *et al.*, 1985; Gillig *et al.*, 1988; Devinsky *et al.*, 1989a, b).

References

Betts TA. Depression, anxiety and epilepsy. In *Epilepsy and Psychiatry* (Reynolds EH, Trimble MR, eds). Edinburgh: Churchill Livingstone, 1981, pp. 60–71.

Bruens JH. Psychoses in epilepsy. *Psychiat Neurol Neurochir* 1971; **74**: 175–92.

Currie S, Heathfield KWG, Henson RA, Scott DF. Clinical causes and prognosis of temporal lobe epilepsy: a survey of 666 patients. *Brain* 1971; **94**: 173–90.

Devinsky O, Feldmann E, Burrowes K, Bromfield E. Autoscopic phenomena with seizures. *Arch Neurol* 1989a; **46**: 1080–8.

Devinsky O, Putnam F, Bromfield E, Grafman J, Theodore WH. Dissociative states and epilepsy. *Neurology* 1989b; **39**: 835–40.

Flor-Henry P. Psychosis and temporal lobe epilepsy: A controlled investigation. *Epilepsia* 1969; **10**: 363–95.

Gillig P, Sackellares JC, Greenberg HS. Right hemisphere partial complex seizures: Mania, hallucinations, and speech disturbances during ictal events. *Epilepsia* 1988; **29**: 26–9.

Gundmunsson G. Epilepsy in Iceland. *Acta Neurol Scand* 1966; **13**: 1–124 (Suppl 25).

Hermann BP, Chhabria S. Interictal psychopathology in patients with ictal fear. *Arch Neurol* 1981; **37**: 667–8.

Hurwitz TA, Wada JA, Kosaka BD, Strauss EH. Cerebral organization of affect suggested by temporal lobe seizures. *Neurology* 1985; **35**: 1335–7.

Jensen I, Larsen JK. Psychoses in drug resistant temporal lobe epilepsy. *J Neurol Neurosurg Psychiat* 1979; **42**: 948–54.

Kenna JC, Sedman. Depersonalization in temporal lobe epilepsy and the organic psychoses. *Br J Psychiat* 1965; **111**: 293–9.

Kristensen O, Sindrup EH. Psychomotor epilepsy and psychosis. I. Physical aspects. *Acta Neurol Scand* 1978a; **57**: 361–9.

Kristensen O, Sindrup EH. Psychomotor epilepsy and psychosis. II. Electroencephalographic findings. *Acta Neurol Scand* 1978b; **57**: 370–9.

Kristensen O, Sindrup EH. Psychomotor epilepsy and psychosis. III. Social and psychological correlates. *Acta Neurol Scand* 1979; **59**: 1–9.

Landolt H. Serial electroencephalographic investigations during psychotic episodes in epileptic patients during schizophrenic attacks. In: *Lectures on Epilepsy* (Lorentz de Haas, ed.). New York: Elsevier, 1958, pp. 91–133.

Lindsay J, Ounsted C, Richards P. Long-term outcome in children with temporal lobe epilepsy: III. Psychiatric manifestations in adult life. *Dev Med Child Neurol* 1979; **21**: 630–6.

Mayer-Gross W, Slater E, Roth M. *Clinical Psychiatry*. Baltimore, MA: Williams & Wilkins 1968, p. 405.

Parnas J, Korsgaard S, Krautwald O, Jensen P. Chronic psychosis in epilepsy: A clinical investigation of 29 patients. *Acta Psychiatrica Scand* 1982; **66**: 282–93.

Perez MM, Trimble MR. Epileptic psychoses: Diagnostic comparisons with process schizophrenia. *Br J Psychiat* 1980; **137**: 245–9.

Perini G, Mendius R. Depression and anxiety in complex partial seizures. *J Nerv Ment Dis* 1984; **172**: 287–90.

Ramani V, Gumnit RJ. Intensive monitoring of interictal psychosis in epilepsy. *Ann Neurol* 1982; **11**: 613–22.

Sherwin I. Psychosis associated with epilepsy: Significance of the laterality of the epileptogenic focus. *J Neurol Neurosurg Psychiat* 1981; **44**: 83–5.

Sjobring H. Ixophreni. In: *Psykologisk-pedagogisk uppslagsbok* (Bd 2). Stockholm, 1944. Quoted and translated by Gundmunsson (1966).

Slater E, Beard AW, Glithero E. The schizophrenia-like psychoses of epilepsy. *Br J Psychiat* 1963; **109**: 95–150.

Stevens JR. Interictal clinical manifestations of complex partial seizures. In: *Advances in Neurology* (volume 11) (Penry JK, Daly DD, eds). New York: Raven Press, 1975, pp. 85–112.

Taylor DC. Mental state and temporal lobe epilepsy. A correlative account of 100 patients treated surgically. *Epilepsia* 1972; **13**: 727–65.

Taylor DC. Factors influencing the occurrence of schizophrenia-like psychosis in patients with temporal lobe epilepsy. *Psychol Med* 1975; **5**: 249–54.

Trimble MR, Perez MM. Quantification of psychopathology in adult patients with epilepsy. In: *Epilepsy and Behavior, 1979* (Wopsassepy I, Kulig BM, Meinhardi H, Stores G, eds). Lisse: Swets and Zeitlingerbr, 1980.

von Meduna L. General discussion of the cardiozol therapy. *Am J Psychiat* 1938; **94**: 40–50 (suppl).

Whitman S, Hermann BP, Gordon A. Psychopathology in epilepsy: How great is the risk? *Biol Psychiat* 1984; **19**: 213–6.

Wilson SAK. *Neurology*. Baltimore, MA: Williams & Wilkins, 1940, p. 1486.

75.   *Depression is a serious psychiatric concomitant of epilepsy, but often goes unrecognized or untreated*

Hippocrates first proposed a relationship between epilepsy and depression. Recent surveys and controlled studies of patients with epilepsy in England (Pond and Bidwell, 1959/60; Currie *et al.*, 1971; Kogeorgos *et al.*, 1982;), Iceland (Gundmundsson, 1966) and Los Angeles (Mendez *et al.*, 1986) have demonstrated an increased incidence of depression that averages about 25 to 30 percent. Up to 80 percent of patients with epilepsy complain of 'depression' when specifically questioned (Mittan and Locke, 1982). Kogeorges *et al.* (1982) found depression to be both more prevalent and more severe in an outpatient epilepsy population than in a control group with chronic neurological illnesses. Mendez *et al.* (1986) observed a nearly two-fold increase in the frequency of depression and a four-fold increase in the rate of attempted suicide in patients with epilepsy relative to individuals with comparable disabling disorders. These studies suggest that the increased prevalence of depression in patients with epilepsy is more than simply a reaction to chronic illness; biological factors also contribute.

The phenomenology of depression in patients with epilepsy is consistent with both endogenous and reactive mechanisms (Mendez *et al.*, 1986; Hermann and Whitman, 1989; Robertson, 1989). Epilepsy is accompanied by psychosocial handicaps, including (1) neurological impairment in patients with structural pathology and/or frequent seizures; (2) social bias and stigma leading to restrictions on employment, living situations and companion-ship; and (3) and disturbed family relations (e.g. dependency, overprotec-tion, rejection, negative self-image), which all act to reduce an individual's capacity to enjoy life and experience personal growth (Ward and Bower, 1978; Long and Moore, 1979; Ziegler, 1981; Hermann and Whitman, 1989). Antiepileptic medications, especially the barbiturates, also contribute to interictal depression in some patients (Robertson *et al.*, 1987).

Biological factors contributing to development of interictal depression include a family history of depression and a left-sided seizure focus (Nielsen and Kristensen, 1981; Perini and Mendius, 1984; Robertson *et al.*, 1987; Altshuler *et al.*, 1990). Left-sided lesions and left carotid amobarbital injections induce greater depressive reactions than those on the right side (Terzian, 1964; Robinson and Szetela, 1981; Robinson *et al.*, 1984). The interictal hypometabolism in patients with complex partial seizures is ipsi-lateral to the seizure focus (Theodore *et al.*, 1983), suggesting that this may represent the physiologic correlate of a left hemisphere 'lesion' (Altshuler *et al.*, 1990). Bilateral frontal hypometabolism has been correlated with depression in patients with epilepsy (Bromfield *et al.*, 1990).

However, the increased incidence of suicide attempts in epilepsy patients is related mainly to interictal psychopathology, as seen in border-line personality and psychosis, rather than to psychosocial stressors, seizure variables or antiepileptic drugs (Matthews and Barabas, 1981; Men-dez *et al.*, 1989).

Depression in patients with epilepsy is a serious problem. When added to the complex behavioral web of medication side effects, neurological and cognitive impairment, and psychosocial disability, depression may have a devastating effect.

Yet depression often goes unrecognized or untreated in patients with epilepsy. Neurologists are more likely to test them for nystagmus and unsteady tandem gait than to inquire about their spirits (Feldmann *et al.*, 1988). This is unfortunate. There are effective treatments for depression. Epilepsy is not an absolute contraindication for the use of antidepressants. Although antidepressants may lower the seizure threshold (Chadwick, 1981; Blain and Stewart-Wynn, 1985), most patients tolerate these medi-cations with no increase in seizure frequency (Ojemann *et al.*, 1987).

References

Altshuler LL, Devinsky O, Post RM, Theodore W. Depression, anxiety and tem-poral lobe epilepsy: Laterality of focus and symptomatology. *Arch Neurol* 1990; **47**: 284–8.

Blain PG, Stewart-Wynne E. Neurologic disorders. In Davies DM (ed), *Textbook of Adverse Drug Reactions*, 3rd ed. Oxford Univ Press, Oxford, 1985.

Bromfield EB, Altshuler L, Leiderman DB, Balish M, Ketter TA, Devinsky O, Post RM, Theodore WH. Cerebral metabolism and depression in patients. *Epilepsia* 1990; **31**: 625 (Abs).

Chadwick DW. Convulsions associated with drug therapy. *Adverse Drug React Bull* 1981; **87**: 316–332.

Currie S, Heathfield KWG, Henson RA, Scott DF. Clinical course and prognosis of temporal lobe epilepsy: A survey of 666 cases. *Brain* 1971; **94**: 173–90.

Feldmann E, Devinsky O, Bromfield E. Somatic and affective complains in patients with complex partial seizures. *Neurology* 1988; **38**: 333 (Abs) (Suppl 1).

Gundmundsson G. Epilepsy in Iceland: A clinical and epidemiological investigation. *Acta Neurol Scand* 1966; **43**: 1–124 (Suppl 25).

Hermann BP, Whitman. Psychosocial predictors of interictal depression. *J Epilepsy* 1989; **2**: 231–7.

Kogeorgos J, Fonagy P, Scott DF. Psychiatric symptom patterns of chronic epileptics attending a neurological clinic: A controlled investigation. *Br J Psychiat* 1982; **140**: 236–43.

Long CG, Moore JL. Parental expectations for their epileptic child. *J Child Psychol Psychiat* 1979; **20**: 299–312.

Matthews WS, Barabas G. Suicide and epilepsy: A review of the literature. *Psychosomatics* 1981; **22**: 515–24.

Mendez MF, Cummings JL, Benson DF. Depression in epilepsy: significance and phenomenology. *Arch Neurol* 1986; **43**: 766–70.

Mendez MF, Lanska DJ, Manon-Espaillat R, Burnstine TH. Causative factors for suicide attempts by overdose in epileptics. *Arch Neurol* 1989; **46**: 1065–8.

Mittan RJ, Locke GE. The other half of epilepsy: Psychosocial problems. *Urban Hlth* 1982; Jan/Feb: 38–89.

Nielsen H, Kristensen O. Personality correlates of sphenoidal EEG-foci in temporal lobe epilepsy. *Acta Neurol Scand* 1981; **64**: 289–300.

Ojemann LM, Baugh-Bookman C, Dudley DL. Effect of psychotropic medications on seizure control in patients with epilepsy. *Neurology* 1987; **37**: 1525–7.

Perini G, Mendius R. Depression and anxiety in complex partial seizures. *J Nerv Ment Dis* 1984; **172**: 287–90.

Pond DA, Bidwell BH. A survey of epilepsy in 14 general practices: II. Social and psychological aspects. *Epilepsia* 1959/60; **1**: 285–99.

Robertson MM. The organic contribution to depressive illness in patients with epilepsy. *J Epilepsy* 1989; **2**: 189–230.

Robinson RG, Kubus KL, Starr LB *et al*. Mood disorders in stroke patients: importance of location of lesion. *Brain* 1984; **42**: 441–7.

Robinson RG, Szetela B. Mood changes following left hemispheric brain injury. *Ann Neurol* 1981; **9**: 447–53.

Robertson MM, Trimble MR, Townsend HRA. Phenomenology of depression in epilepsy. *Epilepsia* 1987; **28**: 364–72.

Terzian H. Behavioral and EEG effects of intracarotid sodium amytal injection. *Acta Neurochir* 1964; **12**: 230–9.

Theodore WH, Newmark ME, Sato S *et al*. Fluorodeoxyglucose positron emission tomography in refractory complex partial seizures. *Ann Neurol* 1983; **14**: 429–37.

Ward F, Bower BD. A study of certain social aspects of epilepsy in childhood. *Dev Med Child Neurol* 1978; **39**: 1–50 (Suppl).

Ziegler RG. Impairments of control and competence in epileptic children and their families. *Epilepsia* 1981; **22**: 339–46.

76.   Interictal personality changes occur in some patients with epilepsy and are characterized by both positive and negative features

The study of personality and behavioral changes in epilepsy has focused largely on the abnormal and perverse. The assumption is often made, *a priori*, that altered behavior in epilepsy must be maladaptive or fit traditional psychiatric categories. However, epilepsy has been associated with positive attributes, such as profound philosophical or religious writing, artistic creativity and military genius (Bryant, 1953; Lennox, 1960; Alajouanine, 1963).

Gibbs *et al.* (1948) reported that patients with temporal lobe epilepsy have a much higher incidence of psychopathology than patients with other focal or generalized seizures. Gastaut and Collomb (1954) and Gastaut *et al.* (1955) noted that 75 percent of patients with psychomotor epilepsy – complex partial seizures with automatisms – had a global decline in excitability that impaired motor, intellectual, affective and sexual functions. However, half of these patients would paroxysmally shift from their abnormally placid state into an irritable condition without significant provocation. These behaviors were the opposite to those produced by bilateral temporolimbic lesions in the Kluver–Bucy syndrome (Maxim 60).

A collection of positive and negative interictal personality changes most frequently observed in temporal lobe epilepsy led Waxman and Geschwind (1975) to propose the existence of a syndrome. They defined this interictal behavioral syndrome of temporal lobe epilepsy, including the behavioral changes of deepened emotions, circumstantiality, altered religious and sexual concerns, and hypergraphia. Deepening of emotions is a central feature characterized by intense interpersonal contact and sustained intense affect. Emphasizing that the features were not necessarily maladaptive or negative, they stressed behavioral change rather than behavioral disorder. Bear and Fedio (1977) later expanded this syndrome to 18 traits, based on a literature review, and found an increased prevalence of all 18 traits in patients with temporal lobe epilepsy when compared with normal or neurological controls. The interictal behavioral traits described by Bear and Fedio, together with several others reported in the literature, are summarized in Table 76.1.

For numerous reasons, it is not surprising that some patients experience interictal changes in behavior. Animal and human studies have revealed that the limbic area plays an essential role in modulation of emotion. Both electrical stimulation of limbic areas and partial seizures cause affective, cognitive and psychic symptoms (Halgren *et al.*, 1978; Gloor *et al.*, 1982). These findings strengthen the association between epilepsy and interictal behavioral changes among certain patients, since epileptogenic foci in patients with partial seizures are most often found in limbic areas of the

Table 76.1 Interictal behavioral traits attributed to patients with epilepsy.

Trait	Clinical observations
Aggression	Irritability, labile temper, anger, overt hostility, rage attack
Altered sexual interest	Loss of libido, hyposexualism, fetishism, transvestism, exhibitionism, hypersexual episodes
Circumstantiality	Loquacious, pedantic, overly detailed, peripheral
Decreased emotionality	Emotional indifference, lack of initiative, dullness, hyperexcitability
Dependence, passivity	Helplessness, 'at hand of fate', always requires assistance
Elation, euphoria	Grandiosity, exhilarated mood, diagnosis of bipolar disorder
Emotional lability	Prominent mood changes with minor or no stimuli
Guilt	Tendency to self-scrutiny and self-recrimination
Humorless, sobriety	Overgeneralized ponderous concern, humor lacking or idiosyncratic
Hypergraphia	Keeping extensive diaries, detailed notes, writing autobiography or novel
Hypermoralism	Attention to rules with inability to distinguish significant from minor infraction, desire to punish
Hypomoralism	Lack of attention to rules, lack of understanding or concern of 'good' and 'bad'
Increased emotionality	Deepening emotions, sustained intense affect, increased sensitivity, brooding
Obsessionalism	Ritualism, orderliness, compulsive attention to detail
Paranoia, jealousy	Suspicious, overinterpretation of motives and events; diagnosis of paranoid schizophrenia
Philosophical interest	Nascent metaphysical or moral speculations, cosmological theories
Religiosity	Holding deep religious beliefs often idiosyncratic, multiple conversations, mystical states
Sadness	Hopelessness, discouragement, self-deprecation, diagnosis of depression, suicide attempts
Sense of personal destiny	Egocentricity, personal events highly charged, divine guidance ascribed to many features of patient's life
Viscosity	Stickiness, tendency to repetition

temporal and frontal lobes. In addition, positron emission tomography demonstrates interictal hypometabolism in partial seizure foci (Theodore *et al.*, 1984), suggesting that the functions of these critical areas are altered between seizures. These observations lend further support to the extensive number of case reports, clinical series and controlled studies that span more than a century and indicate that some patients with partial seizures experience interictal behavioral changes.

Nonetheless, the controversy over personality and epilepsy continues. No one doubts that, in some patients, interictal behavior changes develop after the onset of epilepsy. What is debated is the spectrum of behavioral changes, the frequency of specific traits and the factors contributing to such changes. Both methodological and theoretical issues prevent a resolution.

Another central issue in this controversy is the concept of a syndrome. Is there, indeed, a specific group of interictal behaviors in temporal lobe epilepsy? On the one hand, many of these behaviors are also found in patients with generalized or frontal lobe seizure foci (Hermann and Whitman, 1984; Weiser, 1986), and psychiatric controls also possess many of the 'interictal behavioral traits' (Mungas, 1982). Therefore, specificity is relative at best. On the other hand, the lack of specificity of an individual trait does not negate the concept of a syndrome – syndromes are defined by a complex of signs and symptoms (Maxim 64). Similarly, while the isolated features are not pathognomonic, the syndrome is comprised of the simultaneous occurrence of multiple features that would rarely be found together. For example, hyposexuality, deepened emotions, circumstantiality and hypergraphia constitute an unusual constellation of behaviors not typically found in psychiatric or neurological disorders.

The most extensively studied and best-documented behavioral changes in epilepsy are hyposexuality, which is characterized by decreased libido and impotence; hypergraphia; deepened emotions; and viscosity, a cohesive social tendency favoring prolonged verbal contacts (e.g. patients talk repetitively, circumstantially and pedantically) (Gastaut and Collomb, 1954; Blumer and Walker, 1967; Waxman and Geschwind, 1974; Bear and Fedio, 1977; Mayeux *et al.*, 1980; Sachdev and Waxman, 1981; Fenwick *et al.*, 1985; Hermann *et al.*, 1988; Rao *et al.*, 1992). The frequency of various interictal behavioral traits varies widely in different studies, and many of the traits, including hypergraphia, increased religious and philosophical interests and paranoia, are uncommon. When these traits develop, they usually follow the onset of seizures and are intense.

Sir Charles Symonds (1962), in discussing Beard and Slater's (1962) study of temporal lobe epilepsy and schizophrenia-like psychosis, presented a neglected but eloquent explanation of 'the epileptogenic disorder of function' that may apply to many forms of behavioral change with epilepsy:

> If then neither the fits nor the temporal lobe damage can be held directly responsible for the psychosis, what is the link? . . . Epileptic seizures and epileptiform discharge in the EEG are epiphenomena. They may be regarded

as occasional expressions of a fundamental and continuous disorder of neuronal function. The essence of this disorder is loss of the normal balance between excitation and inhibition at the synaptic junctions. From moment to moment there may be excess either of excitation or inhibtition – or even both at the same time in different parts of the same neuronal system. The epileptogenic disorder of function may be assumed to be present continuously but with peaks at which seizures are likely to occur.

Symonds' hypothesis may explain some aspects of interictal behavior. Thus, while the seizure is a transient disorder, the underlying epileptogenic disorder is a continuous process that causes a sustained alteration of behavior. The neurobiological changes related to epilepsy (the epileptogenic disorder of function) may result from neuronal hyperconnection, excitation or inhibition.

Interictal behavioral traits are not usually altered by antiepileptic medications. These behaviors are most often stable patterns, or personality traits, which resist manipulation. The dramatic response of interictal behaviors to antiepileptic drugs has been reported, but this phenomenon is the exception, not the rule (Geschwind *et al.*, 1980).

References

Alajouanine T. Dostoiewski's epilepsy. *Brain* 1963; **86**: 209–18.

Bear DM, Fedio P. Quantitative analysis of interictal behavior in temporal lobe epilepsy. *Arch Neurol* 1977; **34**: 454–67.

Beard AW, Slater E. The schizophrenic-like psychoses of epilepsy. *Proc Roy Soc Med* 1962; **55**: 311–14.

Blumer D, Walker EA. Sexual behavior in temporal lobe epilepsy. *Arch Neurol* 1967; **16**: 37–43.

Bryant JE. *Genius and Epilepsy*. Concord, MA: Ye Old Depot Press, 1953.

Fenwick PBC, Toone BK, Wheeler MJ, Nanjee MN, Grant R, Brown D. Sexual behavior in a center for epilepsy. *Acta Neurol Scand* 1985; **71**: 428–35.

Gastaut H, Collomb H. Etude du comportement sexuel chez les epileptiques psychomoteurs. *Ann Med Psychol* 1954; **112**: 657–96.

Gastaut H, Morin G, Leserve N. Study of the behavior of psychomotor epileptics during the interval between seizures. *Ann Med Psychol* 1955; **113**: 1–27.

Geschwind N, Shader RI, Bear D, North B, Levin K, Chetham D. Behavioral changes with temporal lobe epilepsy: Assessment and treatment. *J Clin Psychiat* 1980; **41**: 89–95.

Gibbs FA, Gibbs EL, Fuster B. Psychomotor epilepsy. *Arch Neurol Psychiat* 1948; **60**: 331–9.

Gloor P, Olivier A, Quesney LF, Andermann F, Horowitz S. The role of the limbic system in experiential phenomena of temporal lobe epilepsy. *Ann Neurol* 1982; **12**: 129–44.

Halgren E, Walter RD, Cherlow DG, Crandall PH. Mental phenomena evoked by electrical stimulation of the hippocampal formation and amygdala. *Brain* 1978; **101**: 83–117.

Hermann BP, Whitman S. Behavioral and personality correlates of epilepsy: A review, methodological critique, and conceptual model. *Psychol Bull* 1984; **95**: 451–97.

Hermann BP, Whitman S, Wyler AR, Richey ET, Dell J. The neurological, psychosocial and demographic correlates of hypergraphia in patients with epilepsy. *J Neurol Neurosurg Psychiat* 1988; **51**: 203–8.

Lennox WG. *Epilepsy and Related Disorders*. Boston, MA: Little, Brown and Company, 1960, pp. 700–11.

Mayeux R, Brandt J, Rosen J, Benson DF. Interictal memory and language impairment in temporal lobe epilepsy. *Neurology* 1980; **30**: 120–5.

Mungas D. Interictal behavior abnormality in temporal lobe epilepsy: A specific syndrome or nonspecific psychopathology. *Arch Gen Psychiat* 1982; **39**: 108–11.

Rao SM, Devinsky O, Grafman J, Hauser P, Usman MN, Theodore WH. Viscosity in complex partial seizures: Relationship to cerebral laterality and seizure duration. *J Neurol Neurosurg Psychiat* 1992; **55**: 149–152.

Sachdev HS, Waxman SG. Frequency of hypergraphia in temporal lobe epilepsy: An index of interictal behavior syndrome. *J Neurol Neurosurg Psychiat* 1981; **44**: 358–60.

Symonds C. Discussion. *Proc Roy Soc Med* 1962; **55**: 314–15.

Theodore WH, Newmark ME, Sato S, De LaPaz R, DiChiro G, Brooks R, Patronas N, Kessler RM, Manning R, Margolin R, Channing M, Porter RJ. 18F-fluorodeoxyglucose positron emission tomography in refractory complex partial seizures. *Ann Neurol* 1984; **14**: 429–37.

Waxman SG, Geschwind N. Hypergraphia in temporal lobe epilepsy. *Neurology* 1974; **24**: 629–31.

Waxman SG, Geschwind N. The interictal behavior syndrome in temporal lobe epilepsy. *Arch Gen Psychiat* 1975; **32**: 1580–6.

Weiser HG. Selective amygdalohippocampectomy: Indications, investigative technique and results. *Adv Tech Stand Neurosurg* 1986; **13**: 39–133.

77. Non-convulsive status epilepticus presents with confusion, lethargy or bizarre behavior and often requires an EEG for diagnosis

Continuous or repetitive seizure activity may impair mental function without causing 'loss of consciousness' or convulsive movements. There are two principal forms of non-convulsive status epilepticus: absence, or *petit mal*, and complex partial. Both forms present diagnostic problems and are easily mistaken for one another or confused with psychiatric illnesses, systemic disorders and medication toxicity.

Absence status is the most common form of non-convulsive status epilepticus and usually occurs in patients with a history of absence seizures (Porter and Penry, 1983). The initial attack of absence status can occur at any age and may occur in adults who have no history of seizures (Schwartz and Scott, 1971). Precipitating factors include discontinuation of anti-epileptic medications, sleep deprivation, stress, menstruation and metrizamide myelography (Andermann and Robb, 1972; Vollmer *et al.*, 1985; Guberman *et al.*, 1986).

Confusion and lethargy are prominent in most patients with absence status and may resemble catatonia. Patients are either disoriented or oriented only to person (Guberman *et al.*, 1986), and they are mute or have speech that is slow, dysprosodic and limited to yes – no answers or short phrases. Automatic behavior is often preserved; in such cases, patients can walk, follow simple commands after a delay, eat and void. Blinking is common. In rare cases, patients may show only slight decline in mental acuity (Andermann and Robb, 1972), although the diagnosis of absence status in such patients is controversial.

The EEG in absence status usually reveals continuous spike-and-wave or polyspike-and-wave discharges at a frequency of 1 to 6 per second, although generalized slowing with or without intermixed spikes has also been described (Niedermeyer and Khalifeh, 1965; Porter and Penry, 1983; Lee, 1985; Guberman *et al.*, 1986). In most cases, behavioral symptoms and EEG abnormalities respond promptly to intravenous doses of diazepam or lorazepam.

Complex partial status epilepticus results from repetitive (rarely continuous) partial seizures that lead to prolonged impairment of consciousness. Complex partial status is most common in patients with long-standing, medically intractable partial seizures in the setting of antiepileptic drug withdrawal (Treiman and Delgado-Escueta, 1983; Williamson *et al.*, 1985).

Complex partial status epilepticus is easily diagnosed if such auto-matisms such as lip smacking, chewing and repetitive hand movements are present. However, when agitation, sexual automatisms, confusion or psychotic behavior occur during or between repetitive seizures, mis-diagnosis is common (Van Rossum *et al.*, 1985; Williamson *et al.*, 1985). The EEG findings during complex partial status epilepticus are variable. Common findings during the ictus include slowing that is focal (tem-poral or frontal) or diffuse, rhythmic or arrhythmic, and with or without intermixed sharp waves and spikes, as well as bilateral spike-and-wave discharges. Generalized or focal slowing is common between seizures.

Although it is not a life-threatening emergency, complex partial status epilepticus should be treated promptly. Persistent disorders of memory, cognition or behavior may follow complex partial status (Engel *et al.*, 1978; Krumholz *et al.*, 1986).

Epilepsia partialis continua is a continuous partial seizure discharge that alters behavior causing focal motor or sensory, affective, autonomic or psychic symptoms, but does not impair consciousness. While epilepsia partialis continua is not always convulsive, the convulsive, motor variant is most common. Continuous, non-convulsive simple partial seizures often present diagnostic problems. For example, isolated fear lasting longer than an hour is almost always psychiatric, but may rarely be epileptic (McLach-lan and Blume, 1980; Zapoli *et al.*, 1983). Non-convulsive forms of simple partial status can also present as simple and complex auditory hallucina-tions, cognitive impairment, speech arrest and both anterior and posterior aphasias (De Pasquet *et al.*, 1976; Dinner *et al.*, 1981; Sacquegna *et al.*, 1981;

Nakada *et al.*, 1984; Wieser *et al.*, 1985). Epilepsia partialis continua usually occurs in patients with acute or subacute processes, such as stroke, encephalitis or tumor. It is often refractory to antiepileptic drugs (Juul-Jensen and Denny-Brown, 1966; Thomas *et al.*, 1977; Delgado-Escueta and Treiman, 1987).

References

Andermann F, Robb JP. Absence status: a reappraisal following review of thirty-eight patients. *Epilepsia* 1972; **13**: 177–87.

Delgado-Escueta AV, Treiman DM. Focal status epilepticus: Modern concepts. In: *Epilepsy: Electroclinical Syndromes* (Luders H, Lesser RP, eds). Berlin, New York: Springer-Verlag, 1987, pp. 347–91.

De Pasquet E, Gaudin E, Bianchi A, De Mendilaharsu S. Prolonged and monosymptomatic dysphasic status epilepticus. *Neurology* 1976; **25**: 244–7.

Dinner DS, Lueders H, Lederman R, Gretter TE. Aphasic status epilepticus: a case report. *Neurology* 1981; **31**: 888–91.

Engel JJ, Ludwig BI, Fetell M. Prolonged partial complex status epilepticus: EEG and behavioral observations. *Neurology* 1978; **28**: 863–9.

Guberman A, Cantu-Reyna G, Stuss D, Broughton R. Nonconvulsive generalized status epilepticus. *Neurology* 1986; **36**: 1284–91.

Juul-Jensen P, Denny-Brown D. Epilepsia partialis continua. *Arch Neurol* 1966; **15**: 563–78.

Krumholz A, Fisher RS, Weiss HD. Persistent neurological deficits following complex partial status epilepticus (CPSE). *Epilepsia* 1986; **27**: 614.

Lee SI. Nonconvulsive status epilepticus: Ictal confusion in later life. *Arch Neurol* 1985; **42**: 778–81.

McLachlan RS, Blume WT. Isolated fear in complex partial status epilepticus. *Ann Neurol* 1980 **8**: 639–41.

Nakada T, Lee H, Kwee IL, Lerner AM. Epileptic Kluver–Bucy syndrome: case report. *J Clin Psychiat* 1984; **45**: 87–8.

Niedermeyser E, Khalifeh R. *Petit mal* status ('spike-wave stupor'). *Epilepsia* 1965; **6**: 250–62.

Porter RJ, Penry JK. *Petit mal* status. In: *Advances in Neurology* (volume 34) *Status Epilepticus* (Delgado-Escueta AV, Wasterlain CG, Treiman DM, Porter RJ, eds). New York: Raven Press, 1983, pp. 61–7.

Sacquegna T, Pazzaglia P, Baldrati A, DeCarolis P, Gallassi R, Maccheroni M. Status epilepticus with cognitive symptomatology in a patient with partial complex epilepsy. *Eur Neurol* 1981; **20**: 319–25.

Schwartz MS, Scott DF. Isolated *petit-mal* status presenting *de novo* in middle age. *Lancet* 1971; **ii**: 1399–401.

Thomas JE, Reagan TJ, Klass DW. Epilepsia partialis continua: A review of 32 cases. *Arch Neurol* 1977; **34**: 266–75.

Treiman DM, Delgado-Escueta AV. Complex partial status epilepticus. In: *Advances in Neurology* (volume 34) *Status Epilepticus* (Delgado Escueta AV, Wasterlain CG, Treiman DM, Porter RJ, eds). New York: Raven Press, 1983, pp. 69–81.

Van Rossum J, Groeneveld-Ockhuysen AAW, Arts RJHM. Psychomotor status. *Arch Neurol* 1985; **42**: 989–93.

Vollmer ME, Weiss H, Beanland C, Krumholz A. Prolonged confusion due to absence status following metrizamide myelography. *Arch Neurol* 1985; **42**: 1005–8.

Wieser HG, Hailemariam S, Regard M, Landis T. Unilateral limbic epileptic status activity: stereo-EEG, behavioral and cognitive data. *Epilepsia* 1985; **26**: 19–29.

Williamson PD, Spencer DD, Spencer SS, Novelly RA, Mattson RH. Complex partial status epilepticus: A depth-electrode study. *Ann Neurol* 1985; **18**: 647–54.

Zappoli R, Zaccara G, Rossi L, Arnetoli G, Amantini A. Combined partial temporal and secondary generalized status epilepticus. Report of a case with fear bouts followed by prolonged confusion. *Eur Neurol* 1983; **22**: 192–204.

78.   Directed aggression is extremely rare during seizures

Aggressive behavior in patients with epilepsy may occur before, during or after seizures. Jackson (1879) speculated that the 'violence and outrageousness of the seizure depend doubtless very much on the natural disposition of the patient', and Jackson and Gowers (1885) recognized that patients with epilepsy may develop postictal paroxysmal outbursts of aggressive behavior and, if the ictal symptoms are subtle, the relationship of these outbursts to epilepsy may not be recognized.

During the postictal period, restraint often evokes an aggressive reaction. In his explanation of such behavior, Jackson (1881, 1888) theorized that the postictal patient is less of his higher, and more of his lower, self, and he interpreted postictal mania as a release of lower centers from the regulatory influences of higher cerebral centers. Therefore, the aggressive responses evoked by restraint are akin to those seen in wild animals; evolution has endowed us with the instinct to avoid capture.

Disorientation, confusion and amnesia are common after complex partial and generalized tonic–clonic seizures. During this period, patients are usually lethargic, but some may attempt to get up and go, as if they were 'escaping.' In either instance, restraint may evoke an aggressive response. During a generalized tonic–clonic seizure, the patient's head should be protected and, if possible, he should be placed on his side with his head facing down to prevent aspiration. After the seizure, if the patient resists supportive measures and is in no danger of harming himself or others, it is best to simply watch and avoid physical contact. During and after complex partial seizures, restraint may also precipitate aggressive responses that abate when physical restraint is removed (Rodin, 1973).

Ictal and interictal violence are far more controversial than postictal aggression. Ictal aggression is extremely rare and usually consists of spontaneous, non-directed, stereotyped aggressive behavior directed at objects or individuals (Delgado-Escueta *et al.*, 1981). For example, the patient may pick up a glass and throw it against a wall. However, rare case reports suggest that serious violent behavior may occur during seizures (Mark and Ervin, 1970; Ashford *et al*, 1980). In some cases, the ictal nature of violence was documented with depth electrode recording (Saint-Hilaire *et al.*, 1980). The incidence of ictal violence is difficult to assess accurately since most epilepsy centers will not admit patients with a history of serious aggressive behavior because of the potential dangers and expenses (Fenwick, 1991).

Interictal aggressive behavior is often reported in patients with epilepsy, especially temporal lobe epilepsy. However, few prospective or controlled studies have examined the association between interictal aggression and behavior. Lindsay *et al* (1979) prospectively followed 100 consecutive, unselected children with temporal lobe seizures for 13 years and found that 36 percent had rage episodes. Risk factors for rage episodes included first seizure during the first year of life, low IQ, male sex, hyperactivity and disordered home conditions (Ounsted, 1969). An increased incidence of aggressive behavior in children with temporal lobe epilepsy was also found by Nuffield (1961) and Keating (1961).

In adults, evidence linking epilepsy, especially of the temporal lobe, with interictal aggression is very controversial. Gibbs' (1948) and Gastaut's (1954, 1955) anecdotal observations that psychopathology and aggression are more common among patients with temporal lobe epilepsy stimulated interest and fomented heated debates.

Numerous epidemiological studies examining temporal lobe epilepsy and aggression followed. None of the seven studies comparing patients who had temporal lobe epilepsy to patients with other types of epilepsy or with neurological or psychiatric disorders found increased aggression in temporal lobe epilepsy (Hermann and Whitman, 1984). However, most of these studies did observe that the incidence of aggression among all patient groups was higher than the expected rate in the general population. In addition, consecutive but highly selected neurosurgical series, including many referrals from psychiatric facilities, report pathological aggression in 27 to 36 percent of patients (Serafetinides, 1965; Taylor, 1969). This high observed incidence may be largely due to selection bias.

However, case reports document interictal aggression in patients without developmental or sociological risk factors for aggression after the development of an epileptic focus localized clinically or electroencephalographically to the limbic system (Devinsky and Bear, 1984).

Experimental and surgical evidence also supports the theoretical link between increased incidence of aggressiveness and temporal lobe epilepsy. Experimental temporal lobe seizure foci increase aggressive behavior in several animal models (Pinel *et al.*, 1977; Adamec and Stark-Adamec, 1983; Siegel *et al.*, 1985–86; Brutus *et al.*, 1986; Griffith *et al.*, 1987). Resection of temporolimbic areas in humans and animals reduces aggressive behavior (Kluver and Bucy, 1939; Vaernet and Madsen, 1970; Kiloh *et al.*, 1974). Furthermore, the reversibility of aggression in more than 35 percent of violent patients by temporal lobectomy suggests that the dysfunctional temporal lobe contributes to aggressive behavior in some patients (Falconer, 1973).

Despite this body of supportive evidence, the association of temporal lobe epilepsy and aggression remains controversial and uncertain. The controversy results from both social and scientific issues. Patients with epilepsy have been unfairly stigmatized, and of all the behaviors they have been accused of, violence carries perhaps the greatest stigma. Further, since serious aggressive behavior is rare among patients with epilepsy, it is understandable why there is tremendous sensitivity over this issue. However, despite the social issues, epilepsy appears to carry a risk of increased aggressive behavior that may be a product of factors related directly to the epileptogenic process, as well as of medication, psychosocial effects and structural lesions.

Less pathological forms of aggressive behavior, such as irritability and anger, have been less systematically studied. However, when patients with partial or generalized seizures are systematically questioned, almost 30 percent report intense, paroxysmal irritability or moodiness during the interictal period compared with 2 percent in normal or non-brain injured neurological controls (Devinsky et al., 1991).

References

Adamec RE, Stark-Adamec C. Limbic control of aggression in the cat. *Prog Neuropsy-chopharmacol Biol Psychiatr* 1983; **7**: 505–12.

Ashford JW, Schulz SC, Walsh FO. Violent automatism in a partial complex seizure. *Arch Neurol* 1980; **37**: 120–2.

Brutus M, Shaikh MB, Edinger H, Siegel A. Effects of experimental temporal lobe seizures upon hypothalamically elicited aggressive behavior in the cat. *Brain Res* 1986; **366**: 53–63.

Delgado-Escueta AV, Mattson RH, King L, Goldensohn ES, Spiegel H, Madsen J, Crandall P, Dreifuss F, Porter RJ. Special report: The nature of aggression during epileptic seizures. *N Engl J Med* 1981; **305**: 711–16.

Devinsky O, Bear D. Varieties of aggressive behavior in temporal lobe epilepsy. *Am J Psychiat* 1984: **141**; 651–6.

Devinsky O, Feldmann E, Bronfield E, Emoto S, Raubertis R. Structured interview for partial seizures: Clinical phenomenology and diagnosis. *J Epilepsy* 1991; **4**: 107–16.

Falconer MA. Reversibility by temporal-lobe resection of the behavioral abnormalities of temporal-lobe epilepsy. *New Engl J Med* 1973; **289**: 451–5.

Fenwick. P. Aggression and epilepsy. In: *Epilepsy and Behavior* (Devinsky O, Theodore WH, eds). New York: Alan R Liss, 1991, pp. 85–96.

Gastaut H, Collomb H. Etude du comportement sexuel chez les epileptiques psychomoteurs. *Ann Med Psychol (Paris)* 1954; **112**: 657–96.

Gastaut H, Morin G, Leserve N. Etude du comportement des epileptiques psychomoteurs dans l'intervalle de leurs crises. *Ann Medico-Psychol* 1955; **113**: 1–27.

Gibbs FA, Gibbs EL, Foster B. Psychomoter epilepsy. *Arch Neurol Psychiat* 1948; **60**: 331–9.

Griffith N, Engel J, Bandler R. Ictal and enduring interictal disturbances in emotional behavior in an animal model of temporal lobe epilepsy. *Brain Res* 1987; **400**: 360–4.

Hermann BP, Whitman S. Behavioral and personality correlates of epilepsy: A review, methodological critique, and conceptual model. *Psychol Bull* 1984; **95**: 451–97.

Jackson JH. Lectures on the diagnosis of epilepsy. *Med Times Gaz* 1879; **1**: 29, 85, 141, 223.

Jackson JH. Remarks on dissolution of the nervous system, as exemplified in certain post-epileptic conditions. *Med Press Circ* 1881; **i**: 329–33.

Jackson JH. On post-epileptic states: A contribution to the comparative study of insanities. *J Ment Sci* 1888; **34**: 349–65.

Jackson JH, Gowers WR. *Epilepsy and Other Chronic Convulsive Disorders*. New York: William Wood and Company, 1885.

Keating LE. Epilepsy and behavior disorder in schoolchildren. *J Ment Sci* 1961; **107**: 161–80.

Kiloh LG, Gye RS, Rushworthy RG *et al*. Stereotactic amygdalotomy for aggressive behavior. *J Neurol Neurosurg Psychiat* 1974; **37**: 437–44.

Kluver H, Bucy P. Preliminary analysis of functions of the temporal lobes in man. *Arch Neurol Psychiat* 1939; **42**: 979–1000.

Lindsay J, Ounsted C, Richards P. Long-term outcome in children with temporal lobe seizures. III: Psychiatric aspects in childhood and adult life. *Dev Med Child Neurol* 1979; **21**: 630–6.

Mark VH, Ervin FR. *Violence and the Brain*. New York: Harper and Row, 1970.

Nuffield EJA. Neurophysiology and behavior disorders in epileptic children. *J Ment Sci* 1961; **107**: 438–58.

Ounsted C. Aggression and epilepsy: Rage in children with temporal lobe epilepsy. *J Psychosom Res* 1969; **13**: 237–42.

Pinel JPJ, Treit D, Rovner LI. Temporal lobe aggression in rats. *Science* 1977; **197**: 1088–9.

Rodin EA. Psychomotor epilepsy and aggressive behavior. *Arch Gen Psychiat* 1973; **28**: 211–13.

Saint-Hilaire JM, Gilbert M, Bouner G. Aggression as an epileptic manifestation: Two cases with depth electrodes. *Epilepsia* 1980; **21**: 184.

Serafetinides EA. Aggressiveness in temporal lobe epileptics and its relation to cerebral dysfunction and environmental factors. *Epilepsia* 1965; **6**: 33–42.

Siegel A, Brutus M, Shaikh, Edinger H. Effects of temporal lobe epileptiform activity upon aggressive behavior in the cat. *Int J Neurol* 1985–86; **19–20**: 59–73.

Taylor DC. Aggression and epilepsy. *J Psychosom Res* 1969; **13**: 229–36.

Vaernet K, Madsen A. Stereotaxic amygdalatomy and basofrontal tractotomy in psychotics with aggressive behavior. *J Neurol Neurosurg Psychiat* 1970; **33**: 858–63.

79. *Memory disorders are common in patients with epilepsy*

Impairment of memory may occur during, after or between seizures. Ictal amnesia occurs with absence, complex partial and generalized tonic–clonic seizures. Because absence seizures are often unrecognized and may be frequent, affected children often miss important bits of information at school and at home. An EEG with four minutes of hyperventilation can help to determine whether a child is simply daydreaming, ignoring adults or having absence seizures; most patients with absence seizures will have generalized spike-and-wave discharges during hyperventilation, especially if they are not taking antiepileptic drugs. Complex partial and generalized tonic–clonic seizures can impair memory consolidation and storage immediately before, during and after the seizure. Although postictal amnesia usually lasts less than 30 minutes, it may persist more than 24 hours, especially after prolonged or repetitive seizures.

Romberg (1853) recognized that 'it is characteristic to find a loss of memory' between seizures in epilepsy patients. In fact, memory loss is the most common interictal cognitive disorder in epilepsy. Patients often complain of difficulty recalling recently learned information, especially names and details. For some, reading is difficult because information from the last page or paragraph cannot be recalled and integrated with what is currently being read. The same problems may impair recall and comprehension of conversations.

The pathophysiology of interictal memory impairment is multifactorial and includes chronic dysfunction from neuronal loss or hypofunction, interictal epileptiform discharges and antiepileptic medications (Fenwick, 1988; Loiseau *et al.*, 1988; Smith, 1988). Unfortunately, therapy for one of these problems may worsen memory impairment due to another cause.

The limbic portion of the temporal lobe is the most common focus for partial seizures and is a critical memory area. Bilateral lesions in this area cause a devastating loss of short-term memory, resembling Korsakoff's disease (Milner, 1966). Lesions, such as mesial temporal sclerosis, may be associated with both impaired memory and partial seizures. Prolonged seizures can cause selective neuronal death in temporolimbic areas, such as the hippocampus. The medial temporal lobes, as well as other areas involved in memory processes, are involved in the spread of seizure discharges during both complex partial and generalized tonic–clonic seizures. In some patients, seizure control is accompanied by a significant improvement in short-term memory.

Furthermore, interictal positron emission tomography reveals decreased glucose and oxygen utilization in the region of the seizure focus, which may result from a combination of structural and functional changes (Theodore *et al.*, 1984). This hypometabolism may be a physiological correlate of hypofunction and thereby represents a marker of impaired function. It is uncertain to what extent control of seizures reverses interictal hypometabolism.

The interictal period has been associated with a variety of other cognitive disorders, including mental slowing and impaired attention, language, visuospatial and frontal lobe functions (e.g. planning, changing mental set, abstraction) (Brown, 1991; Perrine *et al.*, 1991).

Interictal epileptiform activity can reduce consciousness or selectively impair cognitive functions. Schwab (1947) recognized that brief, generalized spike-and-wave discharges were accompanied by transient increases in reaction time or by failure to respond to a stimulus. In this case, it is best to consider these discharges as ictal. In addition, Aarts *et al.* (1984) found that focal interictal epileptiform discharges can selectively impair cognition. Left-sided discharges caused more errors with a verbal learning task and right-sided discharges caused more errors with a non-verbal learning task. Patients who are handicapped by transient cognitive impairment in association with epileptiform discharges may improve when these discharges are suppressed with antiepileptic medication.

Rarely, control of seizures and interictal epileptiform activity may be associated with the development of psychosis, a phenomenon known as *forced normalization* (Landolt, 1958). Forced normalization occurs with both partial and primary generalized seizure disorders and is most common after the introduction of effective antiepileptic drugs, although it may occur spontaneously (Wolf, 1986).

Antiepileptic drugs are a well-recognized cause of reversible cognitive impairment in patients with epilepsy. These drugs are double-edged swords: they reduce seizures, postictal dysfunction and changes from interictal epileptiform activity on the one hand, but impair mental function on the other. The following guidelines are helpful: (1) although any drug can impair cognitive function, the most common culprits are the barbiturates, followed by the benzodiazepines; (2) polytherapy is more likely to impair cognitive function than monotherapy; (3) high serum antiepileptic drug levels are associated with increased risk of cognitive impairment.

The clinician must try to identify the factors contributing to memory and cognitive dysfunction in each patient. For example, a patient with absence seizures who is taking only valproic acid and is experiencing lethargy and memory dysfunction should have an EEG to assess the frequency of spike-and-wave discharges and tests for serum valproic acid level, serum ammonia level and liver function. Patients who have cognitive dysfunction while taking barbiturates may benefit from replacement with a less sedating antiepileptic drug (Theodore and Porter, 1983). The assistance of a neuropsychologist may prove rewarding in quantifying and isolating cognitive dysfunction and measuring cognitive changes with intervention.

References

Aarts JHP, Bimmin CD, Smit AD, Wilkins AJ. Selective cognitive impairment during focal and generalized epileptiform EEG activity. *Brain* 1984; **107**: 293–308.

Brown E. Cognitive disorders in epilepsy. *Sem Neur* 1991; **11**: 167–74.

Fenwick PBC. Seizures, EEG discharges and behavior. In: *Epilepsy, Behavior and Cognitive Function* (Trimble RM, Reynolds EH, eds). New York: John Wiley and Sons, 1988, pp. 51–66.

Landolt H. Serial electroencephalographic investigations during psychotic episodes in epileptic patients and during schizophrenic attacks. In: *Lectures on Epilepsy* (Lorentz de Haas, Am., ed.). Amsterdam: Elsevier, 1958, pp. 91–133.

Loiseau P, Strube E, Signoret JL. Memory and epilepsy. In: *Epilepsy, Behavior and Cognitive Function* (Trimble MR, Reynolds EH, eds). New York: John Wiley and Sons, 1988, pp. 165–76.

Milner B. Amnesia following operations on the temporal lobes. In: *Amnesia* (Whitty CWM, Zangwill OL, eds). Oxford: Butterworth, 1966.

Perrine K, Gershengorn J, Brown E. Cognitive disorders in epilepsy. In: *Epilepsy and Behavior* (Devinsky O, Theodore WH, eds). New York: Alan R Liss, 1991.

Romberg MD. A manual of the nervous diseases of man (Sieveking EH, transl). London: Sydenham Society, 1853, p. 203.

Schwab RS. Reaction time in *petit mal* epilepsy. *Assoc Res Nerv Men Dis* 1947; **26**: 339–41.

Smith DB. Anticonvulsants, seizures and performance. In: *Epilepsy, Behavior and*

Cognitive Function (Trimble MR, Reynolds EH, eds). New York: John Wiley and Sons, 1988, pp. 67–78.

Theodore WH, Newmark ME, Sato S, DeLaPaz R, DiChiro G, Brooks R, Patronas N, Kessler RM, Manning R, Margolin R, Channing M, Porter RJ. 18F-fluorodeoxyglucose positron emission tomography in refractory complex partial seizures. *Ann Neurol* 1984; **14**: 429–37.

Theodore WH, Porter RJ. Removal of sedative-hypnotic antiepileptic drugs from the regimens of patients with intractable epilepsy. *Ann Neurol* 1983; **13**: 320–4.

Wolf P. Forced normalization. In: *Aspects of Epilepsy and Psychiatry* (Trimble MR, Bolwig TG, eds). New York: John Wiley and Sons, 1986, pp. 101–12.

80.   *Paroxysmal changes in behavior result from a diverse group of neurological, medical and psychiatric disorders*

Epileptic seizures are defined as spontaneous, paroxysmal episodes of altered behavior due to excessive neuronal activity. Clinical features of epileptic seizures include weird, indescribable feelings; hallucinations and illusions in all sensory modalities; psychic phenomena, such as 'forced thinking' and *déjà vu*; affective and autonomic symptoms; impairment of consciousness; and involuntary movements. Non-epileptic paroxysmal disorders are very common and can mimic almost all forms of epileptic seizures (Table 80.1).

The correct diagnosis of paroxysmal behavior is critical. Failure to recognize seizures can prevent prompt diagnosis of curable tumors, lead to accidental death from impaired consciousness while driving, and cause significant educational and employment losses. Alternatively, an incorrect diagnosis of epilepsy can cause permanent loss of self-esteem, employment and driving privileges, and can obscure diagnosis and treatment of the true disorder. Syncope, panic attacks and psychogenic seizures (Maxim 81) are often confused with seizures.

Differentiation of syncope from seizures is a common problem (Porter, 1989). Both disorders are frequent and occur in all age groups. Syncope is a transient loss of consciousness from an acute decrease in cerebral blood flow. The diagnosis of syncope is supported if the episodes: (1) occur exclusively while standing or sitting; (2) are precipitated by anxiety or pain; (3) are associated with facial pallor and sweating; (4) are not associated with tonic–clonic movements and tongue biting; and (5) are not followed by confusion, lethargy and headache.

Prodromal symptoms such as epigastric sensation, fear, flushing, dizziness and feelings of unreality occur with both seizures and syncope (Engel, 1962). Symptoms such as formed auditory or visual hallucinations, olfactory hallucinations, *déjà vu*, or focal sensory or motor phenomena are more specific for partial seizures. The greatest source of error in distinguishing between seizures and syncope is failure to recognize that slight stiffening or clonic jerking may occur in syncope. When neurologists are shown a video-EEG recording of a syncopal episode with minor convulsive move-

Table 80.1   Non-epileptic paroxysmal disorders.

Cardiovascular
Syncope
   Reflex (vasovagal, carotid sinus, glossopharyngeal)
   Respiratory (cough, valsava)
   Decreased cardiac output
      Decreased left ventricular filling
         Hypovolemia/dehydration (orthostatic)
         Pulmonary embolism
      Arrhythmias
      Aortic stenosis
   Decreased systemic venous resistance–autonomic
      dysfunction (neurogenic, medication)
Breath holding spells (cyanotic, noncyanotic)
Mitral valve prolapse

Cerebrovascular (transient ischemic attacks)

Migraine

Movement disorders
Tics, Tourette's syndrome
Myoclonus
Startle attacks (hyperexplexia)
Chorea and paroxysmal choreoathetosis
Shuddering attacks
Spasmus mutans

Sleep disorders
Narcolepsy
Night terrors (parvor nocturnus)
Somnambulism
Benign sleep jerks
Periodic leg movements (nocturnal myoclonus)
REM behavior disorder

Metabolic–Toxic
Endocrine
Drug ingestion

Gastrointestinal disorders

Psychiatric disorders

ments, the vast majority mistakenly diagnose an epileptic seizure. If syncopal episodes are associated with prolonged anoxia, especially in children, generalized tonic–clonic seizures can occur, i.e. convulsive syncope (Battaglia *et al.*, 1989). The patient's medical history and a physical examination, particularly for orthostatic blood pressure changes, is usually sufficient to distinguish syncope and seizures, although routine as well as ambulatory 24-hour ECG and EEG studies may be required for diagnosis.

Panic disorder is characterized by recurrent attacks of intense fear or terror occurring in situations not normally associated with anxiety. Early in the course, fear typically occurs without any provoking stimulus. Later, panic is provoked by specific settings or actions, such as flying, driving or crowded places. Attacks are usually accompanied by autonomic (palpitations, diaphoresis, abdominal or chest discomfort, nausea, vomiting, diarrhea), neurological (numbness, paresthesia, dizziness, unsteadiness, trembling) or psychic (depersonalization, derealization) phenomena. Exhaustion may follow episodes, and patients often present with somatic or neurological complaints (Schofield and Duane; 1987). Katon (1984) found that almost 90 percent of patients with panic disorder present with somatic complaints and are frequently misdiagnosed, often for months or years. There is an increased incidence of depression and suicide attempts in patients with panic disorder (Weissman *et al.*, 1989). Panic disorder is common in women aged 16 to 40 years, with a lifetime prevalence of 1.5 to 2 percent in the general population. However, patients with panic disorder may comprise up to 15 percent of the patient population presenting to some general medical and psychiatric clinics.

Diagnostic confusion arises between panic attacks and partial seizures, in which fear is a prominent feature (Devinsky *et al.*, 1989). Several features help to distinguish these disorders. The intensity of fear often builds over minutes in psychiatric patients, whereas in seizures, symptom intensity may peak within seconds. The most helpful differentiating feature is the duration of the episode: ictal fear often lasts seconds and rarely lasts more than two or three minutes; panic attacks usually last at least 5 minutes. In most patients with ictal fear, some of the episodes are followed by impairment of consciousness with automatisms (complex partial seizures) or generalized convulsions. During panic attacks, patients often feel confused and complain of difficulty concentrating, but responsiveness is not impaired as it is in complex partial seizures – unless they faint! Hyperventilation may occur in association with panic attacks, and when vigorous, can cause syncope (Cowley and Roy-Byrne, 1987). Finally, the EEG during or between panic attacks does not show epileptiform abnormalities – although normal variants or patterns of uncertain clinical significance (Table 80.2) may occur, and their overinterpretation can lead to misdiagnosis.

Table 80.2   Normal EEG variants and patterns of clinical significance.

Mu rhythm
Positive occipital sharp transients of sleep
Lambda waves
Benign epileptiform transients of sleep
Rhythmical mid-temporal discharge (psychomotor variant)
14 and 6 Hz positive spikes
Subclinical rhythmical EEG discharge of adults
Wicket spikes
Temporal theta in the elderly

References

Battaglia A, Guerrini R, Gastaut H. Epileptic seizures induced by syncopal attacks. *J Epilepsy* 1989; **2**: 137–46.

Cowley DS, Roy-Byrne PP. Hyperventilation and panic disorder. *Am J Med* 1987; **83**: 929–37.

Devinsky O, Sato S, Theodore WH, Porter RJ. Fear episodes due to limbic seizures with normal ictal scalp EEG: A subdural electroencephalographic study. *J Clin Psychiat* 1989; **50**: 28–30.

Engel GL. *Fainting*. Springfield, IL: Charles C Thomas, 1962.

Katon W. Panic disorder and somatization. *Am J Med* 1984; **77**: 101–6.

Porter RJ. *Epilepsy: 100 Elementary Principles*. New York: WB Saunders, 1989.

Schofield A, Duane MMA. Neurologic referrals to a psychiatric consultation–liason service: A study of 199 patients. *Gen Hosp Psychiat* 1987; **9**: 280–6.

Weisman MM, Klerman GL, Markowitz JS, Ouellette R. Suicidal ideation and suicide attempts in panic disorder and attacks. *New Engl J Med* 1989; **321**: 1209–14.

81. *Atypical clinical features, normal EEG and ineffectiveness of antiepileptic drugs suggest psychogenic seizures*

Psychogenic seizures, also called hysterical or pseudoseizures, are one of the most common symptoms of conversion disorder, occurring in 10 to 20 percent of these patients. The disorder is most common in women (Lesser, 1985; Lempert and Schmidt 1990). Among patients with medically refractory seizure disorders, approximately 10 percent of patients actually have only psychogenic seizures and an additional 10 percent have both psychogenic and epileptic seizures. While the incidence of isolated psychogenic seizures is unknown, such attacks are not uncommon.

The psychogenic seizure as a conversion symptom

Conversion symptoms are characterized by a loss or alteration of physical function that suggests organic disease but results from psychological conficts or needs (Maxim 93). Although stress, including sexual and physical abuse, is often identified as the precipitating factor for psychogenic seizures, often no psychological cause can be found (LaBarbera and Dozier, 1980; Cascino *et al.*, 1987; Schofield and Duane, 1987; Gates *et al.*, 1991). Patients with psychogenic seizures and other conversion symptoms do not willfully feign epilepsy, as in factitious disorder or malingering (Maxim 94). When seizures begin after minor head-injury litigation has begun, the possibility of intentional deceit should be considered.

In patients predisposed to conversion, the specific symptoms are largely determined by previous experience. A past or current history of epilepsy is found in 10 to 30 percent of patients with psychogenic seizures (Lesser,

1986; Lempert and Schmidt, 1990). In many other cases, seizures have been observed at home or work. Indeed, the early 19th century European asylum doctors separated mental and epileptic patients, because epilepsy was 'contagious' (Temkin, 1979).

Isolated psychogenic seizures often occur in the setting of severe psychological stress. Recurrent psychogenic seizures may occur in association with less intense stressors, such as an argument with a boyfriend or relative. However, one should not diagnose a seizure as psychogenic because it was preceded by stress. Many patients with epilepsy report that stress can precipitate seizures (Fenwick, 1991). Stress also leads to sleep deprivation, another seizure-provoking factor.

Other associated psychiatric disorders

Among patients with psychogenic seizures, there is a high incidence of previous psychiatric treatment and suicide attempts (Roy, 1979; Stewart *et al.*, 1982). Depression is particularly common and has been reported in 24 to 86 percent of patients (Roy, 1979; Stewart *et al.*, 1982; Krumholz and Niedermeyer, 1983; Lempert and Schmidt, 1990). Anxiety disorders, mental retardation, dementia and personality disorders are also associated with psychogenic seizures (Stewart *et al.*, 1982; Krumholz and Niedermeyer, 1983; Gumnit and Gates, 1986; Lempert and Schmidt, 1990). In cases with epilepsy and other psychiatric disorders, treatment should be directed at the primary psychopathology, with appropriate pharmacotherapy as indicated. When psychotropic medications are used, non-epileptogenic agents should be chosen. Antiepileptic medications, especially barbiturates, may exacerbate affective disorders and should be avoided (Thompson and Trimble, 1982; Trimble 1986). When affective disturbances and psychogenic seizures coexist with epilepsy, antiepileptic drug monotherapy is desirable since polytherapy more often exacerbates affective disorders (Thompson and Trimble, 1982; Trimble, 1986).

Diagnosis of psychogenic seizures

The diagnosis of psychogenic seizures is often difficult. Seizures refractory to therapy or with atypical features are cause for suspicion. There is no single clinical finding that reliably distinguishes psychogenic from epileptic seizures (Porter, 1989). A complete history of the seizure pattern is essential. While a careful description of the episode by the patient and a trustworthy witness should be obtained, the recollections may be inaccurate and misleading.

Ask about the following critical points: (1) precipitating features – examples include stress or sleep deprivation; and highly specific stressors (e.g. English class) may suggest psychogenic seizures; (2) suggestibility – if the subject can be talked into or out of a seizure, or attacks can be produced and stopped with normal saline, psychogenic seizures are likely; (3) mode of onset – onset is often gradual in psychogenic seizures and almost always sudden in epilepsy; (4) duration of attacks – attacks often last more than five minutes in psychogenic seizures, but are usually less than three minutes in epilepsy (beware, some patients confuse ictal and postictal states); (5) stereotypy of episodes – frequently changing ictal features are common when the origin is psychological, while epileptic episodes are nearly identical; (6) ictal features – note whether they are typical or atypical for partial and generalized seizures; (7) ability to recall events during a seizure with impaired consciousness or abnormal movements of all extremities – this suggests psychogenic seizures; (8) urinary incontinence or bodily injury (e.g. biting the side of the tongue) during seizure suggests epilepsy; and (9) postictal state – confusion and lethargy suggest epilepsy (Table 81.1).

The combination of various clinical features may allow a fairly confident diagnosis of psychogenic seizures. Attacks that are always precipitated by stress, begin gradually and fluctuate, are initiated and terminated volitionally, last longer than 10 minutes and consist of atypical clinical features (Table 81.1) are inconsistent with epilepsy. Unfortunately, the available history is often unclear and combines features that suggest epileptic and psychogenic seizures.

The common concurrence of epileptic and psychogenic seizures can pose a particularly difficult dignositic and therapeutic dilemma. Additional investigation with video-EEG monitoring is often required to clarify the nature of specific episodes (see below) (Desai *et al.*, 1982; Gates *et al.*, 1991).

Psychogenic seizures are most often confused with complex partial and generalized tonic–clonic seizures. Complex partial seizures are usually accompanied by sudden involuntary changes in facial expression (e.g. blank stare, grimace) and automatisms, and patients are amnesic for the episode. Automatisms in such seizures are stereotypic and classified as (1) oral–alimentary (lip smacking, chewing, swallowing); (2) upper extremity–gestural (hand clasping, grabbing, picking, tapping, dystonia); (3) lower extremity–ambulatory (walking, running, kicking); (4) vocalization (grunts, repetition of words or phrases); and (5) sexual (pelvic thrusting, masturbatory movements). The first two types of automatisms are the most common. Postictal disorientation, confusion and lethargy occur in most cases, but vary in degree. Occasionally, complex partial status epilepticus occurs, presenting as prolonged confusion or bizarre behavior, and may be misdiagnosed as a psychiatric fugue state. Rare cases of postictal poriomania (prolonged wandering with amnesia) have been reported. However, the vast majority of fugue states are psychiatric.

During psychogenic seizures, facial expression often appears to be under volitional control and automatic behaviors are rarely typical oral–alimentary, or upper extremity–gestural, phenomena. Postictally, patients can often recall their automatisms and are usually alert and oriented.

Table 81.1 Comparisons between psychogenic and epileptic seizures.

Psychogenic seizures	Epileptic seizures
Seizures can be precipitated by stress or specific settings (school, work, spouse)	Seizures can be precipitated by stress
Frequent seizures despite therapeutic plasma levels of antiepileptic drugs	Toxicity of antiepileptic drugs (especially phenytoin and carbamazepine) may exacerbate seizures or cause symptoms confused with seizures
Gradual onset of ictus (> 1 min)	Seizures begin suddenly but are often preceded by an aura (usually > 1 min) or premonitory symptoms (irritability, depression > 1 hour)
Prolonged duration (often 5 min)	Brief duration (usually < 5 min)
Thrashing, struggling, crying, pelvic thrusting, side-to-side rolling, wild movements	Bizarre, complex motor automatisms occur with frontal lobe complex partial seizures
Intermittent arrhythmic, out-of-phase jerking	Rhythmic, in-phase jerking slows before stopping in generalized tonic–clonic seizures
Bilateral motor activity with preserved consciousness	Bilateral motor activity with preserved consciousness may occur with supplementary motor area seizures
Clinical features of seizures fluctuate	Seizures are usually stereotypic
No postictal confusion or lethargy	Postictal confusion may occur with frontal lobe, and less often, temporal lobe complex partial seizures
Postictal crying or shouting of obscenities	Aggressive verbal and physical behavior may occur if patients are restrained postictally

Generalized tonic–clonic seizures are characterized by sudden loss of consciousness. This is followed by a tonic phase, as seen by a single involuntary cry or shriek, unilateral head deviation, or tonic spasm of most body muscles, then a clonic phase, in which the bilateral, symmetrical tonic contractions are interrupted by periods of relaxation. Typically, there is a single and final, large clonic jerk followed by flaccidity and brief coma. During coma, memory, pupillary light reflex, corneal reflexes and responsiveness to noxious stimuli are absent. The ictal phase usually lasts less than two minutes and the postictal phase often blends into sleep lasting several hours. Cyanosis, tongue biting (especially the sides of the tongue and cheek), urinary incontinence and progressive slowing in the rate of clonic contractions as the seizure ends are rarely mimicked in psychogenic attacks. With psychogenic seizures, patients often recall events occurring during the period of bilateral motor activity, jerking movements are out-of-phase (e.g. the left arm flexes while the right arm extends), and there is often pelvic thrusting, rolling or thrashing from side to side (Gates *et al.*, 1985).

Diagnostic problems

Some patients with psychogenic seizures have sophisticated medical knowledge. This information is acquired through a personal history of epilepsy, observation of seizures in others, extensive reading and attendance at epilepsy self-help groups. Further, if they have had a diagnosis of psychogenic seizures, one or more physicians may have told them 'what they did wrong'. Occasionally, patients may injure themselves or urinate during psychogenic *grand mal* or display typical epileptic automatisms during psychogenic attacks. Psychogenic episodes during apparent sleep are uncommon, but not rare.

Another important caveat is that epileptic seizures may evoke bizarre behaviors (Williamson *et al.*, 1985). While the vast majority of seizures are associated with typical ictal phenomena, certain seizures have unusual behavioral manifestations and, because of this, are incorrectly diagnosed as hysterical or psychogenic (Table 81.2). Frontal lobe complex–partial seizures, supplementary motor area seizures, temporal lobe seizures and the syndrome of hypothalamic hamartomas with gelastic (laughing) seizures are most likely to be misdiagnosed. Patients with frontal or temporal lobe partial seizures, as well as those with hypothalamic lesions, can develop interictal personality changes or depression that may suggest psychogenic illness. The EEG may not show ictal or interictal epileptiform activity, making diagnosis more difficult.

Before making the diagnosis of psychogenic seizures on clinical features alone, it is humbling to remember that among patients diagnosed with neurological conversion symptoms at academic centers, 20 to 40 percent are subsequently found to have organic disorders, such as epilepsy, lupus or multiple sclerosis (Maxim 93) (Merskey and Buhrich, 1975).

EEG and video-EEG studies

A diagnosis of psychogenic seizures cannot be based solely on the EEG findings. A normal interictal EEG is not uncommon in patients with epilepsy. Conversely, the presence of interictal epileptiform activity does not confirm the diagnosis. In addition to normal patterns that may be incorrectly considered epileptogenic (Table 80.2), true epileptiform transients occur in 1 to 2 percent of the normal population. Finally, because some patients with psychogenic seizures have epileptic seizures, interictal or ictal epileptiform activity does not prove that all seizures are epileptic.

Table 81.2   Epileptic seizures misdiagnosed as psychogenic seizures.

Frontal lobe complex partial seizures
Frequent stereotyped seizures, often in clusters
Brief duration (< 1 min)
Minimal postictal confusion and lethargy
Complex motor automatisms
    Kicking, rocking, thrashing, rubbing, scratching, genital manipulation,
    head nodding, vocalization (hum, squeals, shouting obscenities)
Urinary incontinence
Frequent episodes of complex partial status epilepticus

Supplementary motor area seizures
Unilateral head and/or eye deviation, arm abduction, elbow flexion (head
    looks at the hand – 'fencer's posture')
Bilateral upper and/or lower extremity tonic or clonic acitivity with
    preserved consciousness
Vocalization (grunts, hum)
Speech arrest

Temporal lobe simple partial seizures
Forced thinking
Autoscopy (out-of-body experiences; seeing one's double)
Depersonalization (alteration in one's sense of personal reality and
    experience of self; autoscopy is a form)
Derealization (alteration in one's sense of external reality)
Fear, panic
Depression
Complex visual or auditory hallucinations

Temporal lobe complex partial seizures
Laughing, rarely crying
Walking
Continuation of ongoing behavior

Hypothalamic hamartomas and seizures
Laughing
(Interictal aggressive behavior)

Familiarity with *EEG patterns* during the ictal and postictal periods is
essential for accurate assessment of seizures. *Simple partial seizures* often
show no ictal changes in the background activity, but focal epileptiform or
rhythmical slowing may be found (Devinsky *et al.*, 1988). *Temporal lobe
complex partial seizures* most often show unilateral or bilateral temporal
slowing ictally. *Frontal lobe complex partial seizures* show ictal epileptiform
transients, slow activity, or no background changes. With *generalized tonic-
clonic seizures*, the ictal and postictal EEG is always abnormal. During the
tonic phase, a build-up of generalized low-voltage fast activity evolves into
a high-voltage generalized polyspike discharge. When muscles relax in
the clonic phase and postictally, there is generalized suppression and slowing of EEG activity. In addition, muscle artifact often obscures cerebral

electrographic seizure discharges during general tonic–clonic seizures and, less often, complex partial seizures.

Background changes that follow all generalized tonic–clonic seizures and most complex partial seizures are characterized by slowing of frequency and decreased voltage. In many cases, the background changes are more prominent over the side from which the seizure discharge arose. Although not pathognomonic, absence of background depression and slowing or immediate return of the alpha rhythm after generalized tonic–clonic seizures or prolonged, complex partial seizures strongly suggests psychogenic seizures.

Simultaneous video-EEG monitoring allows more confident differentiation between epileptic and psychogenic seizures. Correlation of clinical and EEG phenomena can be made with repeated review of individual events. In patients with multiple types of episodes, recorded seizures can be shown to family members or care-givers for comparison with events observed outside the hospital. Because patients with psychogenic seizures are often treated for prolonged periods with high doses of antiepileptic drugs – while the needed psychologic therapy is not provided – the benefits of video-EEG monitoring clearly outweigh the costs.

Other diagnostic tests

Provocative testing to initiate and terminate an attack using suggestion (as in 'this can provoke seizures'), alcohol wipes over the region of the carotid artery or saline injection during video-EEG monitoring is a highly effective method for confirming that certain attacks are psychogenic. Ethical considerations and detrimental consequences for the physician–patient relationship must be weighed against the value of the information.

Serum prolactin levels increase after almost all generalized tonic clonic seizures, most complex partial seizures, and some simple partial seizures (Sperling *et al*, 1986; Yerby *et al* 1987). Postictal levels (20–150 ng/ml) peak within 15 minutes after the seizure and return to baseline levels (5–10 ng/ml) after approximately 30 to 60 minutes. Prolactin levels are not significantly increased after psychogenic seizures. Fingerstick prolactin levels can be used (Fisher *et al.*, 1991). Baseline values are essential for correct interpretation of postictal values. As with individual clinical and EEG criteria, absence of postictal prolactin elevation is not by itself a reliable indicator of a psychogenic attack.

Treatment

The diagnosis of psychogenic seizures, although difficult, is often easier than treatment. A psychiatrist or psychologist should be enlisted to help in the treatment program.

Rapport must be established between the patient and physician before treatment is begun. Then one should initiate a non-confrontational discussion of the patient's symptoms and life situation. Suggestion is a powerful therapeutic tool – emphasize that episodes often resolve with time and that recurrence does not represent a therapeutic failure. A majority of patients will exhibit an immediate decrease in the frequency of events (Shen *et al.*, 1990). If the patient's intelligence and motivation are adequate, psychotherapy may be beneficial.

Patients with recurrent psychogenic seizures often pose a therapeutic dilemma. No matter how gentle the explanation, some patients react violently, accusing the staff of labeling them as 'crazy'. In such cases, it may be helpful to show the videotape of an episode to the patient and family, making sure that the episode recorded in the hospital or clinic is the same as the typical attacks at home and pointing out atypical clinical and EEG features (Lesser, 1984; Gates *et al.*, 1991). However, some patients will use this information to make their next seizures more difficult to diagnose. Similarly, confronting them with the results of a suggestion–saline test will make them more knowledgeable when they present to another physician.

Prognosis

Isolated psychogenic seizures precipitated by grave stress (e.g. rape) usually do not recur if psychotherapy is started promptly. Long-term follow-up studies reveal that approximately one-third to one-half of all patients with recurrent psychogenic seizures experience resolution of conversion symptoms and improved psychosocial status (Krumholz and Niedermeyer, 1983; Gumnit and Gates, 1986; Lempert and Schmidt, 1990). In some patients, psychogenic seizures are the most prominent feature of Munchausen's syndrome, which is refractory to treatment. (Savard *et al.*, 1988).

References

Cascino G, Woodard A, Hohnson M. Sexual and/or physical abuse occurring in association with psychogenic seizures. *Epilepsia* 1987; **28**: 632.

Desai BT, Porter RJ, Penry JK. Psychogenic seizures: A study of 42 attacks in six patients with intensive monitoring. *Arch Neurol* 1982; **39**: 202–9.

Devinsky O, Kelleg K, Porter RJ, Theodore WM. Clinical and electroencephalographic features of simple partial seizures. *Neurology* 1988; **38**: 1347–82.

Fenwick P. The influence of mood on seizure activity. In: *Epilepsy and Behavior* (Devinsky O, Theodore WH, eds). New York: Alan R Liss, 1991.

Fisher RS, Chan DW, Bare M, Lesser RP. Capillary prolactin measurement for diagnosis of seizures. *Ann Neurol* 1991; **29**: 187–90.

Gates JR, Luciano D, Devinsky O. Treatment of psychogenic seizures. In: *Epilepsy and Behavior* (Devinsky O, Theodore WH, eds). New York: Alan R Liss, 1991.

Gates JR, Ramani V, Whalen S, Loewenson R. Ictal characteristics of pseudoseizures. *Arch Neurol* 1985; **42**: 1183–7.

Gumnit RJ, Gates JR. Psychogenic seizures. *Epilepsia* 1986; **27**: S124–S129 (Suppl 2)

Krumholz A. Psychogenic seizures: a clinical study with follow-up data. *Neurology* 1983; **33**: 498–502.

Krumholz A, Niedermeyer E. Psychogenic seizures: A clinical study with follow-up data. *Neurology* 1983; **33**: 498–502.

LaBarbera JD, Dozier JE. Hysterical seizures: the role of sexual exploitation. *Psychosomatics* 1980; **21**: 897–903.

Lempert T, Schmidt D. Natural history and outcome of psychogenic seizures: a clinical study in 50 patients. *J Neurol* 1990; **237**: 35–8.

Lesser RP. Psychogenic seizures. *Neurology* 1986; **27**: 823–9.

Lesser RP. Psychogenic seizures. In: *Recent Advances in Epilepsy* (volume 2) (Pedley TA, Meldrum B, eds). Edinburgh: Churchill Livingstone, 1985, pp. 273–96.

Merskey H, Buhrich NA. Hysteria and organic brain disease. *Br J Med Psychol* 1975; **48**: 359–66.

Porter RJ. *Epilepsy: 100 Elementary Principles*. New York: WB Saunders, 1989.

Roy A. Hysterical seizures. *Arch Neurol* 1979; **36**: 447.

Savard G, Andermann F, Teitelbau J, Lehmann H. Epileptic Munchausen's syndrome: A form of pseudoseizures distinct from hysteria and malingering. *Neurology* 1988; **38**: 1628–9.

Schofield A, Duane MMA. Neurologic referrals to a psychiatric consultation-liason service: A study of 199 patients. *Gen Hosp Psychiat* 1987; **9**: 280–6.

Shen W, Bowman ES, Markand ON. Presenting the diagnosis of pseudoseizure. *Neurology* 1990; **40**: 756–9.

Sperling MR, Pritchard PB, Engel J, Daniel C, Sagel J. Prolactin in partial epilepsy: an indicator of limbic siezures. *Ann Neurol* 1986; **20**: 716–22.

Stewart RS, Lovitt R, Stewart RM. Are hysterical seizures more than hysteria? A research diagnostic criteria, DSM-III, and psychometric analysis. *Am J Psychiat* 1982; **139**: 926–8.

Temkin O. *The Falling Sickness*. Baltimore, MA: Johns Hopkins University Press, 1979.

Thompson P. Trimble MR. Anticonvulsant drugs, cognitive function and behavior. *Epilepsia* 1982; **24**: 21–2. (Suppl 18).

Trimble MR. Pseudoseizures. *Neurol Clin* 1986; **4**: 531–48.

Williamson PD, Spencer DD, Spencer SS, Novelly RA, Mattson RH. Complex partial seizures of frontal lobe origin. *Ann Neurol* 1985; **18**: 497–504.

Yerby MS, Van Belle G, Friel PN, Wilensky AJ. Serum proclatins in the diagnosis of epilepsy: Sensitivity, specificity, and predictive value. *Neurology* 1987; **37**: 1224–6.

14
Movement disorders

82. *Lesions in the extrapyramidal motor system cause disorders of movement, cognition, and affect*

The role of the basal ganglia – the heart of the extrapyramidal system – remains mysterious, but medical attention has focused on this area's motor functions. Marsden (1982) postulated that the basal ganglia are responsible for the automatic execution of learned motor programs. However, patients with bilateral lesions in the basal ganglia often develop cognitive, affective and personality changes that coexist with motor abnormalities.

Extrapyramidal movement disorders include both negative and positive symptoms. The functional deficits include loss of motor spontaneity and initiative (akinesia), impaired postural reflexes, an absence of motor planning and a decrease (hypokinesia) and slowing (bradykinesia) of all movements. With unilateral caudate lesions, contralateral hypokinesia may be accentuated by bilateral simultaneous movements (i.e. motor extinction) (Valenstein and Heilman, 1981). Positive symptoms, probably due to loss of inhibition, include rigidity, tremor, dystonia, dyskinesia, chorea, athetosis and ballismus.

As with motor symptoms, behavioral symptoms may be categorized as negative or positive. Negative symptoms include reduced attention, mental inertia, lack of spontaneity, reduced affective range, and inability to formulate plans and strategies (Marsden, 1982). Positive behavioral symptoms include obsessive–compulsive phenomena, irritability, aggressiveness, sexual promiscuity, delusions and hallucinations in somatosensory, auditory and visual modalities (Marsden, 1982; Laplane *et al.*, 1989).

Depression is the most common affective disorder in patients with basal ganglia disorders (e.g. Parkinson's disease, Huntington's disease, progressive supranuclear palsy, Sydenham's chorea and idiopathic basal ganglia calcifications). In these patients, depressive symptoms include behavioral withdrawal, apathy, emotional disinterest, pessimism and hopelessness.

Parkinson's disease and Huntington's disease are the basal ganglia disorders in which cognitive and affective changes have been most extensively studied (Maxims 84 and 85). However, non-motor behavioral changes also occur with other pathological processes.

The pathological and anatomical correlates of these behaviors are not well understood. The most prominent and enduring behavioral manifestations usually occur only with bilateral striatal lesions. However, unilateral caudate lesions to either side can cause abulia, agitation and hyperactivity, while right caudate lesions can cause left-sided neglect and left caudate lesions may produce language disorders (Caplan *et al.*, 1990). The basal ganglia receive massive input from most areas of the cerebral cortex and many brainstem and thalamic nuclei. Output is directed predominantly into the thalamus and brainstem, with secondary connections from these areas to the cortex and spinal cord. Thus, the basal ganglia is uniquely 'wired' to subserve complex integrative functions. Discrete lesions in the basal ganglia of experimental animals produce deficits similar to those caused by lesions of cortical areas supplying afferents to that region of the basal ganglia (Rosvold and Szwarcbart, 1964; Oberg, 1979).

Behavioral effects of basal ganglia lesions in humans closely resemble signs and symptoms of the frontal lobe syndrome (Laplane *et al.*, 1989). Behavioral changes accompany relative preservation of intellectual functions and include inertia, loss of drive, apathy, emotional dulling and impulsivity. Difficulty initiating and maintaining a behavioral set are characteristic of both basal ganglia and frontal lobe disorders. In patients with bilateral basal ganglia lesions, prominent behavioral changes and minimal motor symptoms, positron emission tomography studies demonstrate prefrontal hypometabolism (Laplane *et al.*, 1989). Furthermore, the well-documented behavioral symptoms that follow discrete caudate strokes in the absence of any cortical lesions (Caplan *et al.*, 1990) argue strongly that lesions restricted to the basal ganglia can alter behavior.

References

Bowen FP. Behavioral alterations in patients with basal ganglia lesions. In: *The Basal Ganglia* (Yahr MD, ed.). New York: Raven Press, 1976, pp. 169–77.

Caine ED, Shoulson I. Psychiatric syndromes in Huntington's disease. *Am J Psychiat* 1983; **140**: 728–33.

Caplan LR, Schahmann JD, Kase CS, Feldmann E, Baquis G, Greenberg JP, Gorelick PB, Helgason C, Hier DB. Caudate infarcts. *Arch Neurol* 1990; **47**: 133–43.

Goutieres F, Aicardi J. Acute neurological dysfunction associated with destructive lesions of the basal ganglia in children. *Ann Neurol* 1982; **12**: 328–32.

Laplane D, Levasseur M, Pillon B, Dubois B, Baulac M, Mazoyer B, Dinh ST, Sette G, Danze F, Baron JC. Obsessive–compulsive and other behavioral changes with bilateral basal ganglia lesions. *Brain* 1989; **112**: 699–725.

Lishman WA. *Organic Psychiatry*. Oxford, Boston, MA: Blackwell Scientific Publications, 1978, pp. 446–9.

Marsden CD. The mysterious motor function of the basal ganglia: The Robert Wartenberg Lecture. *Neurology* 1982; **32**: 514–39.

Oberg RGE, Divac I. 'Cognitive' functions of the neostriatum. In: *The Neostriatum* (Divac I, Oberg RGE, eds). Oxford: Pergamon Press, 1979, pp. 291–313.

Rosvold HE, Szwarcbart MK. Neural structures involved in delayed response per-

formance. In: *The Frontal Granular Cortex and Behavior* (Warren JM, Akert K, eds).
New York: McGraw Hill, 1964, pp. 1–15.
Valenstein E, Heilman KM. Unilateral hypokinesia and motor extinction. *Neurology*
1981; **31**: 445–8.

83. *Tourette's syndrome of chronic motor and vocal tics is often associated with obsessive–compulsive and attention deficit disorders*

A motor tic is an involuntary, rapid, non-rhythmical movement, while vocal tics consist of noises and sounds. Tics may be classified as simple or complex. Simple motor tics include eye blinks, grimaces, and head or arm jerks. Complex motor tics are often related to compulsive acts and include grooming behaviors, sequential touching of objects and body parts, and aggressive actions directed against oneself or others. Simple vocal tics include grunts, throat clearing, clicking, snorting and animal sounds, such as barking or quacking. Complex vocal tics consist of words and phrases that are often repeated. Commonly, complex vocal tics take the form of obscenities, or coprolalia, that describe sexual acts or body elimination functions. Coprolalia and other 'forbidden' words may occur at inappropriate times. For example, a patient may shout 'F--ing oink-oink' when passing a policeman (Devinsky and Geller, 1992). Coprolalia is often the most socially disabling symptom. Patients often describe an irresistible 'itch to tic' (Bliss, 1980).

Tic disorders form a continuum along a spectrum from rare tics in 'normal' persons, in whom they are often considered mannerisms or habits, to Tourette's syndrome. In primary tic disorders, other neurological problems are absent. Transient tic disorder, which occurs in up to 15 percent of children and adolescents, is characterized by simple motor or vocal tics that last from two weeks to one year (American Psychiatric Association, 1987). Eye blinks and sudden head movements are most common. The tics may briefly recur during adulthood, especially during periods of stress. In chronic motor tic disorder, the tics last longer than one year and occur almost every day, but do not include vocal tics. Tics are often exacerbated by stress, anxiety or fatigue and are diminished during activities requiring mental concentration and in sleep.

In addition to primary tic disorders, tics may also occur in other neuropsychiatric disorders, including Huntington's chorea, dystonia musculorum deformans, neuroacanthocytosis, and infectious or postinfectious diseases of the central nervous system (e.g. encephalitis, Sydenham's chorea). Tics can result from medications, including amphetamines, methylphenidate, cocaine, levodopa, carbamazepine and phenytoin. Tardive tics (i.e. tics which first develop after medication has been discontinued) occur after the use of dopamine-blocking medications. Tics may follow head trauma, stroke, carbon monoxide poisoning, static perinatal encephalopathy and degenerative disorders (Devinsky and Geller, 1992).

In Tourette's syndrome, diagnosis requires all five of the following criteria (American Psychiatric Press, 1987):

1. Both multiple motor and one or more vocal tics have been present at some time during the illness, although not necessarily concurrently.

2. Tics occur many times a day (usually in bouts), nearly every day or intermittently throughout a period of more than one year.

3. The anatomical location, number, frequency, complexity and severity of the tics changes over time.

4. The tics begin before the age of 21 years.

5. Tics do not occur exclusively during psychoactive substance intoxication or known central nervous system disease, such as Huntington's chorea or postviral encephalitis.

There is a 3:1 male predominance among sufferers of Tourette's syndrome. Symptoms first occur between 2 and 15 years of age (mean: 7 years) in more than 90 percent of patients. The initial symptom is most often a tic in the upper body, commonly involving the eyes or some other part of the face. Vocal tics are among the initial manifestations in approximately 30 percent of cases and begin within three years of onset in most others (Shapiro et al., 1978; Lees, 1985). Simple vocal tics usually occur first, but progress to include coprolalia in about 60 percent of cases. Tourette's syndrome is usually a lifelong illness, but the intensity of symptoms varies.

Patients with Tourette's syndrome usually have normal intelligence. Their IQ parallels that of the general population (Shapiro et al., 1978), but some patients may have difficulties with reading, writing and arithmetic (Jankovic, 1987). Although Tourette's syndrome has been described as 'psychosis with multiple tics', there is no evidence that psychosis is more prevalent in Tourette's syndrome. The patients' emotional response to external stimuli, their experience of affects, and their perception of other people's affect appear entirely normal. Instead, the syndrome may represent a disorder in the expression of affect (Devinsky and Geller, 1992).

Patients with moderate-to-severe Tourette's syndrome suffer from devastating social stigma. Patients are often called 'bizarre', 'crazy', or 'comical' because of their tics, especially vocal tics which often limit social and employment opportunities. Secondary depression is fairly common and is often overlooked.

In addition to motor and vocal tics, patients with Tourette's syndrome have a variety of behavioral symptoms that sometimes cause still greater morbidity. More than half of the patients under the age of 20 years have attention deficit disorder (ADD) with hyperactivity. Unfortunately, therapy for ADD with amphetamines or methylphenidate may exacerbate the tics. Obsessions and compulsions, including obtrusive sexual and aggressive thoughts and actions, occur in roughly half of patients. Mahler and Rangell (1943) described the inability to inhibit sexual and aggressive impulses as 'emotional incontinence'.

Antidopaminergic compounds such as haloperidol and pimozide are highly efficacious for the tics and may relieve obsessive–compulsive phenomena (Mesulam and Petersen, 1987; Devinsky and Geller, 1992). However, the side effects of these medications must be weighed against their therapeutic benefits (even though tardive movement disorders due to neuroleptics are rare among Tourette patients). Clonidine may be used as a first-line agent to treat vocal tics and clonazepam is often used to treat motor tics. Dopamine-depleting agents such as reserpine and tetrabenazine can also be effective in treating tics. Other therapies that help limit associated obsessions and compulsions include clonidine and chloripramine, as well as behavioral therapy.

Additional disorders associated with Tourette's syndrome include (roughly in decreasing order of frequency): sleep disorder; palilalia, which is repeating of one's own sounds or words (most often the last or first syllable) with increasing speed; echolalia, or the repeating of sounds or words from an external source; echopraxia, or repeating movements made by another person; and copropraxia, characterized by such obscene gestures as simulating masturbation or gesturing with the middle finger extended.

References

American Psychiatric Association. *Diagnostic and Statistical Manual of Mental Disorders (DSM – IIIR)* (3rd edition, revised). Washington, DC: American Psychiatric Association Press, 1987.

Bliss J. Sensory experiences of Gilles de la Tourette's syndrome. *Arch Gen Psychiat* 1980; **37**: 1343–7.

Devinsky O, Geller BD. Gilles de la Tourette's syndrome. In: *Disorder of Movement in Psychiatry and Neurology* (Joseph AB, Young RR, eds). Oxford, Cambridge, MA: Blackwell Scientific Publications, Inc., (1992).

Jankovic J. The neurology of tics. In: *Movement Disorders 2* (Marsden CD, Fahn S, eds). Oxford: Butterworths, 1987.

Lees AZ. *Tics and Related Disorders*. Edinburgh, New York: Churchill Livingstone, 1985.

Mahler MS, Rangell L. A psychosomatic study of *maladie des tics* (Gilles de la Tourette's disease). *Psychiatr Q* 1943; **17**: 579–603.

Mesulam M-M, Petersen RC. Treatment of Gilles de la Tourette's syndrome: Eight-year practice-based experience in a predominantly adult population. *Neurology* 1987; **37**: 1828–33.

Shapiro AK, Shapiro ED, Brunn RD *et al. Gilles de la Tourette Syndrome*. New York: Raven Press, 1978, pp. 115–45.

84.   *Parkinson's disease is often accompanied by depression and cognitive impairment*

Parkinsonism is a common neurological syndrome characterized by progressive slowness of movement (bradykinesia), rigidity, tremor most prominent at rest, and abnormal posture and gait. Bradykinesia is often the most troubling symptom. Patients are aspontaneous and have difficulty initiating and executing movements. Rigidity predominates in flexor muscles of the limbs and trunk and, as in other extrapyramidal disorders, this increased muscle tone tends to be equal throughout passive limb excursion ('lead-pipe rigidity') and is not accompanied by increased tendon reflexes. In contrast, spasticity from pyramidal lesions is characterized by increased tone that is maximal during initial limb movement, with increased reflexes. 'Cogwheel rigidity' refers to ratchet-like interruptions in passive movements that are due to rigidity with superimposed tremor. The coarse tremor of parkinsonism is most prominent during rest and is diminished with voluntary movements. The trunk progressively flexes over the waist and walking is difficult to initiate, with small steps and decreased arm swings. Postural instability causes some patients to walk more and more rapidly; in some cases, they require a wall to stop.

These primary symptoms of Parkinson's disease (PD) are often accompanied by expressionless facial features, diminished voice volume, dysarthria, small handwriting (micrographia), sleep disorder, oily seborrheic skin, excessive salivation and constipation.

The pathology of idiopathic PD is degeneration of the dopaminergic substantia nigra and other pigmented brainstem nuclei (noradrenergic locus ceruleus, serotonergic dorsal raphe). Other causes of parkinsonism – such as antipsychotic drugs, encephalitis, and carbon monoxide poisoning – either destroy the dopaminergic nigral cells or the basal ganglia nuclei upon which they terminate, or they block postsynaptic dopamine receptors. Treatment with dopaminergic replacement drugs (e.g. levodopa, bromocriptine) improves bradykinesia, rigidity and gait, but has less consistent effect on tremor. Therefore, this movement disorder is largely due to decreased dopaminergic activity.

Before dopaminergic agents became available, signs and symptoms of parasympathetic overactivity (especially in postencephalitic patients) led to the predominance of anticholinergic drugs for parkinsonism therapy. While anticholinergic therapy is only effective for mild motor symptoms in idiopathic PD, it is highly effective for the parkinsonism syndrome resulting from antipsychotic medications. This is probably because anticholinergics are potent inhibitors of dopamine reuptake, and nigral cells are still producing normal amounts of dopamine in these patients (Coyle and Snyder, 1969). Such clinical observations led to the dopamine–acetylcholine balance theory of parkinsonism (Van Woert *et al.*, 1972). In this simplified construct, dopaminergic deficiency leads to cholinergic hyperactivity in the striatum. Thus, drugs that either increase dopaminergic activity or decrease cholinergic activity will 'restore the balance'.

Although James Parkinson's original 1817 essay on 'the shaking palsy' held that intellectual functions are unaltered until delirium intervenes, shortly before death, it is now well recognized that mental changes often accompany PD. Schwab *et al.* (1951) described several psychiatric disorders in PD, including reactive depression, medication side effects and paroxysmal disorders specifically related to PD. The non-epileptic paroxysmal disorders were most common in patients with postencephalitic parkinsonism who also had oculogyric crises, and they included compulsive thoughts, depression, anxiety and paranoia.

In assessing affective and cognitive disorders in PD, one must differentiate these problems from deficits due to impaired motor performance and somatic complaints (Levin *et al.*, 1988). Tests with time limits or those requiring motor responses are biased against patients with a movement disorder.

Depression has been reported in 30 to 90 percent of PD patients (Mayeux, 1982; Levin *et al.*, 1988). Bradykinesia and bradyphrenia in PD may simulate depression, as the patient is slow in thought and action, and their faces betray little emotion. It is important specifically to assess cognitive and vegetative features of depression (Maxim 95). In Parkinson's disease, depression is accompanied by decreased drive and motivation, concerns over health and somatic complaints, pessimism and hopelessness. Suicidal thoughts are common but completed suicide is rare in PD.

The pathogenesis of depression is probably related to both psychosocial adjustment and neurobiological changes (Robins, 1976; Hoehn *et al.*, 1976; Mindham *et al.*, 1976; Mayeux *et al.*, 1984; Taylor *et al.*, 1988). Gotham *et al.* (1986) found no differences in scores on a standardized depression scale when comparing patients with PD with patients who had arthritis, another progressive and physically disabling illness. However, Horn (1974) found an increased incidence of depression in PD patients compared with an age-matched disabled group. A reactive etiology for depression is supported by studies showing that severity of depression tends to parallel severity of disordered movement in PD (Gotham *et al.*, 1986; Mayeux *et al.*, 1981). Others have not found an association between the severity of depression and PD, suggesting that biological mechanisms, rather than reaction to a disabling illness may account for depression (Celesia and Wanamaker, 1972; Horn, 1974; Robins, 1976; Mayeux *et al.*, 1984).

The monoamine hypothesis of endogenous depression (Garver and Davis, 1979; Schildkraut, 1973) has been extended to account for some of the affective changes in PD (Hoehn *et al.*, 1976; Robins, 1976). Santamaria *et al.* (1986) found that among newly diagnosed PD patients, depression more frequently afflicted younger and less disabled individuals. Therefore, they proposed that there is a subgroup of PD patients in whom the first clinical manifestation is affective and results from abnormal monoaminergic transmission. Mayeux *et al.* (1984) found decreased levels of the serotonin metabolite 5-HIAA in the cerebrospinal fluid of depressed PD patients compared with non-depressed PD patients or controls; these findings await replication. The depression in PD patients probably results from both reactive and endogenous mechanisms, with the relative contributions being highly variable in individual cases. Therapy of depression in PD has not been well studied, although several studies found little or no benefit from levodopa–carbidopa (Damasio *et al.*, 1971; Mindham *et al.*, 1976). Mood and motoric fluctuations may occur together with the 'on–off' phenomenon, but motor disability is almost always more severe than behavioral changes (Delis *et al.*, 1982; Girotti *et al.*, 1986). Antidepressant medication is helpful in some depressed PD patients.

Among patients with idiopathic PD, mania is rare. However, mania was not uncommon among patients with postencephalitic parkinsonism, especially during the initial illness (von Economo, 1931).

Psychiatric complications from drugs for PD are common, especially among the elderly. Levodopa–carbidopa therapy causes hallucinations, paranoia, mania, insomnia, anxiety, nightmares, hypersexuality and depression (Yahr, 1978). Bromocriptine causes similar side effects. Anticholinergic drugs cause delirium, confusion, lethargy, hallucinations and other behavioral reactions that often limit their use.

The frequency, severity, phenomenology and pathogenesis of dementia in PD are controversial issues. Several studies have reported that approximately one-third of PD patients develop dementia (Pollock and Hornabrook, 1966; Martilla and Rinne, 1976; Rajput *et al.*, 1984). However, Brown and Marsden (1984) reviewed the literature and found several important methodologic weaknesses that artificially increased the estimated prevalence of dementia in PD. They suggest that among patients with idiopathic PD who do not have pyramidal or cerebellar signs, only 15 to 20 percent develop dementia. In a consecutive series of 100 PD patients, Taylor *et al.* (1985) found that 8 percent of patients met DSM-IIIR criteria for dementia (12 percent of those 65 years or older). In contrast, Mayeux *et al.* (1988), using the same criteria, found the prevalence rate for dementia was 3.75 times higher in patients with PD than expected for age (Mayeux *et al.*, 1988). If detailed neuropsychological tests are employed, more than 90 percent of patients have cognitive impairment that is usually mild and does not interfere with daily living (Pirozzolo *et al.*, 1982). Visuospatial functions (especially facial recognition) are impaired early in PD (Levin *et al.*, 1991). Dementia is more common in PD patients who also have signs and symptoms of other neurological disorders (Sroka *et al.*, 1981).

During the early stages of PD, intellectual function is usually well preserved, although frontal deficits (e.g. perseverative errors and difficulty shifting conceptual sets) are common and may contribute to mental inflexibility (Lees and Smith, 1983). Impaired facial recognition, a task which requires analysis of complex embedded stimuli, is partially dependent on frontal systems (Luria, 1966). Other features of PD attributed to frontal dysfunction include bradyphrenia, impaired verbal fluency, problems with planning and execution of constructional tasks (Lees and Smith,

1983; Stern *et al.*, 1984; Pillon *et al.*, 1989). Language functions are relatively preserved in the dementia of PD.

Although Mortimer *et al.* (1982) found a significant correlation between motor and intellectual dysfunction, others have not confirmed this relationship (Taylor *et al.*, 1988).

The severity and progression of cognitive dysfunction in PD is age-related: younger patients fair better. Onset of cognitive problems and dementia is delayed and progresses more slowly in younger patients compared to older patients with PD (Lieberman *et al.*, 1979).

The use of anticholinergic drugs in PD has led to concern that these agents may exacerbate memory impairment. Scopolamine, an anticholinergic drug, impairs memory storage in normal subjects without affecting immediate memory (Drachman and Leavitt, 1974). This amnesic effect is blocked by physostigmine, an anticholinesterase that increases cholinergic activity by blocking degradation of acetylcholine (Drachman, 1977). In PD patients with preserved cognition, anticholinergics in standard clinical doses do not impair memory (Levin, personal communication). However, anticholinergic drugs may impair memory in PD patients with cognitive impairment.

The dementia in PD is etiologically heterogeneous, and may include pathological changes of Alzheimer's disease, such as neurofibrillary tangles and senile plaques; subcortical and, in some cases, cortical Lewy bodies; and degeneration in dopaminergic and noradrenergic systems (Hakim and Mathieson, 1979; Lieberman *et al.*, 1979; Jellinger, 1986; Cash *et al.*, 1987). Although cognitive symptoms, especially slowness of thought (brady-phrenia), may improve after dopaminergic therapy, the positive response is usually mild and transient.

References

Brown RG, Marsden CD. How common is dementia in Parkinson's disease? *Lancet* 1984; **ii**: 1262

Cash R, Dennis T, L'Heureux R, Raisman R, Javoy-Agid F, Scatton B. Parkinson's disease and dementia: Norepinephrine and dopamine in the locus ceruleus. *Neurology* 1987; **37**: 42–6.

Celesia GG, Wanamaker WM. Psychiatric disturbances in Parkinson's disease. *Dis Nerv Syst* 1972; **33**: 577–83.

Coyle JT, Snyder SH. Antiparkinsonian drugs: Inhibition of dopamine uptake in the corpus striatum as a possible mechanism of action. *Science* 1969; **166**: 899–903.

Damasio AR, Lobo-Antunes J, Macedo C. Psychiatric aspects in parkinsonism treated with L-dopa. *J Neurol Neurosurg Psychiat* 1971; **34**: 502–7.

Delis D, Direnfeld L, Alexander MP, Kaplan E. Cognitive fluctuations associated with on–off phenomenon in Parkinson disease. *Arch Neurol* 1982; **32**: 1049–52.

Drachman DA. Memory and cognitive function in man: does the cholinergic system have a specific role? *Neurology* 1977; **27**: 783–90.

Drachman DA, Leavitt J. Human memory and the cholinergic system: a relation to aging? *Arch Neurol* 1974; **30**: 113–21.

Garver DL, Davis JM. Biogenic amine hypothesis of affective disorders. *Life Sci* 1979; **24**: 383–94.

Girotti F, Carella F, Grassi MP, Soliveri P, Marano R, Caraceni T. Motor and cognitive performances of Parkinsonian patients in the on and off phases of the disease. *J Neurol Neurosurg Psychiat* 1986; **49**: 657–60.

Gotham AM, Brown RG, Marsden CD. Depression in Parkinson's disease: a quantitative and qualitative analysis. *J Neurol Neurosurg Psychiat* 1986; **49**: 381–9.

Hakim A, Mathieson G. Dementia in Parkinson disease. *Neurology* 1979; **29**: 1209–14.

Hoehn M, Crowley TJ, Rutledge CO. Dopamine correlates of neurological and psychological status in untreated parkinsonism. *J Neurol Neurosurg Psychiat* 1976; **39**: 941–51.

Horn S. Some psychological factors in parkinsonism. *J Neurol Neurosurg Psychiat* 1974; **37**: 27–31.

Jellinger K. Pathology of parkinsonism. In: *Recent Developments in Parkinson's Disease* (Fahn S, ed.). New York: Raven Press, 1986, pp. 33–66.

Lees AJ, Smith E. Cognitive deficits in the early stages of Parkinson's disease. *Brain* 1983; **106**: 257–70.

Levin BE, Llabre MM, Reisman S, Weiner WJ, Sanchez-Ramos J, Singer C, Brown MC. Visuospatial impairment in Parkinson's disease. *Neurology* 1991; **41**: 365–9.

Levin BE, Llabre MM, Weiner WJ. Parkinson's disease and depression: psychometric properties of the Beck Depression Inventory. *J Neurol Neurosurg Psychiat* 1988; **51**: 140–4.

Levin BE. Spatial cognition in Parkinson disease. *Alzheimer Dis Assoc Dis* 1990; **4**: 161–70.

Lieberman A, Dziarolowski M, Kupersmith M *et al*. Dementia in Parkinson's disease. *Ann Neurol* 1979; **6**: 355–9.

Luria AR. *Higher Cortical Functions in Man*. New York: Basic Books, 1966.

Martilla R, Rinne U. Dementia in Parkinson's disease. *Acta Neurol Scand* 1976; **54**: 431–41.

Mayeux R. Depression and dementia in Parkinson's disease In: *Movement Disorders* (Marsden CD, Fahn S, eds). Oxford: Butterworth, 1982, pp. 75–95.

Mayeux R, Stern Y, Cote L, Williams JBW. Altered serotonin metabolism in depressed patients with Parkinson's disease. *Neurology* 1984; **34**: 642–6.

Mayeux R, Stern Y, Rosen J *et al*. Depression, intellectual impairment, and Parkinson's disease. *Neurology* 1981; **31**: 645–50.

Mayeux R, Stern Y, Rosenstein R, Marder K, Hauser A, Cote L, Fahn S. An estimate of the prevalence of dementia in idiopathic Parkinson's disease. *Arch Neurol* 1988; **45**: 260–2.

Mindham RHS, Marsden CD, Parkes JO. Psychiatric symptoms during L-dopa therapy for Parkinson's disease and their relationship to physical disability. *Psychol Med* 1976; **6**: 23–33.

Mortimer JA, Pirozzolo FJ, Hansich EC, Webster DD. Relationship of motor symptoms to intellectual deficits in Parkinson's disease. *Neurology* 1982; **32**: 133–7.

Parkinson J. *An Essay on the Shaking Palsy*. London: Sherwood, Neely and Jones, 1817.

Pillon B, Dubois B, Bonnet AM *et al*. Cognitive slowing in Parkinson's disease fails to respond to levodopa treatment: the 15-object test. *Neurology* 1989; **39**: 762–8.

Pirozzolo FJ, Hansch EC, Mortimer J *et al*. Dementia in Parkinson disease: A neuropsychological analysis. *Brain Cogn* 1982; **1**: 71–83.

Pollock M, Hornabrook RW. The prevalence, natural history, and dementia of Parkinson's disease. *Brain* 1966; **89**: 429–48.

Rajput AH, Offord K, Beard M *et al*. Epidemiological survey of dementia in parkinsonism and control population. In: *Advances in Neurology* (volume 40) (Hassler G, Christ J, eds). New York: Raven Press, 1984 pp. 229–34.

Robins AH. Depression in patients with Parkinsonism. *Br J Psychiat* 1976; **128**: 141–5.

Santamaria J, Tolosa E, Valles A. Parkinson's disease with depression: A possible subgroup of idiopathic parkinsonism. *Neurology* 1986; **36**: 1130–3.

Schildkraut JJ. Neuropharmacology of the affective disorders. *Ann Rev Pharmacol* 1973; **13**: 427–54.

Schwab RS, Fabing HD, Pritchard JS. Psychiatric symptoms and syndromes in Parkinson's disease. *Am J Psychiat* 1951; **107**: 901.

Sroka H, Elizan TS, Yahr MD, Burger B, Mendoza MR. Organic mental syndrome and confusional states in Parkinson's disease: Relationship to computerized tomographic signs of cerebral atrophy. *Arch Neurol* 1981; **38**: 339–42.

Stern Y, Mayeux R, Rosen J. Contribution of perceptual motor dysfunction to construction and tracing disturbances in Parkinson's disease. *J Neurol Neurosurg Psychiat* 1984; **47**: 983–4.

Taylor AE, Saint-Cyr JA, Lang AE. Dementia prevalence in Parkinson's disease. *Lancet* 1985; **i**: 1037.

Taylor AE, Saint-Cyr JA, Lang AE. Idiopathic Parkinson's disease: Revised concepts of cognitive and affective status. *Can J Neurol Sci* 1988; **15**: 106–13.

Van Woert MH, Ambani LM, Bowers MB. Levodopa and cholinergic hypersensitivity in Parkinson's disease. *Neurology* 1972; **22**; 86.

Von Economo C. *Encephalitis Lethargica* (Newman KO, transl). Oxford, New York: Oxford University Press, 1931.

Yahr MD. Overview of present day treatment of Parkinson's disease. *J Neural Transm* 1978; **43**: 227–38.

85.   *In Huntington's disease and Sydenham's chorea behavioral changes may precede abnormal movements*

'Insanity with a tendency to suicide' was one of the three principal features originally described by Huntington (1872). The emotional and intellectual deterioration of this autosomal dominant disorder is feared more than the progressive motor impairment by persons at risk – and their relatives (Stern and Eldridge, 1975). Pathologic changes are maximal in the basal ganglia (Maxim 16).

Common motor symptoms in Huntington's disease include choreiform, 'dance-like' movements as well as dyskinesia, dysarthia and ataxia. Early in the course, chorea appears as 'piano-playing' finger movements, usually observed while walking, or as slight facial grimaces or twitches. In the Westphal variant, extrapyramidal rigidity is the predominant motor disorder (Hayden, 1981).

However, changes in personality are often the first clinical features to develop in patients with Huntington's disease (Dewhurst *et al.*, 1969). Patients are described as 'hard to get along with', impulsive, erratic and disposed to fits of rage or despondency (Martin, 1984). The premorbid personality may be exaggerated or reversed; quiet individuals become introverted and pathetic, extroverts become boisterous, irritable and aggressive, or vise versa (Hayden, 1981). Sleep disorders and appetite changes are often early symptoms. Impaired capacity to function at home and work is common, with diminished spontaneity, lack of insight and initiative, emotional lability, impulsiveness and impaired judgment. Sexual promiscuity and antisocial behavior, including criminal acts, may also occur early in the course (Brothers, 1964; Heathfield, 1967). As the disease progresses, behavioral disorders are more severe; during the latter stages, an apathetic-abulic state with prominent involuntary movements is typical.

Major affective disorders (depression and bipolar disorder) occur in approximately 40 percent of patients with Huntington's disease (Caine and Shoulson, 1983). Depression is much more common than mania, and mood disorders usually develop after personality and motor changes are evident. Apathy is a prominent feature of the depression in Huntington's disease. Chorea often decreases with depression and increases with mania (Whittier *et al.*, 1961; McHugh and Folstein, 1975). Although psychological and social factors may contribute to the development of behavioral changes, especially depression, affective disorders are primarily due to the disease. A biologic – rather than psychosocial – etiology for the affective symptoms is supported by the following findings: development of depression in Huntington's patients prior to diagnosis, as in adopted patients unaware of their risk; the occurrence of manic episodes, which are exceedingly rare in a reactive depression; the episodic nature of depressive symptoms; and the presence of vegetative symptoms, such as anorexia and sleep disorders (McHugh and Folstein, 1975).

Suicide is increased in patients with Huntington's disease. Reed *et al.* (1958) found that, among non-institutionalized patients, 7.8 percent of men and 6.4 percent of women died of suicide. Depression responds to tricyclic antidepressants; mania responds to neuroleptics and may improve with lithium (Whittier *et al.*, 1961; McHugh and Folstein, 1975; Caine and Shoulson, 1983). However, antidepressants often improve the somatic signs of depression without affecting the patients' dysphoric outlook (Caine and Shoulson, 1983).

Schizophreniform psychosis may develop before, concurrently or after motor symptoms. Psychosis affects approximately 10 percent of patients and is more frequent among those who are younger (Heathfield, 1967; Bolt, 1970). Paranoid delusions are the most prominent feature, although auditory and visual hallucinations occur. Neuroleptics are useful in treating both the psychosis and the involuntary movements, but can exacerbate frontal lobe dysfunction, and in the occasional patient with the Westphal variant, can exacerbate rigidity.

Dementia is present in many moderate and advanced cases of Huntington's disease, with mild neuropsychological deficits present during the early stages. Visuospatial and auditory memory deficits are the earliest signs of cognitive impairment (Josiassen *et al.*, 1983), and short-term memory disorder is often the first cognitive deficit observed by family members. Retrieval of information from long-term memory and other symptoms of global cognitive deterioration subsequently develop in many patients.

Sydenham's (rheumatic) chorea probably results from striatal injury, although the neuropathological changes of inflammation and neuronal cell loss also involve the substantia nigra, subthalamic nucleus, and to a lesser degree, the cerebral cortex (Greenfield and Wolfsohn, 1922; Wilson and Winkelman, 1923; Colony and Malamud, 1956). Therefore, the correlation between behavioral symptoms and striatal pathology is imperfect. Also, similar neuropathological changes have been reported in patients with rheumatic fever but without chorea (Bruetsch, 1944; Neubuerger, 1947; Costero, 1949). However, antibodies directed against the cytoplasm of the subthalamic and caudate nuclei are present in almost half of patients with Sydenham's chorea, but in less than a fifth of those with rheumatic fever only, and were absent in controls, suggesting that the basal ganglia are involved in Sydenham's chorea (Husby *et al.*, 1976).

In Sydenham's chorea, the movement disorder may occur with or without joint, skin and cardiac symptoms. Although chorea is the most common and prominent central nervous system manifestation, during the initial stage of the illness, delirium, hallucinations, seizures, depression, mania, paranoia, catatonia, compulsive behavior, tics and aggressiveness can occur (Lewis and Minski, 1935; Bender, 1942; Ch'ien *et al.*, 1978). Long-term sequelae are common and disrupt personality and emotion more than intellect (Bird, 1976; Lishman, 1987) and, again, bear a striking relationship to behavioral changes after frontal lobe injury. Obsessive–compulsive behaviors are also common sequelae (Chapman *et al.*, 1958; Swedo *et al.*, 1989). There is also an increased incidence of motor disorders such as excessive mirror movements, tremor, impaired fine motor control and impaired tandem walking following Sydenham's chorea (Bird, 1976).

References

Bender L. Post-encephalitic behavior disorders in childhood. In: *Encephalitis: A Clinical Study* (Neal JB, ed.). New York: Grune and Stratton, 1942, p. 448.

Bird MT, Palkes H, Prensky AL. A follow-up study of Sydenham's chorea. *Neurology* 1976; **26**: 601–6.

Bolt JM. Huntington's chorea in the West of Scotland. *Br J Psychiat* 1970; **116**: 259–70.

Brothers CRD. Huntington's chorea in Victoria and Tasmania. *J Neurol Sci* 1964; **1**: 405–20.

Bruetsch WL. Late cerebral sequelae of rheumatic fever. *Arch Intern Med* 1944; **73**: 472–6.

Caine ED, Shoulson I. Psychiatric syndromes in Huntington's disease. *Am J Psychiat* 1983; **140**: 728–33.

Chapman AH, Pilkey L, Gibbons MJ. A psychosomatic study of eight children with Sydenham's chorea. *Pediatrics* 1958; **21**: 582–95.

Ch'ien LT, Economides AN, Lemmi H. Sydenham's chorea and seizures: Clinical and electroencephalographic studies. *Arch Neurol* 1978; **35**: 382–5.

Colony HS, Malamud N. Sydenham's chorea: A clinicopathologic study. *Neurology* 1956; **6**: 672–6.

Costero I. Cerebral lesions responsible for death of patients with active rheumatic fever. *Arch Neurol* 1949; **62**: 48–72.

Dewhurst K, Oliver J, Trick KLK, McKnight AL. Neuropsychiatric aspects of Huntington's chorea. *Confin Neurol* 1969; **31**: 258–68.

Greenfield JG, Wolfsohn JM. The pathology of Sydenham's chorea. *Lancet* 1922; **ii**: 603–6.

Hayden MR. *Huntington's Chorea*. Berlin, New York: Springer-Verlag, 1981, pp. 72–4.

Heathfield KWG. Huntington's chorea: investigation into prevalence of this disease in the area covered by the North East Metropolitan Hospital Board. *Brain* 1967; **90**: 203–32.

Huntington G. On chorea. *Med Surg Rep* 1872; **26**: 317–21.

Husby G, van de Ryn I, Zabrisskie JB *et al.* Antibodies reacting with cytoplasm of subthalamic and caudate nuclei neurons in chorea and rheumatic fever. *J Exp Med* 1976; **144**: 1094–110.

Josiassen RC, Curry LM, Mancall EL. Development of neuropsychological deficits in Huntington's disease. *Arch Neurol* 1983; **40**: 791–6.

Lewis AJ, Minski L. Chorea and psychosis. *Lancet* 1935; **i**: 536–8.

Lishman WA. *Organic Psychiatry*. Oxford, Boston, MA: Blackwell Scientific Publications, 1987, pp. 393–400.

Martin JB. Huntington's disease: New approaches to an old problem. *Neurology* 1984; **34**: 1059–72.

McHugh PR, Folstein MF. Psychiatric syndromes of Huntington's chorea. In: *Psychiatric Aspects of Neurologic Disease* (Benson DF, Blumer D, eds). New York: Grune and Stratton, 1975, pp. 275–85.

Neubuerger KT. The brain in rheumatic fever. *Dis Nerv Syst* 1947; **8**: 259–62.

Reed TE, Chandler HJ, Hughes E, Davidson RT. Huntington's chorea in Michigan: demography and genetics. *Am J Hum Genet* 1958; **10**: 201–25.

Stern R, Eldridge R. Attitudes of patients and their relatives to Huntington's disease. *J Med Gen* 1975; **12**: 217–23.

Swedo SE, Rapoport JL, Cheslow DL, Leonard HL, Ayurb EM, Hosier DM, Wald ER. High prevalence of obsessive – compulsive symptoms in patients with Sydenham's chorea. *Am J Psychiat* 1989; **146**: 246–9.

Whittier J, Haydu G, Crawford J. Effect of imipramine on depression and hyperkinesia in Hutington's disease. *Am J. Psychiat* 1961; **118**:79.

Wilson G, Winkelman NW. A clinicopathologic study of acute and chronic chorea. *Arch Neurol* 1923; **9**: 170–7.

15
Sleep Disorders

86. Prescribe only short-term courses of sedative–hypnotic drugs for insomnia

Insomnia is a subjective disorder of inadequate, non-restorative sleep. Difficulty falling asleep is the most common problem in insomnia, but this symptom is often accompanied by awakenings throughout the night and early final awakening (Kales *et al.*, 1984). Insomnia is the most common sleep disorder and annually afflicts approximately a third of adults (Karacan *et al.*, 1976; Bixler *et al.*, 1979). It is more common among women and the elderly (Bixler *et al.*, 1979; Kales *et al.*, 1987) as well as those with psychiatric, substance-abuse and medical disorders (Mellinger *et al.*, 1985; Coleman *et al.*, 1982). Important issues in the sleep history are summarized in Table 86.1.

On the basis of its duration, insomnia may be classified as transient (less than three nights), short-term (three nights to three weeks), and chronic (more than three weeks). This classification is the key factor in the evaluation and treatment of insomnia. Transient and short-term insomnia are common and are usually caused by stress (Table 86.2). In these patients,

Table 86.1 History-taking in patients with sleep disorders.

Define the problem – Obtain history from patient and bedpartner or parent
   Insomnia (disorders of initiating and maintaining sleep)
   Disorder of excessive somnolence
   Disorder of the sleep–wake cycle
   Dysfunction associated with sleep, sleep stages or partial arousals
     (parasomnia)
Patient's 24 hour sleep–wake cycle (inquire about daytime naps)
Onset and duration of disorder
Life situation (inquire about stress, bedtime anxiety and ruminations)
Medical, neurological and psychiatric history
Current medications (prescribed and over-the-counter)
Ethanol, sedative-hypnotic or illicit drug use
Family history of sleep disorder

Table 86.2   Causes of transient and short-term insomnia.

Job-related problems
Interpersonal conflicts
Financial problems
Major life changes (death or termination of close relationship, birth of
   child, marriage)
Hospitalization
Medical problem
Pain
Jet-lag
Altered work shift
Drug or alcohol use
Rebound insomnia after withdrawal of short-acting sedative–hypnotic
   drugs
High altitude

improved sleep can often be achieved by a combination of open discussion of stressful issues with relatives or the physician; relaxation exercises; avoidance of alcohol, caffeine, cigarettes, diet pills and daytime naps; regular, moderate, daytime exercise; a routine for sleep that includes fairly regular bedtime and rising time, and reading but no television before sleeping; an optimal sleep environment of comfortable temperature; and shades and earplugs to block out extraneous light and sound. If these measures fail and the patient finds she continues to 'toss and turn' all night, it may be advisable for her to turn the light on and read, or engage in another activity, until she is sleepy again.

Sedative-hypnotic drugs can be an effective adjunct to these behavioral measures (Editorial, 1984). These drugs should not be prescribed unless the physician has explored the nature and cause of the insomnia, and they should be part of, but *not the entire*, therapeutic strategy. Pharmacologic therapy for insomnia should be initiated only after more obvious causes, such as coffee after dinner, have been addressed and only if the sleep disorder is interfering with social or occupational functions. Despite the widespread use of sedative-hypnotic drugs, up to 85 percent of persons with serious insomnia remain untreated (Mellinger *et al.*, 1985). We may be treating the wrong patients.

Benzodiazepines are the drugs most commonly used to treat insomnia, but antihistamines, barbiturates and chloral hydrate are also effective. The advantages of benzodiazepines for short-term use include their effectiveness, safety (lethal overdoses are rare), minimal side effects, low addictive potential, absence of major withdrawal symptoms, and the lower incidence of patient tolerance to hypnotic effects than encountered with barbiturates, chloral hydrate or antihistamines (Gilin and Byerley, 1990). Table 86.3 shows the pharmacological data for the commonly used benzodiazepines. Only triazolam (Halcion), temazepam (Restoril), flurazepam (Dalmane),

Table 86.3 Commonly used benzodiazepines.

Drug	Dose range for insomnia (mg)	Equivalent dosages	Active metabolite	Half-life (hours)
Short-acting				
Triazolam* (Halcion)	0.125–0.5	0.25	–	3–4
Midazolam		10	–	2–5
Intermediate-acting				
Temazepam* (Restoril)	15–30	15	–	15
Estazopam* (ProSom)	0.5–2.0	1.0	–	15
Oxazepam		15	–	10
Lorazepam		1	–	15
Alprazolam		0.5	–	15
Nitrazepam†		10	–	28
Long-acting				
Flurazepam* (Dalmane)	15–30	15	+	60
Quazepam* (Doral)	7.5–30	15	+	40
Diazepam		5	+	72
Clonazepam		1	+	60

*Marketed in the USA as hypnotics.
†Not marketed in the USA.

quazepam (Doral) and estazopam (ProSom) are technically marketed in the USA as hypnotics, but other benzodiazepines are widely used for this purpose. Benzodiazepines with short half-lives are less likely to accumulate or have sedative or antianxiety effects the following day, but they are more likely to cause rebound insomnia after discontinuation, anterograde amnesia, tolerance to hypnotic effects and early final awakening. The central nervous system side effects of benzodiazepines increase with the patient's age, dose and duration of therapy (Greenblatt *et al.*, 1977, 1991). Triazolam appears to have the highest incidence of side effects (including next day anxiety and irritability, depression, confusion and anterograde amnesia), although its short half-life makes it one of the most popular sleeping pills (Kales *et al.*, 1983; Bixler *et al.*, 1987; Morris and Estes, 1987; Adams and Oswald, 1989). Quazepam is selective for the benzodiazepine omega-1 receptors, and appears to have fewer side effects such as next day sedation or psychomotor slowing, or rebound insomnia (Winsaur *et al.*, 1984; Sauvanet *et al.*, 1988). Benzodiazepines predispose patients to falls and fractures that probably result from ataxia and confusion, which are especially common in the elderly (Ray *et al.*, 1987).

Chronic insomnia leads to conditioned anxiety, with bedtime provoking fear of inability to sleep and of the effects of lost sleep. The non-pharmacological strategies mentioned above are often helpful. Psychiatric disorders are present in approximately half of patients with chronic insomnia, with depression being the most common (American Psychiatric Association, 1987). Alcohol, sedative and illicit drug use, medical and neurological disorders (e.g. hyperthyroidism, dementia), chronic pain, sleep apnea and nocturnal movement disorders (e.g. nocturnal myoclonus, restless-legs syndrome) may all cause chronic insomnia.

Hypnotic drugs are effective only for short-term treatment of insomnia. Nightly reliance on sleeping pills is undesirable; the physician should gradually taper and withdraw hypnotics after several weeks and reassess the patient in the drug-free state. The major problem with nightly sleeping pills is tolerance – higher and higher doses are required to produce the same hypnotic effect. As the dosage of medication is increased, daytime side effects become more likely. Severe anxiety, depression, irritability and other behavioral problems may develop insidiously and are often not attributed to sleeping pills until after the patient and family have suffered considerable hardship. When there is doubt concerning the cause of chronic insomnia, sleep studies, which can be obtained on an outpatient basis, are indicated. Referral to a sleep disorders center should be considered in cases of refractory insomnia.

References

Adams K, Oswald I. Can a rapidly-eliminated hypnotic cause daytime anxiety? *Pharmacopsychiatry* 1989; **22**: 115–19.

American Psychiatric Association. *Diagnostic and Statistical Manual of Mental Disorders (DSM-IIIR)* (3rd edition, revised). Washington, DC: American Psychiatric Association Press, 1987.

Bixler EO, Kales A, Brubaker EM, Kales JD. Adverse reactions to benzodiazepines hypnotics: spontaneous reporting system. *Pharmacology* 1987; **35**: 286–300.

Bixler EO, Kales A, Soldatos CR, Kales JD, Healey S. Prevalence of sleep disorders in the Los Angeles metropolitan area. *Am J Psychiat* 1979; **136**: 1257–62.

Coleman RM, Roffwarg HP, Kennedy SJ. Sleep–wake disorders based on a polysomnographic diagnosis: a national cooperative study. *JAMA* 1982; **247**: 997–1003.

Editorial. Drugs and Insomnia: the use of medications to promote sleep. *JAMA* 1984; **251**: 2410–14.

Gilin JC, Byerley WF. The diagnosis and management of insomnia. *New Engl J Med* 1990; **322**: 239–48.

Greenblatt DJ, Allen MD, Shader RI. Toxicity of high-dose flurazepam in the elderly. *Clin Pharm Ther* 1977; **21**: 355–61.

Greenblatt DJ, Harmatz JS, Sharpiro L, Engelhardt N, Gouthro TA, Shader RI. Sensitivity to triazolam in the elderly. *New Engl J Med* 1991; **324**: 1691–8.

Kales A, Kales JD, Sleep laboratory studies of hypnotic drugs: efficacy and withdrawal effects. *J Clin Psychopharmacol* 1983; **3**: 141–150.

Kales JD, Kales A, Bixler EO. Biopsychobehavioral correlates of insomnia: V. Clinical characteristics and behavioral correlates. *Am J Psychiat* 1984; **141**: 1371–6.

Kales A, Soldatos CR, Kales JD. Sleep disorders: Insomnia, sleepwalking, night terrors, nightmares, and enuresis. *Ann Int Med* 1987; **106**: 582–92.

Karacan I, Thornby JI, Anch M. Prevalence of sleep disturbance in a primarily urban Florida County. *Soc Sci Med* 1976; **10**: 239–44.

Mellinger GD, Malter MB, Uhlenhuth EH. Insomnia and its treatment: prevalence and correlates. *Arch Gen Psychiat* 1985; **42**: 225–32.

Morris HH, Estes ML. Traveler's amnesia: transient global amnesia secondary to triazolam. *JAMA* 1987; **258**: 945–6.

Ray WA, Griffin MR, Schaffner W, Baugh DK, Melton LJ. Psychotropic drug use and the risk of hip fracture. *N Engl J Med* 1987; **316**: 363–9.

Sauvanet JP, Langer SZ, Morselli PL, eds. Imidazopyridines in sleep disorders: a novel experimental and therapautic approach. *L.E.R.S. Monograph Series* (Volume 6). New York: Raven Press, 1988.

Winsaur HJ, O'Hair DE, Valero R. Quazepam: short-term treatment of insomnia in geriatric outpatients. *Curr Ther Res* 1984; **35**: 228–34.

87.   Patients with narcolepsy and certain other sleep disorders have episodes of automatic behavior and amnesia

Narcolepsy is characterized by excessive daytime sleepiness, with sleep attacks that last anywhere from seconds to 30 minutes (Kales *et al.*, 1987b). These irresistible attacks are usually preceded by drowsiness and a struggle to remain awake, and are followed by a refreshed, restored feeling. They are most apt to occur when the patient is bored or engaged in passive, monotonous activities such as listening to a lecture, watching television, or – most dangerously – while driving or flying. Almost all drivers who have narcolepsy report problems, and many have serious accidents (Yoss and Daly, 1963). Although it is less common, sleep attacks also occur in more stimulating situations, such as while eating a meal (face forward into the plate) or even repairing an aortic aneurysm (Daly and Yoss, 1974).

The three ancillary symptoms of narcolepsy are cataplexy, sleep paralysis and hypnogogic hallucinations. Cataplexy is a paroxysmal decrease or loss of muscle tone lasting 2 seconds to 20 minutes, but usually less than 2 minutes. It occurs in three-quarters of patients with narcolepsy. Patients may fall to the ground unable to move, but their consciousness is un-impaired. Cataplectic attacks are typically precipitated by strong emotion such as hearty laughter, surprise or anger. Sleep paralysis and hallucina-tions both on falling asleep (hypnagogic) and on awakening (hypno-pompic) occur during the transitional periods between wakefulness and sleep. Both the paralysis and hallucinations are each present in approxi-mately one-third of patients with narcolepsy (Roth, 1980). With sleep para-lysis, the muscles are suddenly and uncontrollably flaccid from several seconds to a minute and there is usually intense fear. In contrast to the hypnagogic and hypnopompic hallucinations in normal people, narcoleptic patients have intense affective responses, usually terror, in response to the auditory and visual hallucinations perceived as they fall asleep or awaken.

The automatic behavior syndrome in narcolepsy is a fourth auxillary feature that is often overlooked and has not been extensively studied, but occurs in half of patients with narcolepsy. During these episodes, which last minutes or hours, patients perform complex acts such as speaking, driving and sewing in an imperfect, robotic fashion (Guilleminault et al., 1975). Subsequently, there is no memory of the events and actions that occurred during the episodes (Guillemault et al., 1976). These automatic behaviors probably represent a continuation of ongoing activities during deep drowsiness or with multiple microsleeps, without ability to recall (Labar, 1991). Episodes of automatic behavior are often identified upon specific questioning or are reported by the spouse. Automatic behavioral episodes occur with a variety of sleep disorders: narcolepsy, sleep apnea, severe excessive daytime somnolence and sleep deprivation (Wagner, 1991). Differentiation from complex partial or absence seizures is usually made without difficulty, once the history of sleep attacks and other ancillary symptoms is obtained. When the diagnosis is uncertain, patients should be referred for multiple sleep-latency tests.

The most disabling symptom of narcolepsy, usually sleep attacks, should be treated first. Naps are often helpful in reducing the need for medication. Methylphenidate is the drug of choice for sleep attacks and should be given an hour before breakfast or lunch for effective absorption. Stimulants should only be given early in the day to avoid disruption of sleep. Blood pressure should be monitored, especially in patients who also take tricyclic drugs for cataplexy. Imipramine is an effective tricyclic agent for cataplexy, and works at dosages lower than those needed for depression.

Other sleep disorders

Somnambulism

Sleep-walking attacks occur mainly during the first decade of life; they occur in almost 15 percent of normal children (Anders and Weinstein, 1972). The attacks usually occur within several hours of falling asleep as an arousal from stage III or IV non-REM sleep (Kales et al., 1987a). The child appears slightly dazed and is able to engage in complex, seemingly purposeful acts such as leaving the bedroom, walking down a flight of stairs to the kitchen, opening the cupboard and eating biscuits. Alternatively, the child may unlock the front door and wander around the neighborhood. After 2 to 30 minutes, the child will return to sleep, anywhere from the bed to the living room floor to a neighbor's lawn. The child is amnesic for the event. Sleep-walking attacks are not always benign and amusing; injury is common and can be severe (Wagner, 1991). A family history of night terrors or somnambulism is often present.

Somnambulism can occur in adults as a parasomnia or complex partial seizure (Pedley and Guilleminault, 1977; Maselli et al., 1988; Kavey et al.,

1990). As in children, most episodes occur during stages III or IV non-REM sleep, but they are more evenly distributed during the night. Patients may suddenly jump out of bed and appear to be fleeing, scream, kick or verbalize. Patients often recall fragments of a frightening dream. Clonazepam, flurazepam, carbamazepine and phenytoin are effective in treating these episodes (Kavey *et al.*, 1990). Sleep studies with video-EEG recordings are helpful in diagnosis.

Night terrors

Like somnambulism, night terrors occur mainly during the first decade of life and awaken the child within several hours of falling asleep, constituting an arousal from stage III or IV non-REM sleep. This disorder is much less common than somnambulism, occuring in only 2 percent of children; some children have somnambulism, night terrors and enuresis (Kales and Kales, 1974). During the night terror, the child appears horrified and cries for 2 to 15 minutes with intense sympathetic arousal; there is no response to parental comforting or questioning. The child is usually completely amnesic for the attack when they awaken. There is often a family history of night terrors, somnambulism or enuresis.

REM behavior disorder

This recently described parasomnia occurs predominantly in middle-aged men who are spontaneously aroused from REM sleep and engage in vigorous, coordinated motor acts that are often violent in nature (Schenck *et al.*, 1986, 1987). Patients may attack their bed partner, jump off the bed and run into the dresser. Injuries are common and are sustained by both the patient and bed partner. The patient often recalls little or nothing about the attack but may recall a vivid dream, in which he was attacked. Aggressive behavior does not occur during wakefulness.

This disorder has been associated with a variety of neurological conditions: stroke, dementia, multiple sclerosis, alcohol withdrawal, and use of amphetamines and cocaine. However, approximately half of all cases occur without any identified predisposing factor. Clonazepam is effective in most cases (Schenck & Mahowald, 1990).

References

Anders T, Weinstein P. Sleep and its disorders in infants and children – a review. *Pediatrics* 1972; **50**: 312–24.

Daly DD, Yoss RE. Narcolepsy. In: *The Epilepsies: Handbook of Clinical Neurology* (volume 15) (Magnus O, Lorentz de Haas M, eds). Amsterdam: North-Holland, 1974, pp. 836–51.

Guilleminault C, Billiard M, Montplaisir J, Dement WC. Altered states of consciousness in disorders of daytime sleepiness. *J Neurol Sci* 1975; **26**: 377–93.

Guilleminault C, Dement WC, Passouant P. Narcolepsy. In: *Advances in Sleep Research* (volume 3) (Weitzman ED, ed.). New York: Spectrum Publishers, 1976.

Kales A, Constantin R, Soldatos CR, Kales JD. Sleep disorders: insomnia, sleepwalking, night terrors, nightmares, and enuresis. *Ann Int Med* 1987a; **106**: 582–92.

Kales A, Kales J. Sleep disorders: recent findings in the diagnosis and treatment of disturbed sleep. *N Eng J Med* 1974; **290**: 487–99.

Kales A, Vela-Bueno A, Kales JD. Sleep disorders: Sleep apnea and narcolepsy. *Ann Int Med* 1987b; **106**: 434–43.

Kavey NB, Whyte J, Resor SR Jr, Girdo-Frank S. Somnambulism in adults. *Neurology* 1990; **40**: 749–52.

Labar DR. Sleep disorders and epilepsy: Differential diagnosis. *Sem Neurol* 1991; **11**: 128–34.

Maselli RA, Rosenberg RS, Spire J. Episodic nocturnal wanderings in non-epileptic young patients. *Sleep* 1988; **11**: 156–61.

Pedley T, Guilleminault C. Episodic nocturnal wandering responsive to anticonvulsant drug therapy. *Ann Neurol* 1977; **2**: 30–5.

Roth B. *Narcolepsy and Hyersomnia* (revised) (Broughton R, ed.) Basel: Karger, 1980.

Schenck C, Bundlie S, Ettinger M, Mahowald M. Chronic behavioral disorders of human REM sleep; a new category of parasomnia. *Sleep* 1986; **9**: 293–308.

Schenck C, Bundlie S, Patterson A, Mahowald M. Rapid eye movement sleep behavior disorder. *JAMA* 1987; **257**: 1786–9.

Schenck C, Mahowald MW. Polysomnographic, neurologic, psychiatric and clinical outcome report on 70 consecutive cases with the REM sleep behavior disorder. *Cleve Clin J Med* 1990; **57**: 510–524.

Wagner D. Sleep and arousal disorders. In: *Comprehensive Neurology* (Rosenberg R, ed.). New York: Raven Press, 1991.

Yoss RE, Daly DD. Narcolepsy and the automobile. *Trauma* 1963; **5**: 11–20.

88.   *Paramedian thalamic lesions disrupt arousal, attention and memory*

The intralaminar and dorsomedial nuclei are located near the midline of the thalamus and thus comprise the paramedian thalamic region.

The *intralaminar nuclei* are the rostral extension of the ascending reticular activating system (Moruzzi and Magoun, 1949; Weinburger *et al.*, 1965). In humans, extensive bilateral lesions of the intralaminar nuclei reduce the level of consciousness and, in the central herniation syndrome, compression of diencephalic structures produces a depressed level of consciousness, a key diagnostic element in identifying this life-threatening disorder (Plum and Posner, 1980). Depressed or fluctuating levels of consciousness may be the most prominent feature of midline thalamic lesions. In monkeys, intralaminar lesions also cause neglect, that is, failure to attend (Watson *et al.*, 1978).

The large *dorsomedial nucleus* lies just lateral to the intralaminar nuclei and has extensive connections with the frontal lobe and hypothalamus. The Korsakoff amnesic state, along with other clinical observations and animal experiments, demonstrates that lesions in the dorsomedial nuclei produce severe short-term memory impairment (Squire and Moore, 1979; Zola-Morgan and Squire, 1985; Victor *et al.*, 1989).

In humans, paramedian thalamic lesions usually result from infarction (and less often, thalamic tumors or hemorrhage) in the distribution of one or more thalamoperforate branches off the first segment of the posterior communicating artery (also called the basilar communicating or mesencephalic artery) (McKissock and Paine, 1958; Cheek and Taveras, 1966). In some individuals, a single branch supplies the paramedian territory bilaterally (Castaigne *et al.*, 1981). Unilateral and bilateral paramedian lesions cause decreased consciousness, which takes the form of coma, stupor, hypersomnolence or lethargy; confusion; manic delirium with features of the frontal lobe syndrome, which is characterized by confabulations and disinhibition with inappropriate jokes and comments; emotional flattening; hemineglect; visuospatial disorders; anosognosia; and anterograde memory impairment (Watson and Heilman, 1979; Meissner *et al.*, 1987; Bogousslavsky *et al.*, 1988a). With bilateral lesions, behavioral deficits are usually more severe and persistent (thalamic dementia) and patients often have associated impairment in both upward and downward gaze due to involvement of the mesencephalic vertical gaze center (located ventral to the rostral interstitial nucleus of the medial longitudinal fasciculus) (Brodal, 1981). Other neurological findings associated with paramedian thalamic lesions are hemiparesis, face and upper extremity sensory loss (due to involvement of the medial part of ventral posterior nuclear group), ataxia, asterixis, and delayed movement disorders (e.g. dystonic or choreic syndromes) and thalamic pain syndrome.

Impairment of consciousness is the most consistent behavioral feature of paramedian thalamic lesions, especially during the acute stage. With bilateral lesions, hypersomnolence, impaired attention and memory loss are often persistent and produce the syndrome of thalamic dementia (Meissner *et al.*, 1987; Bogousslavsky *et al.*, 1988b). Thalamic neglect almost always follows right-sided or bilateral lesions and can affect motor (as in limb akinesia) or multiple sensory modalities. Patients with sensory deficits demonstrate left-sided extinction on double simultaneous somesthetic, visual or auditory stimulation (Watson and Heilman, 1979). Subcortical neglect syndromes are more often transient than those due to cortical neglect (Ferro *et al.*, 1987).

Level of consciousness can also be reduced by a variety of central nervous system lesions (Plum and Posner, 1980). Lesions of the reticular formation in the pons and midbrain, bilateral hemispheric lesions, and metabolic and toxic disorders that insult the brain diffusely can cause stupor and coma (Brain, 1958; Ingvar and Sourander, 1970; Obrador *et al.*, 1975; Plum and Posner, 1980). Large lesions in the language-dominant hemisphere that cause aphasia can cause stupor (Plum and Posner, 1980).

References

Bogousslavsky J, Ferrazzini M, Regli F, Assal G, Tanabe H, Delaloye-Bischof A. Manic delirium and frontal-like syndrome with paramedian infarction of the right thalamus. *J Neurol Neurosurg Psychiat* 1988a; **51**: 116–19.

Bogousslavsky J, Regli F, Uske A. Thalamic infarcts: Clinical syndromes, etiology, and prognosis. *Neurology* 1988b; **38**: 837–48.

Brain R. The physiological basis of consciousness. *Brain* 1958; **81**: 426–55.

Brodal A. *Neurological Anatomy in Relation to Clinical Medicine* (3rd edition). New York: Oxford University Press, 1981, p. 573.

Castaigne P, Lhermitte F, Buge A, Escourolle R, Hauw JJ, Lyon-Caen O. Paramedian thalamic and midbrain infarcts: clinical and neuropathologic study. *Ann Neurol* 1981; **10**: 127–48.

Cheek WR, Taveras JM. Thalamic tumors. *J Neurosurg* 1966; **24**: 505–13.

Ferro JM, Kertesz A, Black SE. Subcortical neglect: Quantitation, anatomy, and recovery. *Neurology* 1987; **37**: 1487–92.

Ingvar DH, Sourander P. Destruction of the reticular core of the brain stem. *Arch Neurol* 1970; **23**: 1–8.

McKissock W, Paine KWE. Primary tumors of the thalamus. *Brain* 1958; **81**: 41–63.

Meissner I, Sapir S, Kokmem E, Stein SD. The paramedian diencephalic syndrome: A dynamic phenomenon. *Stroke* 1987; **18**: 380–5.

Moruzzi G, Magoun HW. Brainstem reticular formation and activation of the EEG. *EEG Clin Neurophysiol* 1949; **1**: 455–573.

Obrador S, Suarez-Reinoso F, Carbonell J *et al.* Comatose state maintained during eight years following a vascular ponto-mesencephalic lesion. *EEG Clin Neurophysiol* 1975; **38**: 21–26.

Plum F, Posner JB. *The Diagnosis of Stupor and Coma.* Philadelphia: FA Davis Company, 1980.

Squire LR, Moore RY. Dorsal thalamic lesion in a noted case of human memory dysfunction. *Ann Neurol* 1979; **6**: 503–506.

Victor M, Adams RD, Collins GH. *The Wernicke–Korsakoff Syndrome.* Philadelphia: FA Davis Company, 1989, pp. 173–94.

Watson RT, Heilman KM. Thalamic neglect. *Neurology* 1979; **29**: 690–4.

Watson RT, Miller B, Heilman KM. Nonsensory neglect. *Ann Neurol* 1978; **3**: 505–58.

Weinburger NM, Velaxo M, Lindsley DB. Effects of lesions upon thalamically induced electrocortical desynchronization and recruiting. *EEG Clin Neurophysiol* 1965; **18**: 369–77.

Zola-Morgan S, Squire LR. Amnesia in monkeys after lesions of the mediodorsal nucleus of the thalamus. *Ann Neurol* 1985; **17**: 558–64.

89.   *In the Kleine–Levin syndrome, young men eat and sleep morbidly*

This uncommon disorder predominantly affects adolescent or young men and causes periodic episodes of hypersomnolence and hyperphagia. The attacks last between 2 and 30 days, and recur every 1 to 12 months. The episodes usually become less frequent and eventually cease after 5 to 15 years. No precipitating or genetic factors have been identified.

The attacks are usually heralded by a prodromal period of headache, malaise and lethargy, but may develop abruptly (Critchley, 1962). During attacks, the most consistent and dramatic feature is hypersomnolence. Patients often sleep for more than 20 hours a day, and their sleep is usually associated with motor hyperactivity. Although the patient is arousable, when awakened, he often displays behaviors that contrast dramatically

with his usual comportment. He is frequently irritable, resentful and disin-'
hibited with inappropriate verbal, physical and sexual behaviors (Levin,
1936). For example, he may curse, fondle the nurse, or threaten the doctor
to leave him alone 'or else'. Typically, patients will awaken spontaneously
to go to the bathroom and to eat. Under these conditions, the awake patient
may be confused, angry or have 'glazed eyes', as if in a trance state. In
addition, patients may have vivid dreams that continue into the waking
state.

Hyperphagia is another striking feature. This may precede or follow the
onset of hypersomnolence. Patients consume enormous quantities of food
and beverage in a compulsive, robotic fashion, and they often eat all food-
stuffs within sight regardless of quantity or quality; many consume foods
they would not otherwise eat. They may become quite irritable if additional
food is withheld. However, they do not overeat to the point of vomiting.

During the 3- to 30-day attack of hypersomnolence and hyperphagia,
the neurological examination is unremarkable except for mental dullness,
confusion and irritability. The cerebrospinal fluid is normal and the EEG
shows non-specific, diffuse slowing (Critchley, 1962; Green and Cracco,
1970). A thalamic or hypothalamic abnormality has been postulated, but
remains speculative despite preliminary, pathological evidence (Carpenter
et al., 1982). Diencephalic masses, such as tumors, may cause hypersomnolence and hyperphagia (Reeves and Plum, 1969; Beal et al., 1981) and
have led to the speculation that the abnormality in Klein–Levin syndrome
is in this brain region.

A separate syndrome of menstrually related hypersomnia with hyperphagia has been reported and may respond to oral contraceptives (Billiard
et al., 1975; Sachs et al., 1982).

References

Beal MF, Kleinman GM, Ojemann RG, Hochberg FH. Gangliocytoma of the third
ventricle: Hyperphagia, somnolence, and dementia. *Neurology* 1981; **31**: 1224–8.

Billiard M, Guilleminault C, Dement WC. A menstruation-linked periodic hypersomnia: Kleine–Levin syndrome or new clinical entity? *Neurology* 1975; **25**: 436–
43.

Carpenter S, Yassa R, Ochs R. A pathological basis for Kleine–Levin syndrome.
Arch Neurol 1982; **39**: 25–8.

Critchley M. Periodic hyperomnia and megaphagia in adolescent males. *Brain* 1962;
85: 627–57.

Green LN, Cracco RQ. Kleine–Levin syndrome: A case with EEG evidence of
periodic brain dysfunction. *Arch Neurol* 1970; **22**: 166–75.

Levin M. Periodic somnolence and morbid hunger: A new syndrome. *Brain* 1936;
59: 494–504.

Reeves AG, Plum F. Hyperphagia, rage and dementia accompanying a ventromed-
ial hypothalamic neoplasm. *Arch Neurol* 1969; **20**: 616–24.

Sachs C, Persson HE, Hagenfeldt K. Menstruation-related periodic hypersomnia:
A case study with successful treatment. *Neurology* 1982; **32**: 1376–9.

16
Iatrogenic Mental Disorders and Systemic Illness

90. *Iatrogenic mental disorders are common, especially in the elderly, and are usually caused by drugs*

Of the many iatrogenic causes of neurobehavioral disorders, drugs are by far the most common (Table 90.1). Specific patterns of behavioral change are associated with different medications (Table 90.2).

Some patients are exquisitely sensitive to medications. While there is a tendency for physicians to dismiss dramatic complaints of cognitive or behavioral changes after usual or even low dosages of popular medications, reports of behavioral or other medication side effects must always be taken seriously. For example, carbamazepine is usually a well-tolerated drug, especially when it is started at low doses and gradually increased. However, some young and vigorous subjects report moderate lethargy, mental dullness and feeling as if they were a 'zombie' on 200 or 300 mg/day. Although these symptoms tend to resolve after several days or weeks, some people are simply unable to tolerate carbamazepine, even in low doses. Another antiepileptic drug, valproic acid, may cause isolated hyperammonemia (i.e. without elevation of liver function tests) with associated mental status changes that are mistaken for 'subclinical seizures' or drug abuse.

Sensitivity to behavioral side effects of drugs is most apparent in the

Table 90.1 Iatrogenic causes of neurobehavioral disorders.

Drugs, drug withdrawal and drug interactions
Hospitalization (sleep deprivation)
Surgery (trauma/hypoxia/anesthetics)
Infections
Fluid and electrolyte disorders
Radiation therapy
Diagnostic studies (metrizamide myelography, cerebral angiography)

Table 90.2 Neurobehavioral disorders associated with medications.

Delirium–hallucinations

Analgesics: opiates, salicylates

Anticholinergics: amitriptyline (tricyclics), atropine, benztropine, chlorpheniramine (antihistamines), trihexiphenidyl, thioridizine (phenothiazines)

Antiepileptics: phenobarbital, phenytoin, valproate

Anti-infectious agents: acyclovir, amphotericin B, chloroquine, isoniazid, penicillin G procaine, rifampin

Anti-inflamatory: ACTH, glucocorticoids, non-steroidals

Cardiovascular: captopril, clonidine, digoxin, disopyramide, lidocaine, mexilitene, methyldopa, propranolol (beta-blockers), quinidine, procainamide

Dopaminergic: amantadine, carbidopa, levodopa, bromocriptine

Sedative-hypnotic: benzodiazepines, barbiturates, glutethimide

Sympathomimetic: amphetamines, methylphenidate, phenylephrine

Other: aminocaproic acid, aminophylline, chlorpropramide, cimetidine, lithium, metrizamide (myelography), metronidazole, thyroxine, timolol (ophthalmic)

Over-the-counter: Compoz, Excedrin-PM, Sominex

Psychosis–paranoia

Analgesics: opiates, salicylates

Anti-infectious agents: acyclovir, cephalosporins, isoniazid, penicillin G, procaine, trimethoprim-sulphamethaxole

Anti-inflammatory drugs: ACTH, cyclosporine, glucocorticoids, hydroxychloroquine, non-steroidals

CNS drugs: amphetamines, antidepressants (tricyclics and MAOIs), baclofen, benzodiazepines, bromocriptine, carbidopa–levodopa, cyclobenzaprine, phenobarbital, primidone

Cardiac: captopril, disopyramide, lidocaine, tocainide

Other: cimetidine, cisplatinum, clomiphene, cycloserine, disulpharim, thyroxine

Depression

Cardiovascular drugs: clonidine, disopyramide, prazosin, propranolol

CNS drugs: amphetamines, baclofen, barbiturates, benzodiazepines, bromocriptine, levodopa – carbidopa, methyldopa, opiates, reserpine

Other: asparaginase, cimetidine, oral contraceptives, cycloserine, cyclosporine, disulpharim, halothane (postop), non-steroidals, metoclopramide

Over-the-counter: Neosynephrine (nose sprays)

---

elderly (Maxim 20). Delirium and cognitive dysfunction are often caused by medications. In addition, paranoia, agitation, irritability, depression, mania, hallucinations and psychosis can all result from drugs. The problem of drug interactions is also of special importance in the elderly, since poly-pharmacy is so common in this group. When taking a medical history from the patient, always obtain a complete account of all prescription and over-the-counter medications and their dosages. In many cases, supervision of medication intake for several days by a family member may reveal a significant discrepancy between what is supposed to be taken and what actually is being consumed. In addition, some elderly patients accumulate a warehouse of old medications that they periodically take 'as needed'.

When behavioral symptoms develop after starting a medication, precipitation of porphyria should be considered, especially if the drug is a barbiturate, sulfonamide, estrogen, chloroquine or methyldopa and if there is associated abdominal pain, nausea, vomiting, headache, seizures or predominantly motor, peripheral neuropathy (Goldberg, 1968).

Other medical interventions may also produce neurobehavioral disorders. Hospitalization and surgery are both potential precipitants of delirium, paranoia, depression and anxiety, especially in the elderly. In many cases, specific drugs or other factors cannot be identified, but symptoms may resolve with the return home. *Sun-downing* is common when elderly patients with mild cognitive and sensory impairments are hospitalized. As the sun sets, confusion and irritability develop and often lead to a difficult management problem – since the patient's agitated shouting threatens the sleep and sanity of other patients. Avoidance of daytime naps, visits from family and friends, and frequent orientation by nursing staff is helpful in preventing sun-downing; low doses of haloperidol are useful but should be avoided when possible.

Finally, radiation therapy to the brain can cause acute or delayed behavioral symptoms such as personality changes, confusion, aphasia and dementia (Rottenberg *et al.*, 1977, 1980; Rottenberg, 1991; Weingarten and Sze, 1991).

References

Goldberg A. Diagnosis and treatment of porphyrias. *Proc Roy Soc Med* 1968; **61**: 193–6.

Rottenberg DA. Acute and chronic effects of radiation therapy on the nervous system. In: *Neurologic Complications of Cancer Therapy* (Rottenberg DA, ed.). Oxford, Boston, MA: Butterworth–Heinemann, 1991, pp. 3–18.

Rottenberg DA, Chernik NL, Deck MDF, Ellis F, Posner JB. Cerebral necrosis following radiotherapy of extracranial neoplasms. *Ann Neurol* 1977; **1**: 339–57.

Rottenberg DA, Horten Kim J-H, Posner JB. Progressive white matter destruction following irradiation of an extracranial neoplasm. *Ann Neurol* 1980; **8**: 76–8.

Weingarten K, Sze G. Hydrocephalus and dementia as a complication of cancer treatment. In: *Neurologic Complications of Cancer Therapy* (Rottenberg DA, ed.). Oxford, Boston, MA: Butterworth–Heinemann, 1991, pp. 19–36.

91.   *Systemic illnesses often present with behavioral changes*

Neurobehavioral changes are among the earliest symptoms to develop in the course of systemic disease. Virtually any neurological or psychiatric symptom may result from a more generalized disease process. Vascular disorders (such as vasculitis or marantic endocarditis) are most likely to cause focal neurological syndromes (such as Wernicke's aphasia), whereas endocrine disorders are more likely to mimic primary psychiatric illness (Table 91.1). A complete discussion on the central nervous system (CNS) effects of systemic disorders is beyond the scope of this maxim. The inter-

Table 91.1   Systemic disorders that affect the brain.

Metabolic disorders
Hypoxia, severe anemia
Hypoglycemia
Hepatic renal, pancreatic, pulmonary insufficiency
Fluid/electrolyte (Na, K, Ca and Mg) disorders
Porphyria

Endocrine disorders
Hyperinsulinism (hypoglycemia)
Hypo- and hyperthyroidism
Hypopituitarism
Hypo- and hypercortisolism
Hypo- and hyperparathyroidism

Infections

Cancer
Metastases
Leptomeningeal dissemination
Paraneoplastic and neurohumoral factors

Nutritional disorders
Deficiency states: nicotinic acid, thiamine, B_{12}, folate
Hypervitaminosis A or D

Toxins
Drugs (see Tables 13.1 and 90.2)
Poisons (see Table 13.1)

Others
Systemic lupus erythematosus
Hypertensive encephalopathy
Thrombotic thrombocytopenic purpura
Vascular disorders: vasculitis, marantic endocarditis, subacute bacterial
  endocarditis

ested reader is referred to excellent texts by Lishman (1987) and Hales and Yudofsky (1987).

Any patient presenting with neurobehavioral signs and symptoms must be evaluated for concomitant systemic diseases. The extent of the work-up should be guided by the history and physical examination. However, it is useful to screen for common disorders, such as hypothyroidism and hypercalcemia.

Metabolic encephalopathy is the most common systemic disorder affecting the brain. The various metabolic disorders have somewhat distinctive behavioral features, but the similarities are more obvious than the differences. Recognition of metabolic encephalopathy (delirium) is essential, since it can be confused with psychiatric disorders and CNS structural lesions and often requires specific therapy (Maxims 12 and 13). The EEG and evaluation of mental status – as well as respiratory, pupillary, ocular and motor functions – assist in diagnosing the metabolic encephalopathy syndrome (Plum and Posner, 1980). The EEG usually reveals diffuse slowing in metabolic encephalopathy (Markand, 1984). The level of alertness is variable and ranges from hypervigilant mania to somnolence and reduced level of consciousness. Patients are most often withdrawn and apathetic, but they may be agitated or fluctuate between these affective states. The earliest and most consistent behavioral features of metabolic encephalopathy are diminished attention and global cognitive dysfunction. Mental status testing may be insufficient to reveal these symptoms, because results from patients who are easily distracted and are unable to sustain their attention on a conversation or task have limited accuracy. Furthermore, many patients appear quiet and give 'yes–no' answers appropriately. Exploring mental function more fully brings global dysfunction to light; a brief assessment is usually sufficient to uncover a broad range of cognitive deficits.

The spectrum of impairment can encompass deficits in memory, calculations, reading comprehension, writing, performance of multistep commands and abstract thought. Disorientation for time and place, perceptual errors and illusions are also common. Hallucinations, whether visual or combined visual and auditory, may occur and are often only discovered upon specific questioning (Lowe, 1973). Affected patients often mistake hospital staff for friends and the hospital for other familiar places.

Respiration often provides clues to the cause of metabolic encephalopathy. Hyperventilation is usually associated with either metabolic acidosis (diabetes, uremia, lactic acidosis, acidic poisons) or respiratory alkalosis (hepatic or pulmonary disease, salicylism, sepsis or psychogenic hyperventilation) (Plum and Posner, 1980). Hypoventilation is most often due to pulmonary disease and depressed respiration, as seen from sedative-hypnotic drugs and neuromuscular disorders, but it may also reflect compensation for metabolic alkalosis. When patients have a reduced level of consciousness, the findings of posthyperventilation apnea and Cheyne–Stokes respiration are common and non-specific.

Pupillary and oculomotor function are usually normal in metabolic encephalopathy. Roving eye movements are common, and if metabolic coma ensues, conjugate downward gaze may occur. As metabolic coma deepens, doll's eyes (ocular deviation to passive head movements) are lost and, subsequently, response to cold-water caloric stimulation is lost. Pupillary light reflexes are retained until shortly before death. However, certain drug-induced comas – atropine, for example – impair pupillary reactions. Structural brain lesions that cause coma are usually associated with both pupillary and oculomotor dysfunction.

Metabolic disorders are often associated with asterixis, tremor, multifocal myoclonus and other motor disorders. Asterixis is a sudden downward jerk of the hand that is most often elicited in the drowsy patient by extending the patient's arms and dorsiflexing the hands at the wrist ('stopping traffic'). The downward flap results from sudden muscle inactivity and is followed by a compensatory contraction upward (Leavitt and Tyler, 1964). Originally described with hepatic disease (Adams and Foley, 1953), bilateral asterixis occurs with a wide variety of metabolic insults. Unilateral asterixis has been reported as an occasional consequence of focal cerebral lesions (Tarsy et al., 1977; Massey et al., 1979). A coarse and slightly irregular 7–10 Hz tremor seen best with the arms outstretched is often present in cases of metabolic encephalopathy. Multifocal myoclonus consists of isolated non-rhythmic twitches that involve distinct muscle groups in a random distribution. Multifocal myoclonus usually occurs in patients with a reduced level of consciousness due to uremia, hyperosmolarity (hyperglycemia, hypernatremia), or CO_2 narcosis.

Other motor disorders occurring with metabolic, as well as structural, abnormalities include paratonia (gegenhalten; resistance to passive movements that is proportional to the speed of movement), diminished muscle tone, alteration in the deep tendon reflexes, grasp reflex, and partial or generalized seizures.

References

Adams RD, Foley JM. The neurological disorder associated with liver disease. *Res Publ Assoc Res Nerv Ment Dis* 1953; **32**: 198–237.

Hales RE, Yudofsky SC, eds. *Textbook of Neuropsychiatry*. Washington, DC: American Psychiatric Association Press, 1987.

Leavitt S, Tyler HR. Studies in asterixis. *Arch Neurol* 1964; **10**: 360–8.

Lishman WA. *Organic Psychiatry*. Oxford, Boston, MA: Blackwell Scientific Publications, 1987.

Lowe GR. The phenomenology of hallucinations as an aid to differential diagnosis. *Br J Psychiat* 1973; **123**: 621–33.

Markand O. Electroencephalography in diffuse encephalopathies. *J Clin Neurophysiol* 1984; **1**: 357–407.

Massey EW, Goodman JC, Stewart C et al. Unilateral asterixis: motor integrative dysfunciton in focal vascular disease. *Neurology* 1979; **29**: 1188–90.

Plum F, Posner JB. *Stupor and Coma*. Philadelphia: FA Davis Company, 1980, pp. 180–91.

Tarsy D, Lieberman B, Chirico-Post J et al. Unilateral asterixis associated with a mesencephalic syndrome. *Arch Neurol* 1977; **34**: 446–7.

17
Psychiatric Disorders

92. *The diagnosis of conversion disorder should be based on clinical features that are both suggestive of psychiatric disease and inconsistent with organic disease*

Conversion disorder is characterized by a loss or alteration of physical function that suggests organic disease but results from psychological conflicts or needs. Ford and Folks (1985) defined conversion symptoms as 'non-verbal communications facilitated by non-specific factors that inhibit a more articulate verbal expression of ideas and emotions'. The DSM-IIIR diagnostic criteria for conversion disorder are given in Table 92.1 (American Psychiatric Association, 1987).

The greatest problems in diagnosing conversion disorder are proving the absence of physical illness and establishing the etiologic significance of psychological conflict or need. Pitfalls of overdiagnosis and underdiagnosis of conversion disorder are legion. The skilled clinician can usually make the correct diagnosis from the medical history, physical examination and a few ancillary laboratory studies. In some cases, however, repeated exam-

Table 92.1 DSM-IIIR diagnostic criteria for conversion disorder.

A loss of, or alteration in, physical functioning suggesting a physical disorder

Psychological factors are judged to be etiologically related to the symptom because of a temporal relationship between a psychosocial stressor that is apparently related to a psychological conflict or need and initiation or exacerbation of the symptom

The person is not conscious of intentionally producing the symptom

The symptom is not a culturally sanctioned response pattern and cannot, after appropriate investigation be explained by a known physical disorder

The symptom is not limited to pain or to a disturbance in sexual functioning

American Psychiatric Association, 1987 (with permission)

ination, extensive and costly work-ups, therapeutic trials, and the passage of time do not assuage uncertainty.

The clearest cases of conversion disorder are those in which symptoms and signs clearly violate the rules of pathophysiology, symptoms and signs of organic disease are absent, a psychological stressor immediately precedes the occurrence of symptoms, and there is an obvious relation between the specific stressor and symptoms. Each of these components deserves careful consideration.

One of the most common reasons for misdiagnosis of physical disorders as conversion symptoms is a rigid conception of pathophysiology and disease states. A good friend told me that his grandmother, who had not visited a physician in more than 30 years was having severe head pains, 'like her scalp was on fire'. Her internist, a professor of medicine at a major academic center, had done extensive testing. The results were all normal except for anemia and an elevated erythrocyte sedimentation rate. The diagnosis was 'stress headache'. When asked if the disorder could instead be temporal arteritis, the internist responded, 'Definitely not, her temporal arteries are not tender'. When told that temporal artery tenderness is often absent, he replied, 'Not in my experience; every case has had it'. Self-fulfilling prophesies are difficult to dispel. The temporal artery biopsy was positive. Conversion disorder usually begins before age 40 years; this disorder must be diagnosed with extreme caution after this age. However, depression in elderly persons often presents with somatic complaints.

Uncommon presentations of common disorders are frequent. One must not rely on the 'textbook' description, since most patients will violate the classic picture. This principle is especially dear in behavioral neurology. Furthermore, one must be familiar with the uncommon disorders (e.g. Kleine–Levin syndrome, Balint's syndrome, peduncular hallucinosis) that can be easily confused with functional disorders.

The vigor with which organic disease must be ruled out varies from patient to patient. It is extemely difficult to definitively exclude the possibility of physical illness. Furthermore, concomitant systemic or neurologic disorders are not infrequent among patients with conversion disorder (Maxim 93). Certain illnesses such as systemic lupus erythematosus, multiple sclerosis, retrobulbar neuritis and myasthenia gravis, should be considered when specific symptoms are present, since physical findings may be absent and complaints may seem bizarre in these disorders. In the process of systematically excluding physical disorders, one must also consider other mental disorders that can be confused with conversion disorder, especially depression, somatization disorder and schizophrenia. 'Hysteria' is overdiagnosed.

Let us examine one of the oldest conversion symptoms – *globus hystericus* – as an example of how dangerous the diagnosis of conversion disorder can be. The *Oxford University Dictionary* (1794) defined Globus Hystericus as 'a choking sensation, as of a lump in the throat to which hysterical persons are subject' (Malcomson, 1968). Malcomson (1968) reviewed 307 cases previously diagnosed with globus hystericus. Elements of the hysterical personality – emotionality, histrionics, attention-seeking – were absent in most of these cases. Organic lesions were documented on clinical and radiological examination in 79 percent of cases. In contrast to patients with malignancies, patients with 'globus' had no dysphagia or weight loss and the sensation of a lump was more marked between, rather than during, meals. He suggests that the term globus pharyngis replace globus hystericus.

Identifying the specific psychological stressor is sometimes impossible in conversion disorder. Once the diagnosis of conversion disorder is suspected, and if an organic disorder is not supported by clinical evidence, the aid of a psychiatrist or psychologist should be sought. In some cases, the amobarbital interview may uncover important psychological conflicts or needs (Dysken, 1979). Interpretation of stressors can be complicated, as stress is omnipresent and may or may not contribute to disease development. For example, a woman can be victimized by rape and develop a variety of physical complaints such as fatigue, malaise, headache or abdominal discomfort which result from systemic lupus erythematosus or another physical illness, and which are not a psychosomatic reaction to the rape. The development of somatic complaints after a major psychological trauma by no means proves that somatic symptoms are psychological in origin.

Primary or secondary gain usually underlies conversion symptoms. In primary gain, an internal conflict or need is suppressed through the elaboration of a conversion symptom. For example, following rape or physical abuse, the rage and anger may be symbolically expressed as a psychogenic seizure. In secondary gain, the conversion symptom allows patients to receive support from people and social services that they might not get otherwise, or to avoid confronting unpleasant situations. Conversion symptoms can become a conditioned response or coping mechanism learned in childhood that persists into adulthood. For example, a patient may learn as a child to feign sickness to avoid unpleasant obligations, and grow up to complain of severe lower back spasms in order to prevent in-laws from coming over for dinner.

A common misconception is that patients with conversion disorder usually have 'hysterical personalities' or '*la belle indifference*' (Malcomson, 1968; Merskey and Buhrich, 1975; Weintraub, 1983). Hysterical personality is no longer part of the current psychiatric nomenclature, but histrionic personality disorder encompasses what was considered hysterical behavior. This disorder is a pervasive, long-standing pattern of overly emotional, flamboyant and attention-seeking behavior. It is more frequent in women and is often associated with seductive behavior, diminished tolerance for frustration, and constant demands for approval. *La belle indifference* was coined by Janet (1907) to describe a lack of concern regarding such serious bodily dysfunction as hemiparesis. This pattern is often absent in patients with conversion disorder; conversely, it can occur in seriously ill patients who are stoical and seeking to protect family members, or are denying their illness.

Another common misconception is that conversion disorder and organic disease are mutually exclusive. In patients with previously diagnosed neuromedical disorders, conversion symptoms are often superimposed and may be difficult to distinguish from an exacerbation of the underlying illness (Caplan and Nadelson, 1980). Also, patients who present with conversion disorder may harbor or develop organic disease that is 'written off' as hysterical.

Conversion disorder is at least three times more common in women than men and occurs most frequently between 15 and 40 years of age. Rural environment and low socioeconomic and educational status are factors associated with an increased risk of conversion disorder. The incidence and prevalence of this disorder are hard to determine and vary by medical practice and clinical judgment. Although it is commonly said that conversion disorder is rare and becoming rarer with time, in fact, conversion disorder is alive and well in the 1990s. It is not rare.

References

American Psychiatric Association. *Diagnostic and Statistical Manual of Psychiatry* (3rd edition). Washington, DC: American Psychiatric Association Press, 1987.

Caplan LR, Nadelson T. Multiple sclerosis and hysteria. *JAMA* 1980; **243**: 2418–21.

Dysken MW. Clinical usefulness of sodium amobarbital interviewing. *Arch Gen Psych* 1979; **36**: 789–94.

Ford CV, Folks DG. Conversion disorders: An overview. *Psychosomatics* 1985; **26**: 371–83.

Janet P. *The Major Symptoms of Hysteria*. London: MacMillan, 1907.

Malcomson KG. Globus hystericus vel pharyngis. *J Laryngol Otol* 1968; **82**: 219–30.

Merskey H, Buhrich NA. Hysteria and organic brain disease. *Br J Med Psychol* 1975; **48**: 359–66.

Weintraub MI. *Hysterical Conversion Reactions*. New York: Spectrum Publications, 1983.

93.   *Neurological symptoms are common in conversion and somatization disorders*

The somatoform disorders – body dysmorphic disorder, conversion disorder, hypochondriasis, somatization disorder and somatoform pain disorder – present with somatic symptoms that suggest physical illness. However, in these disorders, presenting symptoms are not accompanied by demonstrable objective findings and there is positive evidence, or a strong presumption, that psychological factors are responsible (American Psychiatric Association, 1987). This maxim will focus on the conversion and somatization disorders, although patients with somatoform pain disorder, in which the patient is unduly preoccupied with pain for at least six months, also frequently present to neurologists.

Misdiagnosis between organic and somatoform disorders cuts both ways – physical disorders may be written off as 'hysterical' while many patients with psychogenic disorders are subjected to extensive, expensive and invasive diagnostic work-ups and therapy with potentially dangerous drugs or surgery.

In conversion disorder (Maxim 92), anesthesia, paresthesia, pain, seizures and gait disturbance are the most common neurological symptoms. The sensory loss often involves all modalities and has sharp borders affecting all modalities equally. In contrast, peripheral nerve lesions typically show a gradient in which the area of temperature and light touch sensory loss is less than the area with loss of pin sensation. As with hysterical paralysis, the dominant side is more often involved with functional sensory disturbances. Psychogenic seizures are a common disorder that may give rise to considerable diagnostic confusion (Porter, 1989). Psychogenic attacks are most likely to be mistaken for complex partial and generalized tonic–clonic (grand mal) seizures (Maxim 81). *Astasia-abasia* is the classic conversion gait disorder characterized by lurching, unsteadiness, zigzagging and inconsistent pattern of ambulation.

Somatization disorder is a chronic syndrome of somatic symptoms that are not caused by physical illness (Ford, 1983). Psychosocial stress is often present and patients seek medical attention for their complaints and are often treated with medications. The DSM-IIIR diagnostic criteria for somatization disorder are given in Table 93.1 (American Psychiatric Association, 1987). Somatization disorder has formerly been referred to as hysteria and Briquet's syndrome. It is more common in women, affecting approximately 1 percent. These patients form a disproportionate percentage of those seeking medical attention. In general, patients with somatization disorder present repeatedly to internists or neurologists and are typically misdiagnosed with physical illness for several years prior to recognition of the psychiatric disorder. Many of the symptoms in somatization disorder overlap with those of conversion disorder. The multiplicity and chronicity of symptoms separates somatization disorders from those of conversion.

In somatization disorder, psychogenic amnesia, difficulty swallowing (globus hystericus), and psychogenic seizures are the most common neurological symptoms (Table 93.1). *Psychogenic amnesia* often includes loss of personal identity, which is extremely rare with neurological causes of amnesia (Maxims 39 and 97). *Globus hystericus* (Maxim 92) is a psychogenic swallowing disorder in which patients complain of a choking sensation or painful 'lump' in the throat that can be intermittent or persistent. The results of barium esophagram, upper gastrointestinal series and vocal cord examination are normal. Organic palatal and swallowing disorders are usually not painful or associated with a lump in the throat, but are characterized by a pressure or uncomfortable sensation that is accompanied by

Table 93.1 DSM-IIIR diagnositic criteria for somatization disorder.

A history of many physical complaints or a belief that one is sickly, beginning before the age of 30 years and persisting for several years.

At least 13 symptoms from the list below. To count a symptom as significant, the following criteria must be met:

No organic pathology or pathophysiologic mechanism (e.g. a physical disorder or the effects of injury, medication, drugs or alcohol) to account for the symptom or, when there is related organic pathology, the complaint or resulting social or occupational impairment is grossly in excess of what would be expected from the physical findings

It has not occurred only during a panic attack

It has caused the person to take medicine (other than over-the-counter-pain medication), see a doctor, or alter life-style

Symptom list

Gastrointestinal symptoms
   Vomiting (other than during pregnancy)
   Abdominal pain (other than when menstruating)
   Nausea (other than motion sickness)
   Bloating (gassy)
   Diarrhea
   Intolerance of (gets sick from) several different foods

Pain symptoms
   Pain in extremities
   Back pain
   Joint pain
   Pain during urination
   Other pain (excluding headaches)

Cardiopulmonary symptoms
   Shortness of breath when not exerting oneself
   Palpitations
   Chest pain
   Dizziness

Conversion or pseudoneurological symptoms
   Amnesia
   Difficulty swallowing
   Loss of voice
   Deafness
   Double vision
   Blurred vision
   Blindness
   Fainting or loss of consciousness
   Seizure or convulsion
   Trouble walking
   Paralysis or muscle weakness
   Urinary retention or difficulty urinating

Sexual symptoms for the major part of the person's life after opportunities for sexual activity
Burning sensation in sexual organs or rectum (other than during intercourse)
Sexual indifference
Pain during intercourse
Impotence

Female reproductive symptoms judged by the person to occur more frequently or severely than in most women
Painful menstruation
Irregular menstrual periods
Excessive menstrual bleeding
Vomiting throughout pregnancy

American Psychiatric Association, 1987 (with permission)

Note: The seven items in bold may be used to screen for the disorder. The presence of two or more of these items suggests a high likelihood of the disorder.

changes on clinical and laboratory examination. *Psychogenic seizures* are discussed in Maxim 81.

When functional symptoms are suspected in patients with somatoform disorders, the physician sets out to disprove organicity and searches for positive evidence of conversion. Hysterical signs and symptoms fluctuate from one examination to the next. Conversion signs and symptoms can be elicited with suggestion. These patients often display a lack of effort and 'give way weakness', in which muscles that are 'paralyzed' when tested as prime movers may function normally as synergists; sensory disturbances are extensive, involve all modalities, and have borders that correspond to surface landmarks (e.g. joints) but not nerve distributions (Devinsky and Feldmann, 1988). The physician's identification of inconsistencies on examination is followed by attempts to uncover the psychological conflict. One must exercise caution. It is easy to uncover a recent loss or life stress – whether at work, with the family, with relationships, or with finances – in almost any patient.

The diagnosis of somatoform disorder must be made with great care. Follow-up studies at academic centers of patients who are diagnosed with 'hysteria' reveal a misdiagnosis rate of 20 to 40 percent (Slater, 1965; Merskey and Buhrich, 1975; Ford and Folks, 1985). The most common errors are failure to identify connective tissue disease (e.g. systemic lupus erythematosus) and disorders of the skeleton, musculature, spinal cord, peripheral nerve, as well as demyelinating and partial seizure disorders.

One important reason for the high index of suspicion required when diagnosing somatization or conversion disorder is that presentation in many cases does not conform to physician expectations for 'hysterical' symptoms. The following case exemplifies the potential pitfalls in diagnosis:

A 12-year-old boy was referred for refractory partial seizures. He presented several years earlier with syncopal episodes and was later observed to have 'convulsive movements' after losing consciousness. He was treated with antiepileptic drugs with initial success, but his episodes became refractory to medications. An MRI scan revealed an atypical signal, and he underwent 3 carotid arteriograms for what was finally diagnosed as a normal arterial variant. Video-EEG monitoring of the episodes revealed obvious psychogenic seizures. His episodes began shortly after the death of his grandfather and have since become less frequent with therapy and without antiepileptic drugs.

In addition, the presence of functional disease does not preclude the existence of organic disease; they often coexist. Organic disease is common in hospitalized patients who have conversion disorder. Several studies have found that more than 60 percent of patients diagnosed with conversion disorder also (or only) have some form of neurological or systemic illness (Whitlock, 1967; Merskey and Buhrich, 1975).

Therefore, once diagnosis of conversion or somatization disorder has been made, it is worth reviewing the evidence and considering that the formulation is incorrect or that organic disease is also present. The diagnosis is the child of the doctor and we have great difficulty finding faults in our children.

Signs of conversion are present in many patients with known organic illness, but they are disregarded when magnetic resonance imaging (MRI) shows a large lesion or, in dramatic cases, the behavior is labeled as elaboration.

Finally, patients who have been thoroughly evaluated and have unquestionable conversion disorder may later develop organic disease. To complicate the clinical problem, these patients will often present in a dramatic, hysterical style, thus leading the doctor to lump new symptoms with the old. Beware.

References

American Psychiatric Association. *Diagnostic and Statistical Manual of Mental Disorders* (3rd edition, revised). Washington, DC: American Psychiatric Association, 1987.

Devinsky O, Feldmann E. *Examination of the Cranial and Peripheral Nerves.* New York: Churchill Livingstone, 1988.

Ford CV. *The Somatizing Disorders.* New York: Elsevier, 1983.

Ford CV, Folks DG. Conversion disorders: An overview. *Psychosomatics* 1985; **26**: 371–83.

Merskey H, Buhrich NA. Hysteria and organic brain disease. *Br J Med Psychol* 1975; **48**: 359–66.

Porter RJ. *Epilepsy: 100 Elementary Principles.* London: WB Saunders Company, 1989.

Slater E. The diagnosis of 'hysteria'. *Br Med J* 1965; **1**: 1395–9.

Whitlock FA. The etiology of hysteria. *Acta Psychiat Scand* 1967; **43**: 144–62.

94.   *Patients with factitious disorder (Munchausen's syndrome) are often very knowledgeable about medicine*

In factitious disorder, patients present physical or psychological signs and symptoms that are intentionally produced or feigned. There is a higher incidence of factitious disorder among those individuals who were themselves hospitalized for bona fide physical illness while young or had relatives who were hospitalized during childhood or adolescence; believe that the medical establishment mistreated them; work in the health care environment; or have family members, especially parents, who are physicians. The disorder usually begins in early adulthood and is more common among men.

The pathogenesis of factitious disorder is thought to involve psychodynamic factors, including the need for dependence or control over early deprivation and trauma and the desire to assume the role of patient. Masochistic personality traits are often present, as many of these patients undergo invasive, dangerous diagnostic studies and painful surgical procedures. In contrast to malingering, financial gain is not a motivation among patients with factitious disorder.

The presentation can involve any organ system and is often dramatic (Asher, 1951). The most common forms include the 'acute abdomen', bleeding, dermatological disorders and such neurological syndromes as paroxysmal headache, loss of consciousness or seizures (Asher, 1951; Savard *et al.*, 1988). Pain is often a prominent symptom, and some patients may seek narcotics. These subjects tend to be quite sophisticated and present convincing stories often supported by intentional pathological signs such as blood mixed with urine, anticoagulant ingestion with elevated bleeding time, excoriation, intradermal or intravenous injection of saliva or other non-sterile liquids to cause fever and skin lesions, and feigned seizures with self-induced physical trauma, tongue laceration and urination. In some patients, the symptoms are primarily psychological and include bizarre behavior, depression, hallucinations and dissociative phenomena. Because men are incorrectly assumed to have a high pain threshold and rarely to dramatize illness, physicians almost never consider the possibility of factitious disorder during the early phase of their illness.

Patients often travel from doctor to doctor, hospital to hospital and city to city, learning and refining their signs and symptoms in the process. Textbook histories are typically provided to the unsuspecting physician who is seduced by the 'ease' of diagnosis and 'need' for diagnostic studies and therapeutic interventions. Many patients prefer to live in the hospital and develop new disorders as discharge approaches. Some patients have had more than 400 documented admissions (Maur *et al.*, 1973). In the hospital, these patients often break the rules, as if they were at home, and demand an undue share of medical and nursing attention.

Therapy is usually ineffective, and recognition of the disorder is crucial to prevent additional, dangerous, medical interventions.

Munchausen's syndrome by proxy refers to pediatric cases in which the parents, usually the mother, fabricate clinical histories and signs causing needless and potentially harmful medical investigations, hospitalizations and treatment of the child (Meadow, 1982). Bleeding and neurological symptoms (seizures, ataxia, and drowsiness and coma due to tranquilizers) are among the most common presentations.

References

Asher R. Munchausen's syndrome. *Lancet* 1951; **i**: 339–41.

Maur KV, Wasson KR, DeFord JW *et al*. Munchausen's syndrome. *S Med J* 1973; **66**: 629.

Meadow R. Munchausen syndrome by proxy. *Arch Dis Child* 1982; **57**: 92–8.

Savard G, Andermann F, Teitelbaum J, Lehmann H. Epileptic Munchausen's syndrome: a form of pseudoseizures distinct from hysteria and malingering. *Neurology* 1988; **38**: 1628–9.

95.   *Depression often complicates organic disease*

Depression is extremely common. In the USA, the prevalence of major depression is approximately 4 percent, with a lifetime risk of 5 to 10 percent for men and 20 to 25 percent for women. Cognitive symptoms of depression include feelings of sadness, worthlessness and guilt; diminished interest or pleasure in activities; and difficulty in concentrating. Vegetative symptoms of depression are weight loss or gain, fatigue or lack of energy (anergia), insomnia or hypersomnia, and psychomotor retardation or restlessness. DSM-IIIR criteria for major depression are presented in Table 95.1 (American Psychiatric Association, 1987).

The high prevalence of depression and its wide spectrum of clinical manifestations and presentations (Table 95.2) necessitate heightened vigilance for recognition of this psychiatric syndrome. Furthermore, depression always causes significant morbidity for patients and their families, and it is potentially lethal (Maxim 96).

The pathogenesis of depression is often difficult to define and depends on several, variable factors. Genetic predisposition, recent childbirth or life stress, season of the year, alcoholism or drug abuse, and other organic factors may all contribute. The recognition of neurological and systemic disorders and medications in the etiology of depression is critical. However, it is also essential that depression is recognized in patients with known organic disease.

In fact, depression is often caused by physical illness (Table 95.3) and may be the presenting feature of systemic and neurological disorders. Pan-

Table 95.1 DSM-IIIR diagnostic criteria for major depressive episodes.

A. At least five of the following symptoms have been present during the same two-week period and represent a change from previous functioning; at least one of the symptoms is either (1) depressed mood, or (2) loss of interest of pleasure. (Do not include symptoms that are clearly due to a physical condition, mood-incongruent delusions or hallucinations, incoherence, or marked loosening or association.)

1. Depressed mood (or can be irritable mood in children and adolescents) most of the day, nearly every day, as indicated either by subjective account or observation by others

2. Markedly diminished interest or pleasure in all, or almost all, activities most of the day, nearly every day (as indicated either by subjective account or observation by others of apathy most of the time)

3. Significant weight loss or weight gain when not dieting (e.g. more than 5 percent of body weight in a month), or decrease or increase in appetite, nearly every day (in children, consider failure to make expected weight gains)

4. Insomnia or hypersomnia nearly every day

5. Psychomotor agitation or retardation nearly every day (observable by others, not merely subjective feelings or restlessness or being slowed down)

6. Fatigue or loss of energy nearly every day

7. Feelings of worthlessness or excessive or inappropriate guilt (which may be delusional) nearly every day (not merely self-reproach or guilt about being sick)

8. Diminished ability to think or concentrate, or indecisiveness, nearly every day (either by subjective account or as observed by others)

9. Recurrent thoughts of death (not just fear of dying), recurrent suicidal ideation without a specific plan, or a suicide attempt or a specific plan for committing suicide

B. 1. It cannot be established that an organic factor initiated and maintained the disturbance

   2. The disturbance is not a normal reaction to the death of a loved one (uncomplicated bereavement)

   Note: Morbid preoccupation with worthlessness, suicidal ideation, marked functional impairment or psychomotor retardation, or prolonged duration suggest bereavement complicated by major depression

C. At no time during the disturbance have there been delusions or hallucinations for as long as two weeks in the absence of prominent mood symptoms (i.e. before the mood symptoms developed or after they have remitted)

D. Not superimposed on schizophrenia, schizophreniform disorder, delusional disorder, or psychotic disorder not otherwise specified.

American Psychiatric Association, 1987 (with permission) (DSM-IIIR)

Table 95.2   Clinical manifestations of depression.

Symptom type	Symptom
Affective	Sadness/feeling 'blue' Anxiety Irritability Inability to enjoy life (anhedonia)
Cognitive – psychologic	Hopelessness Helplessness Worthlessness Obsessive thoughts Guilt Suicidal ideation Impaired attention Impaired memory Social withdrawal
Vegetative	Appetite decreased or increased Sleep decreased or increased Libido decreased Fatigue or lack of energy (anergia) Psychomotor retardation, less often agitation Constipation
Somatic	Pain (e.g. headache, back pain) Gastrointestinal complaints
Psychotic	Delusions Hallucinations: most often auditory

creatic carcinoma, Cushing's syndrome, hypothyroidism, Parkinson's disease and systemic lupus erythematosus are commonly associated with depression. When depression precedes the diagnosis or the patient's recognition of other symptoms, its pathogenesis is biological, not psychological. However, depression is often a secondary reaction to physical illness – the more serious the illness (e.g. cancer, myocardial infarction, stroke), the more catastrophic the depressive reaction.

Both neurological and psychosocial factors contribute to the association between depression and such neurological disorders as multiple sclerosis and epilepsy (Maxim 72). In addition, chronic disorders, including rheumatoid arthritis and pain syndromes, are also frequently complicated by depression.

Depression complicates many cerebral disorders (Table 95.3). Approximately half of acute stroke patients have mood disorders, with 25 percent meeting criteria for major depression (Robinson *et al.*, 1983). Patients with left anterior strokes, either cortical or subcortical, are most likely to become

Table 95.3 Common organic causes of depression.

Endocrine disorders
Hypothyroidism
Hyperthyroidism
Cushing's syndrome
Addison's disease/glucocorticoid withdrawal
Hypoglycemia
Diabetes mellitus

Infections
Mononucleosis
Hepatitis
Influenza
AIDS

Vitamin deficiencies
B_{12}
Folate
Niacin

Miscellaneous medical disorders
Pancreatic cancer
Systemic lupus erythematosus

Neurological disorders
Stroke
Multiple sclerosis
Epilepsy
Encephalitis
Parkinson's disease
Huntington's disease
Brain tumor

Drugs
Levodopa–carbidopa
Barbiturates
Benzodiazepines
Phenothiazines
Alpha-methyldopa
Reserpine
Beta-blockers
Glucocorticoids

depressed (Robinson *et al.*, 1983; Starkstein *et al.*, 1987). Other factors predisposing to poststroke depression include severe intellectual and physical impairment, poor quality of social support and young age (Robinson *et al.*, 1983). Antidepressants are effective in treating poststroke depression (Reding *et al.*, 1986). In stroke patients with major depression, antidepressant medication and psychotherapy should be considered.

Medications are an important, and often overlooked, cause of depression

(Table 95.3). In some patients, drug use has been chronic (e.g. propranalol or phenobarbital) and is not recognized as relevant to depressive symptoms of recent onset. Even in these cases, however, drugs can aggravate biologic tendencies and environmental stresses. Some patients on alternate day glucocorticoid therapy become depressed on the 'off' day.

Unfortunately, this common coexistence of depression and organic illness can lead physicians astray. It is extremely common for physicians to overlook diagnosis of depression and thereby withhold treatment – even when patients display classic symptoms. When one cares for patients with known illness, depressed spirits are easily attributed to 'normal reaction to having a disease'. There is a fine line between depression and the appropriate feelings of sadness as one copes with illness or loss. In addition, major depression may be misdiagnosed as a sleep disorder, dementia or a pain syndrome (e.g. headache or low back pain).

One should specifically ask patients about their spirits, but some patients are unaware that they are depressed. To further complicate diagnosis, depression can be masked by somatic complaints. When the chief complaints are lethargy, palpitations, abdominal or chest pains, headache or back pain – and an organic disorder cannot be identified – the physician should always search for vegetative signs of depression. A family history of depression and previous depressive episodes support the diagnosis of depression.

When depression is strongly suspected, whether in isolation or accompanied by organic disease, enlist the help of a psychiatrist. Medical and neurological training does not provide extensive education about the diagnosis, evaluation and treatment of depression. It is unwise either to make a casual diagnosis of depression and prescribe antidepressant medication or to dismiss the symptoms as unimportant. Furthermore, the differential diagnosis of depression includes not only organic disease, but also other associated psychiatric disorders. The psychiatrist can provide important insights into the patient's family and social structure, how these factors influence the patient's response to illness, and how best to begin therapy.

A psychiatrist should also make the decision to use antidepressant medications, and determine which would be the most effective and best tolerated. In addition, electroconvulsive shock therapy (ECT) should only be used after formal psychiatric evaluation. Electroconvulsive shock therapy is 'contraindicated in the presence of increased intracranial pressure, while space-occupying lesions in the brain, a recent history of myocardial infarction, and large aneurysms are relative contraindications' (National Institute of Mental Health Consensus Conference, 1985).

If a patient is depressed and receives only psychotherapy without significant improvement in symptoms, pharmacotherapy should be considered.

References

American Psychiatric Association. *Dragnostic and Statistical Manual of Psychiatry* (3rd edition). Washington, DC: American Psychiatric Association Press, 1987.

National Institute of Mental Health Consensus Development Conference on Electroconvulsive Therapy. *JAMA* 1985; **254**: 2103–8.

Reding MJ, Orto LA, Winter SW, Fortuna IM, Di Ponte P, McDowell FH. Antidepressant therapy after stroke: A double-blind trial. *Arch Neurol* 1986; **43**: 763–5.

Robinson RG, Starr LB, Kubos KL, Priced TR. A two-year longitudinal study of post-stroke mood disorders: Findings during the initial evaluation. *Stroke* 1983; **14**: 736–41.

Starkstein SE, Robinson RG, Price TR. Comparison of cortical and subcortical lesions in the production of poststroke mood disorders. *Brain* 1987; **110**: 1045–59.

96.   *People contemplating suicide often provide clues of their intent*

Suicide is one of the top ten leading causes of death in the USA. The greatest risk of suicide occurs in patients with affective disorder, alcoholism and schizophrenia (Beskow, 1979; Galanter, 1985); all of these groups have an approximately 15 percent incidence of completed suicide. Depression, a common antecedent to suicide, is common in patients with epilepsy during posticital and interictal periods, stroke (especially left frontal) and head trauma. Therefore, neurologists should consider suicidal ideation in patients with depression related to central nervous system disorders. Other patients at increased risk include those with delirium and terminal illnesses (e.g. systemic cancer and AIDS). Epidemiological studies have identified the factors that predict high risk of completed suicide among those who attempt suicide (Table 96.1).

Clues of suicidal intent must be carefully sought (Tuckman and Youngman, 1968). Nearly 80 percent of patients who have completed suicide have communicated their intent to others. Verbal clues include statements about wanting to 'end it all' or 'I'd be better off dead'. Similarly, patients who inquire about how one donates organs or discuss 'a friend' who is contemplating suicide should be considered at risk. Behavioral clues are often most revealing. Patients may suddenly contact their attorney and family to 'put their affairs in order' or give away prized possessions, thus providing messages of their intent. Similarly, small overdoses of prescribed or over-the-counter medication and careless accidents that cause self-injury may be forewarnings. Situational clues include major life stresses, such as loss of a loved one or job and diagnosis of a potentially fatal illness. Among alcoholics, completed suicide often occurs within six weeks of marital dissolution or the death of a loved one.

Table 96.1   Risk factors for completed suicide among those who attempt suicide.

Factor	High risk	Low risk
Age	>45 years	< 45 years
Sex	Male	Female
Race	White	Non-white
Marital status	Separated, divorced, widowed	Single, married
Employment	Unemployed, retired	Employed
Physical health	Poor	Good
Mental health	Mood disorder, alcoholism, schizophrenia	Normal, brief situational reactions
Medical care (within 6 months)	Yes	No
Method	Hanging, firearms, jumping	Cutting, gas, poison
Season	April–September	October–March
Location of attempt	Own or someone else's house	Public, other places
Suicide note	Yes	No
Previous attempt or threat	Yes	No

The vast majority of patients who commit suicide visit a physician during the months before death. Because depression often goes undiagnosed, it is important for psychiatrists and non-psychiatrists to consider this possibility. A helpful screening question is to ask all patients, 'How have your spirits been lately?' This inquiry often provides useful information about affective state, as well as important family or work-related stresses that may have an impact on medical care. If depression is suspected, or if there are clues that suicide is being contemplated, then specific questions should follow: 'Has anyone in your family ever hurt themselves or comitted suicide?', 'Have you ever had thoughts about hurting yourself?', 'Have you ever tried to hurt yourself before?', 'Are you thinking about hurting yourself now or in the near future?', 'Do you have a plan?', 'What is the plan?'

Any patient with suicidal ideation must be taken seriously and referred for psychiatric evaluation and treatment. The decision to hospitalize patients depends on the risk of completed suicide. 'Hysterical' and manipulative patients are often dismissed as trivial risks, but may succeed (often unintentionally) in harming themselves. Patients with poor impulse control, lack of a support structure, major affective disorder, schizophrenia, delirium or alcoholism who express suicidal ideation should be strongly considered for inpatient psychiatric treatment.

References

Beskow J. Suicide and mental disorder in Swedish men. *Acta Psychiatr Scand* 1979; **277**: 1–138 (Suppl).

Galanter M, Castaneda R. Self-destructive behavior in the substance abuser. *Psychiatr Clin N Am* 1985; **8**: 2.

Tuckman J, Youngman WF. A scale for assessing suicide risk of attempted suicides. *J Clin Psychiat* 1968; **24**: 17.

97.   *The dissociative disorders are often confused with other psychiatric and neurological disorders*

The dissociative disorders are characterized by disturbances of one's sense of self and memory. These disturbances of self take the form of psychogenic amnesia, or loss of memory for self-referential information; elaboration of secondary identities, as in psychogenic fugue and multiple personality; and depersonalization, as in feeling like an automaton that is detached from one's mind. Memory changes seen after dissociative states (psychogenic amnesia and fugue) usually take the form of amnesia, which can be complete or partial and disrupts recall of events during the episode. While in dissociative states, patients are often amnesic for important personal data, such as home address or spouse's name. Dissociative disorders may occur suddenly or gradually, and they may be brief or persistent.

Psychogenic amnesia is the sudden inability to recall basic personal information. It usually occurs as an acute response to overwhelming trauma and is common in combat and disasters (Putnam, 1985). With the exception of wartime cases, this disorder is most common in young women. In contrast with psychogenic fugue, the patient does not assume a new identity or travel to a new place. The memory loss is often limited to the period around the trauma, and may be selective for certain events. In some cases, however, the amnesia may be continuous, affecting recollection for all past events of a person's life and all events following the disorder's onset. Patients may wander in a confused and disoriented state, especially when amnesia is continuous. The amnesia usually ends abruptly and recovery is complete. The differential diagnosis of psychogenic amnesia is discussed in Maxim 39, and includes such neurological causes of amnesia as head trauma, epilepsy and limbic lesions, as well as transient global amnesia, alcoholic blackouts, catatonic stupor and malingering.

Psychogenic fugue is the assumption of a new identity with amnesia for one's original identity, in association with sudden travel away from home. The distinction between psychogenic amnesia and fugue is often blurred as patients commonly leave home, traveling to the next town or across the country, and are unable to recall any personal information, giving only a new first name without any associated biographical data. In some cases, elaborate new identities are created, and patients engage in complex social arrangements. The 'new person' is often outgoing and fun-loving, while the original personality was subdued. Fugue often emerges following stress – such as after marital discord, death of a loved one, or personal rejection. It usually lasts less than two days, but may extend for months. As with psychogenic amnesia, recurrences are rare. Psychogenic fugue must be distinguished from multiple personality disorder, psychogenic amnesia, complex partial or absence status epilepticus (Maxim 77), postictal states and malingering. There are occasional patients in whom complex partial seizures are followed by prolonged confusional periods and wandering (poriomania) (Mayeux *et al.*, 1979). In some, these 'postictal' states may be accompanied by persistent epileptiform discharges limited to limbic areas. However, in contrast to psychogenic fugue, these patients are disoriented, often have abnormal language, and have relative preservation of personal memories. The assumption of an independent personal identity in patients with epilepsy is extremely rare (Maxim 77). Wernicke's aphasia may be confused with fugue states.

Multiple personality disorder (MPD) is a chronic dissociative disorder in which two or more distinct personality states, or alters, exchange control over the behavior of the individual (American Psychiatric Association, 1987). Each of the alters posesses its own, relatively enduring pattern of perceiving, relating to and thinking about the environment and self. Alters may also have differing sex, age and widely divergent behavioral features. The relationship between different personalities is complex and their knowledge of each other is variable. Common alters include 'a frightened child', 'a seductive girl or woman', 'a strong protector', and 'a creative artist'. Approximately half of cases have more than 10 alters. Personalities are often aware of time losses and distortions.

Multiple personality disorder often begins in childhood, frequently following severe physical and sexual abuse (Putnam *et al.*, 1986). However, because the diagnosis of MPD is usually made after a prolonged period, these patients are often misdiagnosed with various psychiatric, neurologic and medical disorders, such as depression, epilepsy and hypoglycemia (Coons *et al.*, 1988). Many symptoms reported in MPD are shared by patients with seizure disorders. These include blackouts, fugues, depersonalization, derealization, *déjà vu, jamais vu*, dreamy states, hypergraphia, 'forced thinking', unusual somatic sensations, illusions and hallucinations (Putnam 1986; Putnam *et al.*, 1986). Patients with both MPD and epilepsy have been reported (Mesulam, 1981; Schenk and Bear, 1981; Benson *et al.*, 1986). However, video-EEG monitoring of six consecutive patients with MPD and previously diagnosed epilepsy revealed that the paroxysmal episodes were non-epileptic (Devinsky *et al.*, 1989a), suggesting that the combination is uncommon.

Depersonalization disorder is classified as a dissociative disorder because the sense of oneself is disturbed. However, memory is preserved. The disorder is characterized by recurrent or persistent depersonalization that is severe and causes marked distress (American Psychiatric Association, 1987). Depersonalization refers to an alteration in perception of self such that the subject no longer 'feels like himself'. Out-of-body experiences (i.e. the feeling of leaving one's body and viewing it from another vantage point), feelings of mental detachment and living in a dream, and the feeling that one is an automaton are all depersonalization phenomena. Patients with depersonalization disorder often suffer from derealization (i.e. feeling that the external world is unreal), anxiety, depression, somatic complaints and dizziness. The disorder usually begins in adolescence or early adulthood. Ictal depersonalization is a transient disorder of organic etiology and is usually associated with other seizure symptoms and epileptogenic activity on EEG (Devinsky *et al.*, 1989b).

Other dissociative disorders include Ganser's syndrome, derealization without depersonalization, trance states with apparent wakefulness and diminished environmental responsiveness (e.g. in children following abuse), and dissociative states in subjects who have been brainwashed. Ganser's syndrome is diagnosed in patients who answer questions with 'approximate' answers, and this syndrome is often associated with conversion disorders, amnesia and perceptual disturbances. These patients may be misdiagnosed with dementia, since they show global cognitive impairment on mental status examination.

Recurrent paroxysms or persistent perception the world is unreal can occur without associated disorders of self-identity and memory; i.e. derealizeation without depersonalization. Trance states can follow severe psychic trauma, and patients appear unresponsive or confused. In such cases, differentiation with non-convulsive status may require an EEG, especially when trauma is not identified. Finally, subjects who are indoctrinated into cults or brainwashed by terrorists can develop atypical dissociative disorders.

References

American Psychiatric Association. *Diagnostic and Statistical Manual of Mental Disorders* (3rd edition, revised). Washington, DC: American Psychiatric Association Press, 1987.

Benson DF, Miller BL, Singer SF. Dual personality associated with epilepsy. *Arch Neurol* 1986; **43**: 471–4.

Coons PM, Bowman ES, Milstein V. Multiple personality disorder: a clinical investigation of 50 cases. *J Nerv Ment Dis* 1988; **176**: 519–27.

Devinsky O, Putnam F, Grafman J, Bromfield E, Theodore WH. Dissociative states and epilepsy. *Neurology* 1989a; **39**: 835–40.

Devinsky O, Feldmann E, Burrowes K, Bromfield E. Autoscopic phenomena with seizures. *Arch Neurol* 1989b; **46**: 1080–8.

Mayeux R, Alexander MP, Benson DF, Brandt J, Rosen J. Poriomania. *Neurology* 1979; **29**: 16161–19.

Mesulam M-M. Dissociative states with abnormal temporal lobe EEG. *Arch Neurol* 1981; **38**: 176–81.

Putnam FW. Dissociation as a response to extreme trauma. In: *The Childhood Ante-*

cedents of Multiple Personality (Kluft RP, ed.) Washington, DC: American Psychiatric Association Press, 1985.

Putnam FW. The scientific investigation of multiple personality disorder. In: Split Minds/Split Brains (Quen JM, ed.). New York: New York University Press, 1986.

Putnam FW, Guroff JJ, Silberman EK et al. The clinical phenomenology of multiple personality disorder: review of 100 recent cases. J Clin Psychiat 1986; **47**: 285–93.

Schenk L, Bear D. Multiple personality and related dissociative phenomena in patients with temporal lobe epilepsy. Am J Psychiat 1981; **138**: 1311–16.

98.   Hyperventilation syndrome is diagnosed when typical symptoms are reproduced by three or four minutes of hyperventilation and other causes have been excluded

Gowers' original conception of vasovagal attacks undoubtedly included patients with hyperventilation syndrome:

> The symptoms comprehend subjective gastric, respiratory, and cardiac discomfort . . . often combined with a slight mental change [difficulty thinking or concentrating] and also disturbance of the vasomotor center, causing constriction of the vessels and coldness, especially of the extremities. Associated with the latter may be some sensory impairment and a form of slight tetanoid spasm . . . Women suffer more frequently.
>
> (Gowers, 1907)

Hyperventilation is a common psychophysiological reaction to anxiety or stress, producing somatic symptoms that may become the focus of the patient's and doctor's attention. Unlike the 'normal' reaction to a frightening stimulus, the hyperventilation syndrome is characterized by recurrent episodes and the absence of a stimulus that would be expected to elicit a prominent fear response. Many patients with this syndrome suffer from panic attacks or generalized anxiety disorder.

Patients with hyperventilation syndrome rarely report the occurrence of overbreathing, rather they typically present with neurological, gastrointestinal, respiratory and cardiac complaints (Table 98.1) (Mckell and Sullivan, 1947; Pincus and Tucker, 1985; Perkin and Joseph, 1986). In the vast majority of cases, patients report multiple symptoms, which usually encompass at least two organ systems. Shortness of breath, chest or abdominal discomfort, dizziness, blurred vision and impaired thinking are among the most common symptoms. Patients are often extremely concerned over the symptoms and convinced that they are suffering from a serious illness; they are often seen in emergency rooms.

Neurological manifestations of the hyperventilation syndrome are common and often lead to misdiagnosis. The paroxysmal impairments of consciousness associated with hyperventilation are often mistaken for absence seizures (Lum, 1976). When loss of consciousness occurs, especi-

Table 98.1   Clinical features of the hyperventilation syndrome.

Symptom type	Symptom
Neurological*	Lightheadedness/dizziness
	Paresthesia
	Visual disturbance
	Headache
	Impaired concentration
	Loss of consciousness
	Weakness
	Unsteadiness
	Tremor
	Tinnitus
	Tetanus
Gastrointestinal*	Nausea
	Difficulty swallowing
	Abdominal pains
Cardiorespiratory*	Dyspnea
	Palpitations
	Chest discomfort

*Listed in decreasing order of frequency.

ally with tetanic spasm, other seizure types may be diagnosed. Paresthesiae are most often bilateral, but may be unilateral with a left-sided predominance (Blau *et al.*, 1983; Perkin and Joseph, 1986).

The disorder is most common in girls or women aged 15 to 30 years, but also occurs in males, young children and the elderly (Lum, 1976; Joorabchi, 1977). Patients often undergo extensive diagnostic evaluations and may go years or decades before the syndrome is recognized.

Management of the hyperventilation syndrome begins by reassuring the patient that the somatic symptoms are not serious. The patient must learn to recognize when excessive breathing occurs and use breathing exercises or rebreathe from a paper bag. In chronic cases, treatment is more difficult. Behavioral modification and beta-blockers may be helpful (Folgering *et al.*, 1983).

References

Blau JN, Wiles CM, Solomon FS. Unilateral somatic symptoms due to hyperventilation. *Br Med J* 1983; **286**: 1108.

Folgering H, Rutten H, Roumen Y. Beta-blockage in the hyperventilation syndrome. A retrospective assessment of symptoms and complaints. *Respiration* 1983; **44**: 19–25.

Gowers WR. *The Border-Land of Epilepsy*. Edinburgh: Churchill-Livingstone, 1907, pp. 18–21.

Joorabchi B. Expression of the hyperventilation syndrome in childhood. *Clin Ped* 1977; **16**: 1110–15.

Lum LC. The syndrome of habitual chronic hyperventilation. In: *Modern Trends in Psychosomatic Medicine* (3rd edition) (Hill OW, ed.). Oxford: Butterworths, 1976, pp. 196–230.

McKell TE, Sullivan AJ. The hyperventilation syndrome in gastroenterology. *Gastroenterology* 1947; **9**: 6–16.

Perkin GD, Joseph R. Neurological manifestations of the hyperventilation syndrome. *J Roy Soc Med* 1986; **79**: 448–50.

Pincus JH, Tucker GJ. *Behavioral Neurology*. Oxford, New York: Oxford University Press, 1985, pp. 287–92.

99. *Psychosis and mania may result from neurological and metabolic disorders*

Psychosis is a profound disruption of behavior with some combination of delusions, hallucinations, incoherent thought with loosening of associations, affective poverty or lability, and catatonia. The presence of hallucinations does not by itself indicate psychosis. Psychiatric causes of psychosis include schizophrenia, schizophreniform disorder (similar to schizophrenia with symptoms lasting less than six months), delusional (paranoid) disorder, schizoaffective and affective disorders, and such induced psychotic disorders as *folie à deux*, in which a person with psychotic delusions kindles a similar delusional system in another person with whom he has a close relationship.

Schizophrenia is the most common psychotic disorder and can only be diagnosed when symptoms persist for at least six months. Prodromal symptoms, present in the majority of patients for months or years prior to onset of psychosis, include social withdrawal, impaired ability to function in daily life, bizarre behavior (e.g. collecting garbage) and disorganized speech. In schizophrenia, auditory hallucinations are common; the voices often command or comment about the patient. Visual hallucinations are less common and are equally frequent during day and night, whereas they usually occur at night in patients with affective disorders or delirium. Olfactory, gustatory, vestibular and tactile hallucinations are uncommon; when they occur without auditory hallucinations, an organic disorder is often present. Schizophrenia usually presents in early adulthood, while most cases of psychosis due to structural brain or metabolic disorders occur after the age of 35 years.

There is an emerging body of evidence that structural and physiological changes occur in schizophrenia. Kraeplin's descriptor – dementia praecox – betrays the fact that progressive cognitive deterioration (Johnstone *et al.*, 1978; Taylor and Abrams, 1984) and cerebral atrophy (Andreasen *et al.*, 1982; Narsallah *et al.*, 1983) often occur in schizophrenia, and that this 'functional' disorder has its basis in brain pathology (Stevens, 1982; Andreasen *et al.*, 1986; Benes *et al.*, 1986; Brown *et al.*, 1986), rather than psychologic traits of the parents. Although the psychiatric disorder schizophrenia results in large part from organic brain disease, it is essential to distinguish schizophrenia from psychosis due to other, often reversible, neurological and metabolic disorders.

Whenever psychosis emerges out of a background of normal behavior, an organic etiology should be investigated. Both acute and chronic psychosis may result from neurological and medical disorders and drugs (Table 99.1). Psychosis may be an isolated manifestation of a cerebral disorder or may develop in patients with focal deficits, dementia, delirium and seizures. Patients with organic psychosis often have associated behavioral disorders, such as impaired attention, disorientation for place and time, and anomia; these problems are usually worse at night. Short-term memory is usually impaired in organic psychosis, as is the capacity to judge the passage of time and the temporal sequence of personal or environmental events. Thought processes and psychomotor behavior are often impoverished. Language disorders include word-finding pauses and impairment of fluency, prosody and comprehension. The principle that auditory hallucinations occur with psychiatric disorders, while visual hallucinations occur with organic disorders, is fraught with exceptions. Simple auditory (e.g. tones and buzzes), complex auditory (e.g. voices, music), simple visual (e.g. spots of light, colors) and complex visual (e.g. scenes, faces) hallucinations occur with neurological disorders. While perceptual distortions and hallucinations in neurological disorders are most frequently visual, auditory hallucinations are common and may include voices that threaten or discuss the patient. Furthermore, the combination of auditory and visual hallucinations may be found in both neurological and psychiatric disorders. When hallucinations are associated with an alteration of consciousness, the cause is usually neurological.

In patients with organic psychosis, delusions are common and often focus on fears of persecution, injury or death, and ideas of reference. Delusions may be simple (e.g. husband is cheating, nurses are stealing money) or elaborate, having a complex structure that tends to be more persistent and difficult to treat than simple delusions (Cummings, 1985). Patients often act on delusional beliefs and may endanger themselves or others.

There are no pathognomic signs or symptoms to distinguish between psychiatric and organic causes of psychosis. This differentiation is based on the cluster of clinical features, together with the premorbid background, medical and family histories, and examination. In most cases of acute psychosis, it is impossible to make a definitive etiologic diagnosis. In such patients, repeated neurological assessment is essential. Patients may have normal memory and language during the initial examination, but these functions can become impaired several days later, suggesting a neurological disorder.

Table 99.1 Organic causes of psychosis and mania.

Cause	Condition
Neurological	Epilepsy: postictal or interictal
	Head trauma
	Encephalitis
	Dementia
	Neurosyphilis
	Brain tumor: most often temporal lobe; primary or metastatic
	Stroke
	Korsakoff's psychosis
	Parkinsonism
	Huntington's chorea
	Wilson's disease
	Multiple sclerosis
	Kleine–Levin syndrome (mania)
Medical	Metabolic: hyponatremia, hypercalcemia, hypoglycemia
	Anoxia (psychosis)
	Uremia
	Postpartum
	Systemic lupus erythematosus
	Hyperthyroidism
	Porphyria
	Vitamin B_{12} deficiency
	Pellagra
	Carcinoid (mania)
Medications/drugs	Amphetamines
	Cocaine
	Phencyclidine (PCP)
	Hallucinogens, e.g. LSD
	Dopaminergic agonists, e.g. bromocriptine, levodopa
	Atropine (psychosis)
	Glucocorticoids
	Digitalis glycosides (psychosis)
	Yohimbine
	Indomethacin
	Opiates
	Antidepressants
	Thyroxin
	Baclofen (mania)
	Bromide

Herpes simplex encephalitis (Maxim 67) should always be considered in the differential diagnosis of acute psychosis and when bizarre behavior occurs in a person with no previous history of psychiatric illness or chronic behavioral change. Herpes simplex encephalitis is the most common cause of acute sporadic encephalitis and is neurologically devastating, or even fatal, when left untreated. Acyclovir, a relatively benign drug, is the treatment of choice. The symptoms evolve over several days and include findings that reflect the virus' propensity to infect inferomedial portions of the temporal and frontal lobes (i.e. areas involved in olfactory and gustatory hallucinations, personality changes, psychosis, visual or auditory hallucinations). In addition, more common features of encephalitis such as headache, fever, seizures, confusion, hemiparesis, aphasia and depressed consciousness, are common. The most difficult cases are those in which these typical features of encephalitis are absent or minimal during the early stage of the illness. Computed tomography, magnetic resonance imaging and electroencephalography may be normal during the first several days of illness, although a cerebrospinal fluid pleocytosis is almost always present when symptoms occur.

The treatment of organic psychoses is directed at the underlying disorder. Antipsychotic medications may be required but should be used in lower doses, particularly in elderly patients with neurological and medical disorders. Strongly held delusions may empower patients to act dangerously and require prompt attention to protect both the patient and others.

Mania is an expansive, elevated or irritable mood state accompanied by some combination of grandiosity, diminished attention, decreased need to sleep, excessive and pressured speech, excessive pleasurable activities (spending spree, uncharacteristic sexual proclivities or drug use), racing thoughts, psychomotor agitation or initiation of projects that cannot be realistically completed (American Psychiatric Association, 1987). Delusions and hallucinations can occur with mania. Manic episodes often develop over hours or days, and patients may incur significant social, occupational or financial losses.

Secondary mania can result from cerebral lesions, as well as toxic and metabolic insults (Table 99.1). The diagnosis of secondary mania requires (1) that symptoms last at least one week and are approximately contemporaneous with the somatic disorder (Jamieson and Wells, 1979); (2) an elated or irritable mood; and (3) at least two of the following: pressured speech, flight of ideas, grandiosity, decreased sleep, distractibility and impaired judgment (Krauthammer and Klerman, 1978).

Focal cerebral lesions that cause secondary mania usually involve the right hemisphere (Cummings and Mendez, 1984; Starkstein *et al.*, 1990). Lesions associated with mania have been found in the right temporal, parietal and frontal lobes, as well as the right caudate and thalamus (Oppler, 1950; Rosenbaum and Barry, 1975; Cohen and Niska, 1980; Jampala and Abrams, 1983; Cummings and Mendez, 1984; Starkstein *et al.*, 1990). Left temporal and frontal lesions (Herlihy and Herlihy, 1979; Jampala and Abrams, 1983), as well as hypothalamic and brainstem lesions (Bromberg, 1930; Alpers, 1937; Stern and Dancey, 1942; Malamud, 1967; Trimble and Cummings, 1981) are also associated with secondary mania. Preliminary positron emission tomographic studies have demonstrated glucose hypometabolism in the basal region of the right temporal lobe in patients with mania after brain injury (Starkstein *et al.*, 1990).

The right-sided predominance of cerebral lesions associated with mania is supported by the finding that patients who have partial seizures and develop mania usually have right temporal seizure foci (Flor-Henry, 1969; Rosenbaum and Barry, 1975). Furthermore, intracarotid sodium amobarbital injection preferentially elicits laughter and elated mood following right-sided injections (Lee *et al.*, 1988). Together, these observations suggest that loss of right temporal affective modulation shifts the mood toward a manic state, possibly by 'releasing' or 'disinhibiting' limbic functions in the left hemisphere.

Secondary mania is often associated with transient amnesia and left-sided neglect in patients with right thalamic or hemispheric lesions. In most cases, mania resolves after a period of weeks or months, especially with treatment of the underlying illness. In chronic cases of secondary mania, lithium is usually effective (Rosenbaum and Barry, 1975; Cohn *et al.*, 1977).

References

Alpers BJ. Relation of the hypothalamus to disorders of personality. *Arch Neurol Psychiat* 1937; **38**: 291–303.

American Psychiatric Association. *Diagnostic and Statistical Manual* (3rd edition). Washington, DC: American Psychiatric Association Press, 1987.

Andreasen NC, Narsallah H, Dunn V *et al.* Structural abnormalities of the frontal system in schizophrenia. *Arch Gen Psychiat* 1986; **43**: 136–7.

Andreasen NC, Smith MR, Jacoby CG, Dennert JW, Olsen SA. Ventricular enlargement in schizophrenia: Definition and prevalence. *Am J Psychiat* 1982; **139**: 292–6.

Benes FM, Davidson J, Bird ED. Quantitative cytoarchitectonic studies of the cerebral cortex in schizophrenia. *Arch Gen Psychiat* 1986; **43**: 31–5.

Bromberg W. Mental states in chronic encephalitis. *Psychiat Q* 1930; **4**: 537–66.

Brown R, Colter N, Corsellis N, Crow TJ, Frith CD, Jagoe R, Johnstone EC, Marsh L. *Postmortem* evidence of structural brain changes in schizophrenia. *Am J Psychiat* 1986; **43**: 36–42.

Cohen MR, Niska RW. Localized right cerebral hemisphere dysfunction and recurrent mania. *Am J Psychiat* 1980; **137**: 847–8.

Cohn CK, Wright JR, DeVaul RA. Post head trauma syndrome in an adolescent treated with lithium carbonate – case report. *Dis Nerv Syst* 1977; **38**: 630–1.

Cummings JL. Organic delusions: Phenomenology, anatomical correlations, and review. *Br J Psychiat* 1985; **146**: 184–97.

Cummings JL, Mendez MF. Secondary mania with focal cerebrovascular lesions. *Am J Psychiat* 1984; **141**: 1084–7.

Flor-Henry P. Psychosis and temporal lobe epilepsy. *Epilepsia* 1969; **10**: 363–95.

Herlihy CE Jr, Herlihy CE. Lithium and organic brain syndrome. *J Clin Psychiat* 1979; **40**: 455.

Jamieson RC, Wells CE. Manic psychosis in a patient with multiple metastatic brain tumors. *J Clin Psychiat* 1979; **40**: 280–3.

Jampala VC, Abrams R. Mania secondary to left and right hemisphere damage. *Am J Psychiat* 1983; **140**: 1197–9.

Johnstone EC, Crow TJ, Frith CD *et al.* The dementia of dementia praecox. *Acta Psychiat Scand* 1978; **57**: 305–24.

Krauthammer C, Klerman GL. Secondary mania. *Arch Gen Psychiat* 1978; **35**: 1333.

Lee GP, Loring DW, Meador KJ, Flanigin HF. Emotional reactions and behavioral complications following intracarotid sodium amytal injection. *J Clin Exp Neuropsychol* 1988; **10**: 83–4.

Malamud N. Psychiatric disorders with intracranial tumors of the limbic system. *Arch Neurol* 1967; **17**: 113–23.

Narsallah HA, McCaley-Whitters M, Jacoby CG. Cortical atrophy in schizophrenia and mania: a comparative study. *J Clin Psychiat* 1982; **43**: 439–41.

Oppler W. Manic psychosis in a case of parasagittal meningioma. *Arch Neurol Psychiat* 1950; **64**: 417–30.

Rosenbaum AH, Barry MJ. Positive therapeutic response to lithium in hypomania secondary to organic brain syndrome. *Am J Psychiat* 1975; **132**: 1072–3.

Starkstein SE, Mayberg, HS, Berthier ML, Fedoroff P, Price TR, Dannals R, Wagner HN, Leiguarda R, Robinson RG. Mania after brain injury: Neuroradiological and metabolic findings. *Ann Neurol* 1990; **27**: 652–9.

Stern K, Dancey TE. Glioma of the diencephalon in a manic patient. *Am J Psychiat* 1942; **98**: 716–19.

Stevens JR. Neuropathology of schizophrenia. *Arch Gen Psychiat* 1982; **39**: 1131–9.

Taylor MA, Abrams R. Cognitive impairment in schizophrenia. *Am J Psychiat* 1984; **141**: 196–201.

Trimble MR, Cummings JL. Neuropsychiatric disturbances following brainstem lesions. *Br J Psychiat* 1981; **138**: 56–9.

100.   *Violence scars permanently and kills; physicians must recognize and treat it when appropriate*

Violence is usually the result of interaction between biological and environmental factors. Environmental causes are often important: children who are physically abused or who witness intrafamily violence are more likely to become violent as adults (Pincus and Lewis, 1991); violence observed on television may contribute to subsequent aggressive acts; lower socioeconomic status is associated with increased violence; and increased physical crowding and environmental temperature can raise the risk of violence. In addition, easy access to firearms transforms what would have been assaults into homicides.

Among the biological factors that predispose to violent behavior are neurophysiological dysfunction, as in the postictal state; genetic factors; hormonal changes, such as hypercortisolism, hyperthyroidism and hyperandrogenemia; central neurotransmitter alterations may be a marker for aggressive behavior (low cerebrospinal fluid 5-HIAA levels); neurological disorders, such as mental retardation, stroke, delirium, brain tumor and encephalitis; psychiatric disorders, including schizophrenia and mania; and such drugs as alcohol, phencyclidine, amphetamines, cocaine and hallucinogens. However, distilling the biological and environmental factors that lead to aggressive acts is often impossible.

The relationship between epilepsy and violence is controversial (Maxim 78). Directed ictal violence is extremely rare. However, violence appears to be more common interictally in patients with epilepsy than in patients with other neurological or medical disorders (Taylor, 1969). *While the vast majority of patients with epilepsy are not violent*, rage episodes have been reported in up to one-third of children with temporal lobe epilepsy (Keating, 1961; Lindsay *et al.*, 1979). The unresolved question is whether this violence is actually related to epilepsy or results from other factors, such as structural brain damage, antiepileptic drugs (e.g. primidone and phenobarbital) and social variables. Anterior temporal lobectomy in aggressive adults with epilepsy reduces aggressivity (Vaernet and Madsen, 1970; Falconer, 1973; Kiloh *et al.*, 1974), the same as it does in rhesus monkeys (Kluver and Bucy, 1939).

Regardless of the cause, when physicians are called to deal with a patient who is threatening or engaged in violent behavior, they are expected to take charge of the situation. Unfortunately, in some cases, the only course of action may be to flee and get help, trying to warn others as you flee; for example, one might do well to run from an armed psychotic patient, who is acting under a command hallucination. In most settings, violent patients can be managed and injury avoided. As with other emergencies, the physician must simultaneously assess and treat the violent behavior using a flexible blueprint for action:

1. Be calm and maintain control.
2. Notify security personnel of the location and nature of the problem.
3. Assess the risk and possible severity of violence.
4. Formulate an instant differential diagnosis; patients who are psychotic, intoxicated or suffering from an organic mental disorder will often require restraints for safety, whereas those with personality disorders can often be effectively managed by 'talking them down'.
5. Consider your own safety as you approach the situation. If the patient has a weapon or is physically overpowering and in a rage, wait until police or security personnel arrive.
6. Avoid threatening verbal and non-verbal actions; speak softly; ask understandingly what the problem is.
7. Listen to the patient.
8. Avoid prolonged, direct, eye contact.

If restraint is indicated, a leader should be accompanied by at least four other staff members with a previously reviewed plan of action. If the patient is uncooperative, he is brought to the ground with each staff member holding an extremity and the leader securing the head, preventing biting with one hand under the chin and on the vertex. When confronting a large, strong violent patient, additional staff are required.

Acute medical therapy for violent patients usually consists of a neuroleptic administered intramuscularly. These medications should be used with caution in delirious patients, in those intoxicated by drugs or alcohol, and in those experiencing alcohol or drug withdrawal. In such patients, neuroleptics may aggravate confusion or dangerously depress the level of consciousness. Haloperidol is most often used, administered intramuscularly in a dose of 5 to 10 mg initially, followed by 5 to 10 mg every 30 to 60 minutes as needed. Paradoxical agitation may occur with neuroleptics. Short-acting barbiturates (e.g. amobarbital) or benzodiazepines (e.g. lorazepam) may also be given intramuscularly or intravenously to sedate violent patients; respiratory and cardiovascular status must be closely monitored.

References

Falconer MA. Reversibility by temporal-lobe resection of the behavioral abnormalities of temporal-lobe epilepsy. *N Engl J Med* 1973; **289**: 451–5.

Keating LE. Epilepsy and behavior disorder in schoolchildren. *J Ment Sci* 1961; **107**: 161–80.

Kiloh LG, Gye RS, Rushworthy RG *et al.* Stereotactic amygdalotomy for aggressive behavior. *J Neurol Neurosurg Psychiat* 1974; **37**: 437–44.

Kluver H, Bucy P. Preliminary analysis of functions of the temporal lobes in man. *Arch Neurol Psychiat* 1939; **42**: 979–1000.

Lindsay J, Ounsted C, Richards P. Long-term outcome in children with temporal lobe seizures. III: Psychiatric aspects in childhood and adult life. *Dev Med Child Neurol* 1979; **21**: 630–6.

Pincus JH, Lewis DO. Episodic violence. Behavioral aspects of paroxysmal disorders. *Sem Neurol* 1991; **11**: 146–54.

Taylor DC. Aggression and epilepsy. *J Psychosom Res* 1969; **13**: 229–36.

Vaernet K, Madsen A. Stereotaxic amygdalatomy and basofrontal tractotomy in psychotics with aggressive behavior. *J Neurol Neurosurg Psychiat* 1970; **33**: 858–63.

Index